AMERICA'S
TEST KITCHEN

The Complete
Baby and Toddler
›Cookbook‹

THE VERY BEST PUREES,
FINGER FOODS, AND TODDLER MEALS
FOR HAPPY FAMILIES

sourcebooks
jabberwocky

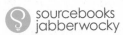

Published by Sourcebooks Jabberwocky, an imprint of Sourcebooks, Inc.

P.O. Box 4410, Naperville, Illinois 60567-4410

(630) 961-3900

Fax: (630) 961-2168

sourcebooks.com

Source of Production: 1010 Printing International, North Point, Hong Kong, China

Date of Production: January 2019

Run Number: 5013727

Printed and bound in China.

OGP 10 9 8 7 6 5 4 3 2 1

AMERICA'S TEST KITCHEN

EDITOR IN CHIEF: Molly Birnbaum

EXECUTIVE FOOD EDITOR: Suzannah McFerran

PEDIATRIC DIETITIAN: Toni Pert, MS, RD, CSP, LDN

MANAGING EDITOR, EDUCATION: Kristin Sargianis

SENIOR EDITORS: Nicole Konstantinakos, Katie Leaird

ASSOCIATE EDITORS: Afton Cyrus, Sasha Marx

PHOTOGRAPHY DIRECTOR: Julie Bozzo Cote

SENIOR STAFF PHOTOGRAPHER: Daniel J. van Ackere

STAFF PHOTOGRAPHERS: Steve Klise, Kevin White

FOOD STYLING: Kendra McKnight, Sally Staub, Catrine Kelty, Elle Simone

PHOTOGRAPHY PRODUCER: Meredith Mulcahy

PHOTOSHOOT KITCHEN TEAM:

    MANAGER: Timothy McQuinn

    LEAD TEST COOK: Jessica Rudolph

    ASSISTANT TEST COOKS: Sarah Ewald, Eric Haessler

IMAGING MANAGER: Lauren Robbins

PRODUCTION AND IMAGING SPECIALISTS: Heather Dube, Dennis Noble, Jessica Voas

SENIOR CONTENT OPERATIONS MANAGER: Taylor Argenzio

COPY EDITOR: Louise Emerick

CHIEF CREATIVE OFFICER: Jack Bishop

EXECUTIVE EDITORIAL DIRECTORS: Julia Collin Davison, Bridget Lancaster

CONTENTS

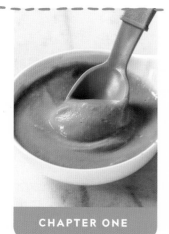
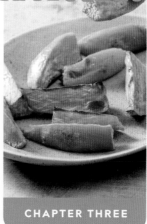
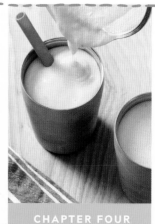
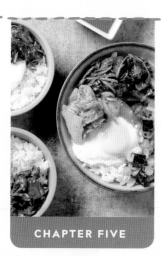
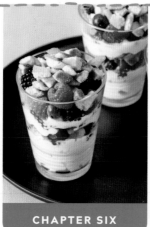
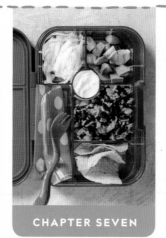
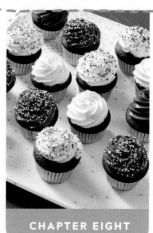

FOREWORD

BY JULIANA DAMON, MD

When I was 9 months old, I was adopted from Korea. When I arrived, my family worried because I was thin and malnourished. But I was lucky enough to live close to both of my grandmothers, both of whom loved to cook. I grew up surrounded by crackers, blueberry muffins, tuna casseroles with potato chips, and steamed broccoli. There was amazing chocolate icing and many batches of oatmeal lace cookies. Every year I chose one of my grandmother's Thanksgiving meals as my birthday dinner: stuffing, potato puree, and gravy. The food was delicious and dependable, and I certainly felt loved eating it. My grandmothers offered "love on a fork," we used to joke.

These days I am a baker and also a pediatrician. My 13-year-old daughter's friends are mystified by this seeming conundrum. But I bake to relax, and I enjoy the end results as well as sharing them with my friends and family. Over many years, I have learned that home-cooked food is more satisfying, healthier, and more economical. Plus, everyone could use a little love on a fork.

In my line of work, there is never a day without parents asking: "How much do I feed my baby?", "What should I start with?", "Have you heard that rice cereal might be bad for babies?" With certainty and experience, I can say that while we pediatricians have certain guidelines for 6-month-old babies (and beyond), there are no correct answers. Much of medicine, like parenting, is ever changing. These days, we encourage parents to feed their babies meat and peanut butter early on, but in a decade, who knows what we will be saying.

Well, what are you new parents to do? Honestly, we dole out advice within a framework of practicality and common sense. Try a few simple foods one at a time. Build upon flavors slowly as your baby shows you what he or she enjoys. Keep rotating foods so your child tolerates change. Variety is good for all people, but some weeks are better than others.

I'm so happy that a cookbook exists with tasty recipes that are flexible enough to please the youngest burgeoning palates. Not only has a nutritionist researched these recipes, but real parents have cooked them at home, helping the test cooks at America's Test Kitchen perfect the techniques, getting the best taste and nutrition. You may have just survived some harrowing months of keeping a newborn alive and well and are ready to explore a new world of taste, color, and smells together. How wonderful to experience food as a baby and toddler, discovering so many new foods and flavors. It might even get you eating better yourself.

I hope you feel similarly moved by these recipes. They are delicious suggestions—not dogmatic advice—and are ready to be tweaked to fit your family's lifestyle and taste. Enjoy and move from the "have to" mind-set to the inspired!

Juliana Damon, MD, FAAP, attended Harvard College studying English, Columbia College of Physicians and Surgeons for medical school, and the University of Massachusetts for residency. Her special interests are adoption, developmental issues, and integrative medicine. She has worked as a pediatrician at East Bay Pediatrics in Berkeley, California, since 2002.

INTRODUCTION

No matter who you are, where you live, or what you do, food is a huge part of daily life. And food can be one of the *best* parts of daily life. It's delicious. It has the power to bring people together. But feeding young children carries with it a lot of responsibility. Are the choices you're making right now going to affect their eating habits, and therefore their health, for the rest of their lives?

How do you guarantee raising a healthy child who loves to eat?

Spoiler: you can't!

What you can do is set the stage for a lifetime of good eating. There will be ups and downs, food on the floor and food in the hair, as well on the plate and in the mouth. But there are three basic things to start with:

✱ **COOK AND EAT TOGETHER.** You might already cook at home a lot. You might just be starting. The goal of this book is, in part, to get you in the kitchen, cooking more meals, and eating them together.

✱ **EAT A VARIETY OF FOODS.** Introducing kids to a variety of flavors, textures, and colors opens the door to a lifetime of adventurous eating. In our puree chapters (page 1 and page 37), we suggest different ways to introduce new spices or herbs or other flavorings to your plain purees. Another powerful tool when it comes to enticing your toddler to eat is choice. In our family meal chapter (page 137), take note of the recipes that incorporate choice into the procedure.

✱ **EAT FOOD THAT TASTES GOOD.** We developed all the recipes for this book with a team of test cooks in our 15,000-square-foot kitchen. We wanted to create a variety of recipes, with many simple and fast options. But, most importantly, we believe that eating food that tastes good from the beginning will set your kids up for a lifetime of good food. So these recipes were all developed to be, first and foremost, tasty. We did this with the help of feedback from more than 3,000 parents, grandparents, and caretakers of little ones, who made our recipes at home and sent us notes via survey. You'll see quotes from our testers throughout the book.

It's important to note that this is not a medical book. We worked with a pediatric dietitian at the Children's Hospital of Philadelphia, Toni Pert, to make sure we developed recipes that respected nutritional standards for this book. Dr. Juliana Damon, a pediatrician in Berkeley, California, provided helpful overall insight. Please always ask your pediatrician if you have questions, worries, or doubts. Every baby and toddler is different.

Other benefits to cooking at home? You'll save money if you cook rather than go out to eat. You'll have fun (especially when you start cooking with your kids!). And you'll know exactly what ingredients (and quality of ingredients) go into your food.

HOW TO USE THIS BOOK

ORGANIZED BY AGE

We have organized this cookbook chronologically by age, starting with food for the youngest kids and moving up from there. Note that the ages in chapter 6 ("Cooking with your Kids," page 187) are the ages we recommend for allowing your child to help with the cooking, and not the recommended age for eating that food.

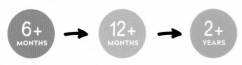

PICK AND CHOOSE

Don't hesitate to pick and choose the types and kinds of recipes you cook. Feel free to skip the purees, if you are interested in baby-led weaning (see page 31). Feel free to combine purees *and* finger foods when you start to introduce solids, if that's what you prefer. Play around with variations, or with how you serve family meals to different ages and personalities.

Fast, Freezer-Friendly, or Allergen-Free? Icons at a Glance

Throughout this book, we have included icons for an at-a-glance look at what to expect from (and in) the recipe.

 FAST: Recipe can be completed in 45 minutes or less.

 FREEZE IT: Recipe freezes well.

 MILK: Recipe contains dairy.

 EGGS: Recipe contains eggs.

 WHEAT: Recipe contains wheat.

 SOY: Recipe contains soy.

 TREE NUTS: Recipe contains tree nuts.

 PEANUTS: Recipe contains peanuts.

 FISH: Recipe contains fish.

SO YOU'RE ABOUT TO START SOLIDS...

WHEN TO START SOLID FOODS

The American Academy of Pediatrics recommends starting to introduce solid foods at 6 months. How do you know if your baby is ready? Your baby should be able to sit up mostly on his or her own and can hold up his or her head for a long while. He or she might also be showing literal interest in food: swiping food off your plate or watching you eat intently. Finally, very young babies have an automatic reflex to push food out of their mouths with their tongues. This reflex slowly fades away and should be gone when babies are ready to start eating solids. Remember that introducing solids does not mean scaling back on breast milk or formula. Pediatricians recommend continuing to feed your baby breast milk or formula, complementing solid food, until they are at least 12 months old.

WHAT TO OFFER

Start simple. You can begin with purees (page 1), finger foods (page 31), or a combination of both. All of the purees in chapter 1 (page 1) consist of one ingredient. While pediatricians are no longer recommending that babies should be fed white rice cereal starting around 4 months old (a recommendation once in vogue!), baby cereals can be a good choice, in moderation. We've developed recipes to make your own baby cereals using various whole grains (page 33).

WHAT TO AVOID

There are two things to avoid feeding babies under 12 months old: added salt and honey. Young babies' kidneys are not yet ready to process a large amount of salt. A small amount, on occasion, is okay. "About 15 to 20 milligrams per serving is fine for babies under 12 months," says pediatric dietitian Toni Pert. We have added zero salt to our purees and limited amounts to family meals that are easily modified for babies. If using canned products (like tomatoes, stock, or beans), we call for low-salt varieties. Honey has a higher risk of botulism and should not be given to babies under 12 months. Also avoid choking hazards. These include whole grapes, hot dogs, large chunks of meat, whole or chopped nuts, large bites of sticky nut butters, popcorn, raisins, crunchy items like raw apples or celery, and hard or gummy candy.

WHAT NOT TO AVOID

Allergens! (Yes, really.) For a long time, the recommendation was to avoid giving your baby anything potentially allergenic until 12 months. However, research has found that introducing allergens earlier can help to prevent the development of lifelong allergies. As of 2017, the recommendation from the American Association of Pediatrics is to introduce allergens before the 12-month mark, even as early as 6 months. Of course, check with your pediatrician before offering any allergens to your baby.

HOW DO FLAVOR PREFERENCES DEVELOP?

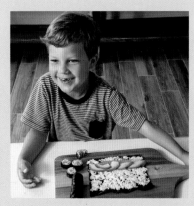

Why do some kids love to eat their veggies and others stick to beige-colored foods? A lot of research has been done on how our flavor preferences develop, but there are still a lot of unknowns.

Some things we do know: What your mother eats while pregnant will influence your taste preferences. What your mother eats while breastfeeding also influences your preferences. Babies innately like the taste of sweet and dislike the taste of bitter. Also, tastes change over time.

Some of this is evolutionary. It makes sense that we're born liking the taste of sweet. Sweet means calories, and calories mean survival. It also makes sense that we're born not liking the taste of bitter. Bitter is the taste of danger, the taste of poisonous plants.

But much of our taste preferences come from experience. "There are innate taste preferences, but you are continually building upon them with experiences that begin prior to birth, extended to nursing period, and then into weaning period," says Gary Beauchamp, emeritus director and president of the Monell Chemical Senses Center. "These experiences set the pathway for some of the most fundamental likes and dislikes that can last for a person's entire life."

What about Picky Eating?

There are many, many different theories for why some people are picky eaters. They range from genetics to a need for control to feelings of depression.

But, really: All toddlers go through picky phases. There isn't much you can do to change it. You can be patient, you can offer well-loved foods, you can try and try and try again.

Research has shown, in short-term studies, that if you expose a child to a novel food or flavor at least 8 or 10 or 12 times, in many cases you can induce them to accept it, and perhaps even come to like it. Focus on developing good habits and don't focus on a single meal that doesn't go well. What your child eats across the day, the week, and the month matters more. A single meal that isn't terribly successful, well...that just happens.

Research has also shown that children who can take part in the process of choosing food at the market, growing food in the garden, or cooking food with you in the kitchen are more likely to try new foods. Being able to choose what they eat at the table is also helpful. This is why we've created a number of recipes in which every diner can choose his or her own toppings or sides, to make the meal feel more like it is in their control. (See Pork Tinga Bowls, page 158, California-Style Fish Tacos, page 164, and Baked Potato Bar, page 175, among others.)

DO YOU NEED A BABY FOOD MAKER?
(And Other Equipment Questions)

Short answer: no! However, if you are looking to outfit your kitchen with new tools, our team at America's Test Kitchen tested popular models of baby food and reusable baby food pouches. Check out www.americastestkitchen.com/kids for more (including a review of bottle brushes).

BABY FOOD MAKERS

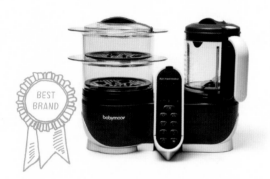

Baby food makers are hands-off machines designed to make purees. We rounded up six of these small appliances, priced from $78.95 to $159.99, and used them to prepare three different purees from this book. There were a lot of drawbacks to the machines, including the fact that most only make small amounts per batch, are a lot of work to use, and are not precise. As a result, we can only fully recommend one baby food maker: **Babymoov Duo Meal Station: 6-in-1 Food Maker ($159.99).** This machine had the most parts (10) and the largest footprint of any machine we tried, but it made silky smooth purees.

REUSABLE BABY POUCHES

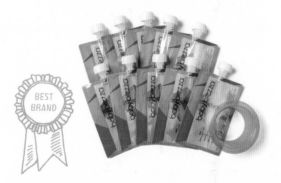

With small spouts and twist-off caps, these lightweight pouches are convenient for babies and young kids to eat on the go. We tested 6 brands of reusable pouches, priced from $0.99 to $13.99 per pouch, that parents can fill with the food of their choice, to serve fresh or freeze for later use. We tested how easy they were to fill, use, and clean, and whether they leaked.

After putting the baby food pouches to use in the test kitchen and at home, an all-around favorite emerged: **Baby Brezza Reusable Baby Food Pouches ($9.99 for ten 7-ounce pouches).** These plastic pouches were the least expensive, had the widest opening of all the models, and they were easy to keep clean, too.

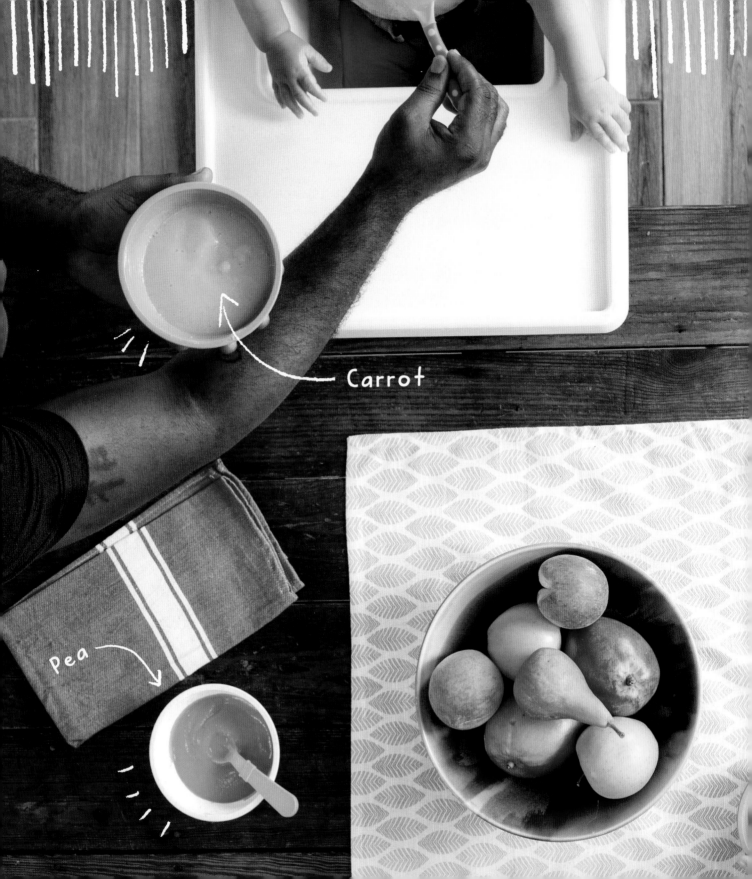

Carrot

Pea

FIRST FRUITS, VEGETABLES, and GRAINS

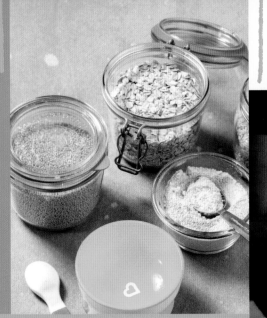

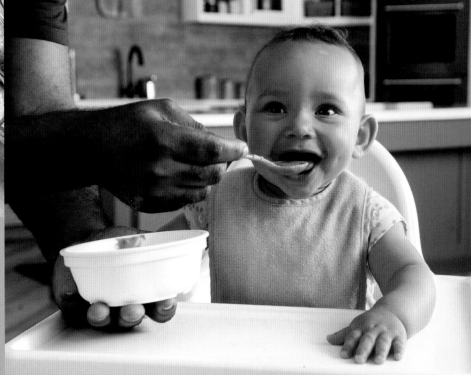

"I love the advice to make ice cubes from the puree. Very easy for baby food."

—Parent of 11-month-old, on Apple Puree

"My child very much liked the peas both warm at the time I made the recipe and cold from the refrigerator the next day."

—Parent of 9-month-old, on Pea Puree

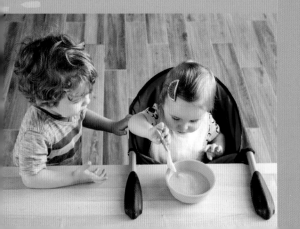

"It was debatable who liked this recipe more: me or my 12-month-old. The cinnamon addition was very good. My daughter was a huge fan."

—Parent of 12-month-old, on Sweet Potato Puree

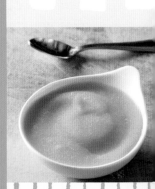

ALL ABOUT FIRST FRUITS, VEGETABLES, AND GRAINS

Welcome to the world of baby purees! Feeding your child food for the first time can go in so many different ways—from fun (smiles of surprise and delight) to lackluster (a casual bite and then a disinterested push away) to disappointing (tears) and every combination in between. It's hard to predict what a baby will like or not like, especially in the very beginning.

We're here to give you options. We can't promise that your baby will love the apple puree, but we can promise that our recipe is tasty, easy, and foolproof for all of you parents (or grandparents or caregivers) of new eaters. We developed these recipes with an eye on nutrition (our pediatric dietitian, Toni Pert, weighed in on all of the healthy benefits of these simple fruits, vegetables, and grains), ease (note the fast icons ⚡ next to recipes that will take 45 minutes or less), and flavor.

Flavor might be the most important part here, at least when it comes to raising a kid who loves to eat. We wanted to create purees that tasted *good*. To start, our test kitchen team tasted all of the supermarket options. We compared them to purees made with a bevy of cooking techniques in order to end up with baby food that has the purest flavor of the ingredient. (Not that there's anything wrong with supermarket purees. We get that convenience is a priority. But it is undeniable: they don't taste as good.)

This is why we roast our sweet potatoes to make an earthy, sweet puree, rather than steam them (see page 29). Steaming, however, gave us a carrot puree with the best carroty flavor (see page 11). Each recipe includes options to add more flavor to the mix with spices or herbs to help expand your baby's palate when you (and your baby) feel ready. During the first 6 months of eating, the majority of your baby's nutrition still comes from breast milk or formula, so it's a good time to try new flavors. None of the recipes in this chapter include added salt, which is not recommended for babies under 12 months. For more on salt, see page vii.

If you're going the baby-led weaning route or offering a combination of finger foods and purees, check out page 31 for some great first finger-food options and to learn more about baby-led weaning. For more advanced finger foods, see chapter 3 (page 77).

A NOTE ABOUT STORAGE

We wanted to make sure that if you're making homemade puree, you'll have enough for at least a few meals. Unless otherwise noted, all purees in this chapter can be refrigerated for up to 3 days. Purees that can be frozen are marked with a snowflake icon ❄. To freeze, divide puree evenly into ice cube tray. Once frozen, pop cubes out of tray and transfer to heavy-duty zipper-lock bag. To serve, defrost in refrigerator overnight or microwave 1 cube for 30 to 45 seconds and stir to recombine.

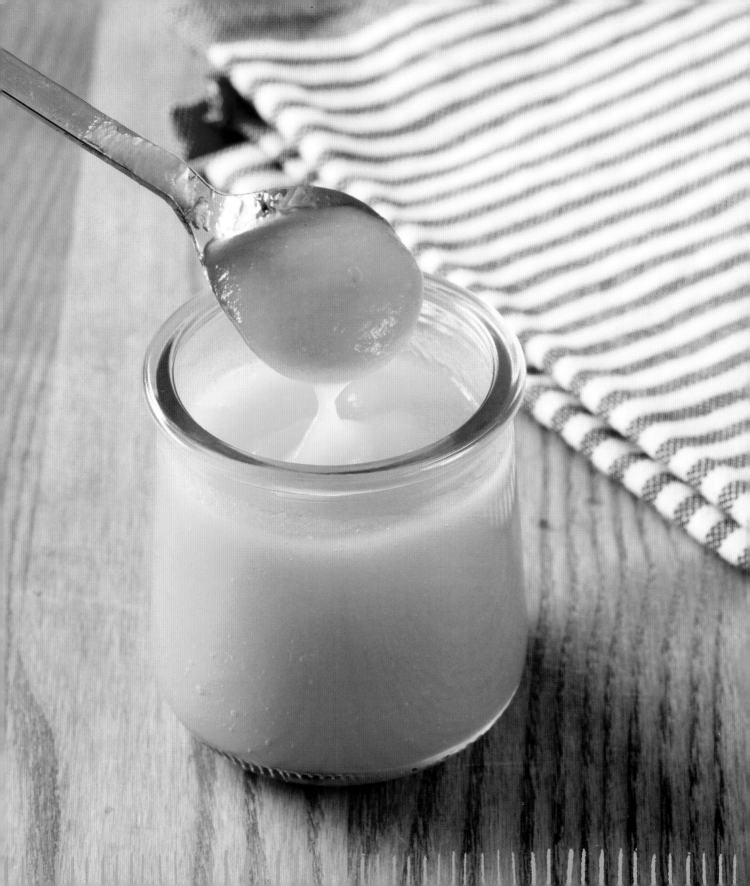

Apple

Makes about 2½ cups
Total Time: 25 minutes

Why This Recipe Works

Apple puree is quintessential kid food—and not just for babies. There's even an applesauce aisle in most supermarkets. But store-bought apple purees are bland (we know; we tried them all). We wanted an apple puree that was smooth, easy to eat, and had real apple flavor. Steaming the chopped, peeled apples for just 8 minutes before pureeing in a blender gave us super smooth, super appley apple puree. And, unlike boiling, steaming keeps most of the nutrients in the puree (not in the cooking water).

Tart apples, like Granny Smith, are more acidic and may not be as appealing to your baby. You can use a food processor instead of a blender, but the puree will not be quite as smooth.

2 pounds Fuji, Gala, or Golden Delicious apples, peeled, cored, and cut into 1-inch pieces

1. Bring 1 inch water to rolling boil in Dutch oven over high heat. Place steamer basket in pot and fill basket with apples. Cover and cook until tender, 8 to 10 minutes.

2. Carefully remove steamer basket from pot and transfer apples to blender, reserving cooking liquid. Add 1 cup cooking liquid to apples and process on high speed for 1 minute. Scrape down sides of blender jar and continue to process until very smooth, about 1 minute.

3. Add additional cooking liquid (or breast milk or formula) as needed to thin puree to desired consistency. Let puree cool to room temperature. Serve or store (see page 3 for storage options).

> ### SPICE IT UP
> Add ¼ teaspoon ground cinnamon or pinch ground cloves or nutmeg to blender along with apples in step 2.

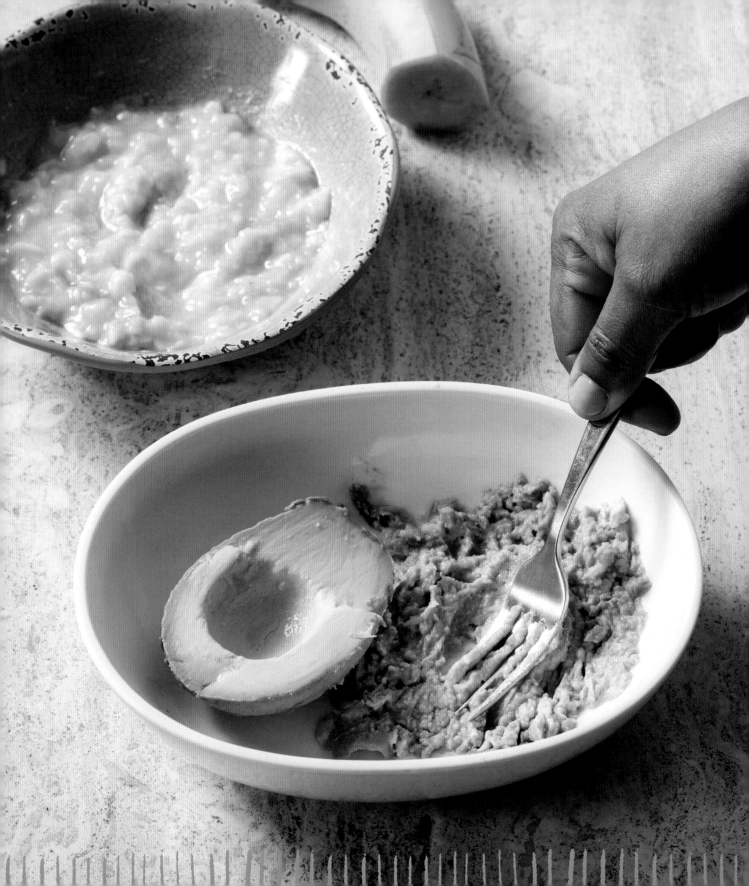

Mashed Avocado or Banana

6+ MONTHS

Makes about ½ cup
Total Time: 5 minutes

Why This Recipe Works

Mashed avocado and mashed banana win the "easiest recipes in the book" award. These purees, which are really just simple mashes, are best eaten right away as they will oxidize and turn progressively browner the longer they sit. (Don't worry, they are still safe to eat when brown.) For a special treat, try combining mashed avocado and mashed banana *together*. Our team dubbed this delicious meal "baby guacamole."

1 avocado, halved, pitted, and peeled, or 1 ripe banana, peeled

1 Place avocado or banana in bowl. Use large fork to mash to desired consistency. Add water (or breast milk or formula) as needed to thin to desired consistency. Serve immediately.

2 For smooth puree, process avocado or banana in blender on high speed for 1 minute, scraping blender jar as needed and adding 2 to 4 tablespoons water (or breast milk or formula) to thin to desired consistency. Serve.

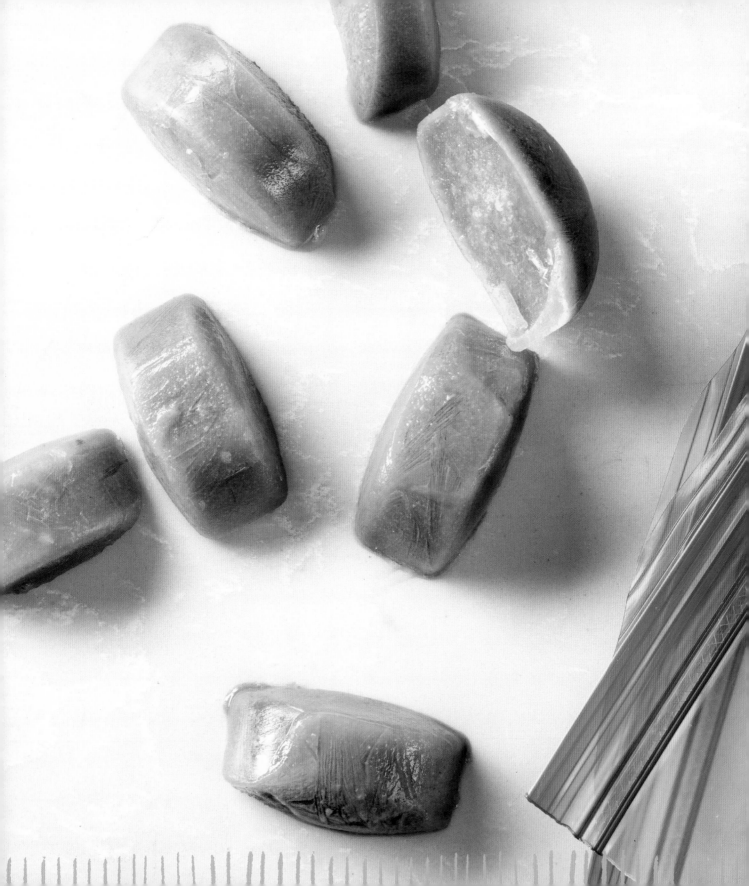

Broccoli

Makes about 2½ cups
Total Time: 25 minutes

Why This Recipe Works

While you may not have great memories of eating broccoli as a kid (whose parents *didn't* overcook it?), this vibrant vegetable makes for a beautiful and tasty puree. We found that a short, 10-minute stovetop steam was sufficient to tenderize broccoli florets without turning them mushy or a drab army green.

You can use 12 ounces thawed frozen broccoli florets in place of fresh broccoli. You can use a food processor instead of a blender, but the puree will not be quite as smooth.

4½ cups broccoli florets (12 ounces), cut into 1-inch pieces

1. Bring 1 inch water to rolling boil in large saucepan over high heat. Place steamer basket in saucepan and fill basket with broccoli. Cover and cook until tender, about 10 minutes.

2. Carefully remove steamer basket from saucepan and transfer broccoli to blender, reserving cooking liquid. Add 1½ cups cooking liquid to broccoli and process on high speed for 1 minute. Scrape down sides of blender jar and continue to process until very smooth, about 1 minute.

3. Add additional cooking liquid (or breast milk or formula) as needed to thin puree to desired consistency. Let puree cool to room temperature. Serve or store (see page 3 for storage options).

> **SPICE IT UP**
> Add ¼ teaspoon ground coriander or pinch ground ginger to blender along with broccoli in step 2.

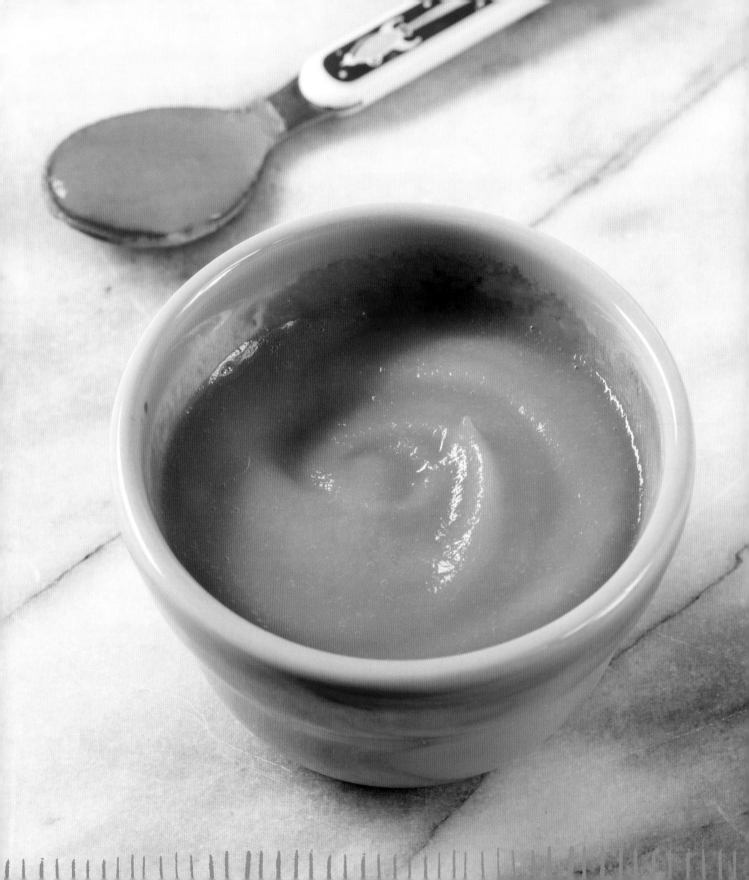

Carrot

Makes about 2½ cups
Total Time: 25 minutes

Why This Recipe Works

There are two great reasons to make baby food out of carrots. First, carrots get sweeter when cooked. Second, they contain very little starch, which means that with just 10 minutes in a steamer basket, they become perfectly soft and puree-able. Bonus: the resulting puree is packed with beta-carotene, a bright-orange pigment that the body converts to vitamin A.

You can use 1 pound thawed frozen sliced carrots in place of fresh carrots (they're already peeled!). You can use a food processor instead of a blender, but the puree will not be quite as smooth.

1 pound carrots, peeled and cut into ½-inch pieces

1. Bring 1 inch water to rolling boil in large saucepan over high heat. Place steamer basket in saucepan and fill basket with carrots. Cover and cook until tender, about 10 minutes.

2. Carefully remove steamer basket from saucepan and transfer carrots to blender, reserving cooking liquid. Add 1½ cups cooking liquid to carrots and process on high speed for 1 minute. Scrape down sides of blender jar and continue to process until very smooth, about 1 minute.

3. Add additional cooking liquid (or breast milk or formula) as needed to thin puree to desired consistency. Let puree cool to room temperature. Serve or store (see page 3 for storage options).

> ### SPICE IT UP
> Add ¼ teaspoon ground cinnamon or pinch ground ginger to blender along with carrots in step 2.

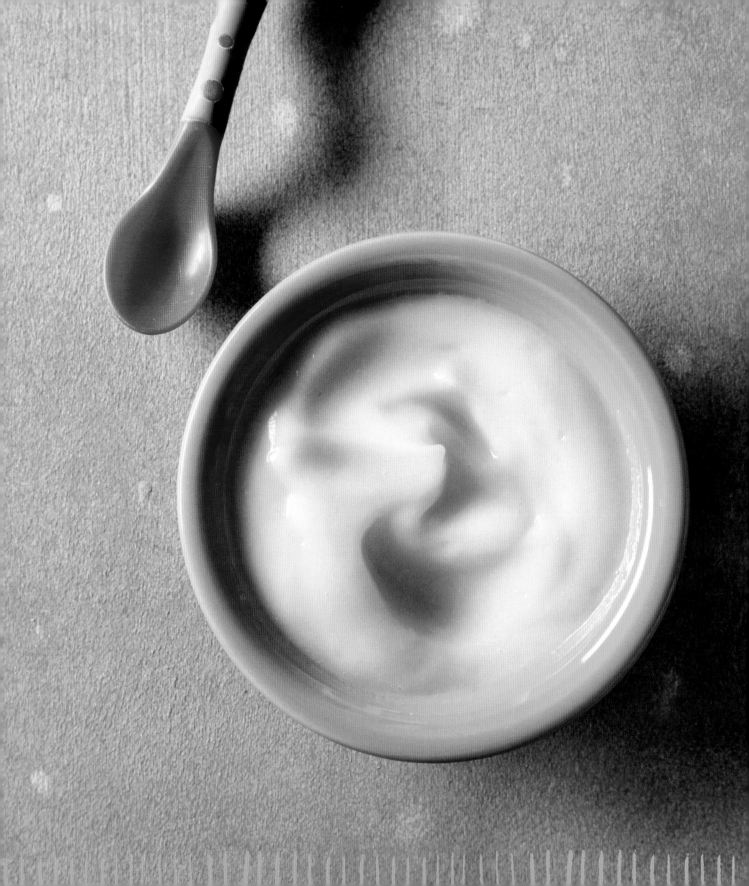

Cauliflower

Makes about 2½ cups
Total Time: 25 minutes

Why This Recipe Works

Cauliflower is another perfect candidate for a super-smooth puree, as it breaks down very, very easily when cooked. We found that steaming florets for just 10 minutes weakened their cell walls enough to make the vegetable extremely tender and easily blended into a silky-smooth consistency with subtly sweet flavor.

You can use a food processor instead of a blender, but the puree will not be quite as smooth.

4½ cups cauliflower florets (12 ounces), cut into 1-inch pieces

1 Bring 1 inch water to rolling boil in large saucepan over high heat. Place steamer basket in saucepan and fill basket with cauliflower. Cover and cook until tender, about 10 minutes.

2 Carefully remove steamer basket from saucepan and transfer cauliflower to blender, reserving cooking liquid. Add 1 cup cooking liquid to cauliflower and process on high speed for 1 minute. Scrape down sides of blender jar and continue to process until very smooth, about 1 minute.

3 Add additional cooking liquid (or breast milk or formula) as needed to thin puree to desired consistency. Let puree cool to room temperature. Serve or store (see page 3 for storage options).

> **SPICE IT UP**
> Add ⅛ teaspoon ground coriander or pinch ground nutmeg to blender along with cauliflower in step 2.

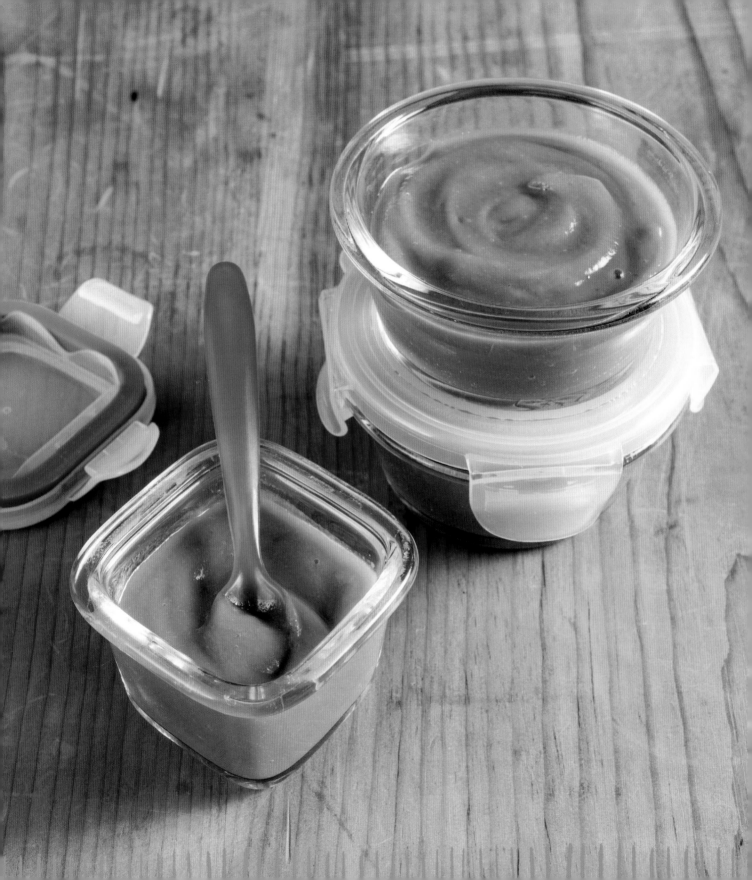

Green Bean

6+ MONTHS

Makes about 2½ cups
Total Time: 30 minutes

Why This Recipe Works

Without the help of a label, it would be hard to tell that commercial green bean baby purees are actually made from this vibrant, chlorophyll-rich legume. Supermarket versions taste about as good as they look: watered down and often slightly sour. (Some producers add citric acid in an attempt to preserve color.) For a better green bean puree, we steamed fresh green beans just until they were tender. The short cooking time translated to a puree with bright color and a deep flavor.

You can use 1 pound frozen cut green beans in place of fresh green beans. You can use a food processor instead of a blender, but the puree will not be quite as smooth.

1 pound green beans, trimmed and cut into 1-inch pieces

1 Bring 1 inch water to rolling boil in large saucepan over high heat. Place steamer basket in saucepan and fill basket with green beans. Cover and cook until tender, about 15 minutes.

2 Carefully remove steamer basket from saucepan and transfer green beans to blender, reserving cooking liquid. Add 1 cup cooking liquid to green beans and process on high speed for 1 minute. Scrape down sides of blender jar and continue to process until very smooth, about 1 minute.

3 Add additional cooking liquid (or breast milk or formula) as needed to thin puree to desired consistency. Let puree cool to room temperature. Serve or store (see page 3 for storage options).

SPICE IT UP
Add ½ teaspoon curry powder or ¼ teaspoon ground coriander to blender along with green beans in step 2.

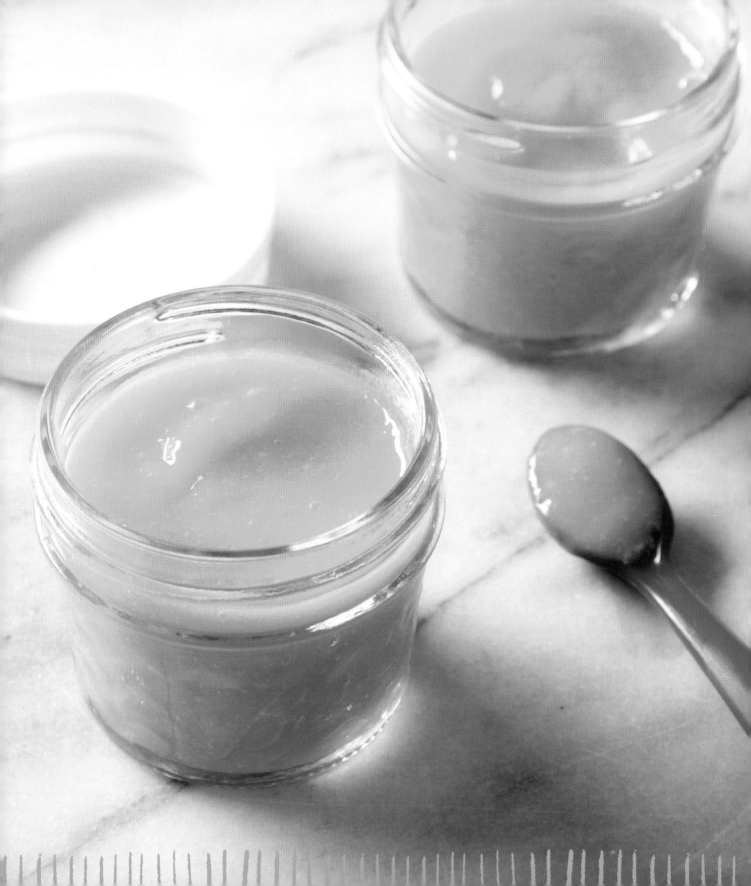

Mango

Makes about 2½ cups
Total Time: 15 minutes

Why This Recipe Works

In the world of recipes, one-ingredient baby purees are some of the easiest to accomplish. Mango puree takes the simplicity one step further. You don't even need to cook it. We set up a side-by-side tasting of pureed steamed versus pureed raw mango, and it was unanimous: raw mango tasted juicy, bright, and fresh, while steamed mango tasted a little washed out. Simply blending the mango with a bit of water yielded a fast, spoonable puree.

You can use 1½ pounds thawed frozen mango chunks in place of the fresh mango. You can use a food processor instead of a blender, but the puree will not be quite as smooth, and you may find that the puree has a more fibrous texture. To make an extra-smooth puree, strain the processed mangoes through a fine-mesh strainer set over a bowl and use the back of a ladle to extract as much puree as possible, discarding solids.

2 pounds mangoes, peeled, pitted, and cut into 1-inch pieces
⅓ cup water

1   Combine mangoes and water in blender. Process on high speed for 1 minute. Scrape down sides of blender jar and continue to process until very smooth, about 1 minute.

2   Add additional water (or breast milk or formula) as needed to thin puree to desired consistency. Serve or store (see page 3 for storage options).

> **SPICE IT UP**
> Add 2 tablespoons coconut milk or pinch garam masala to blender along with mangoes in step 1.

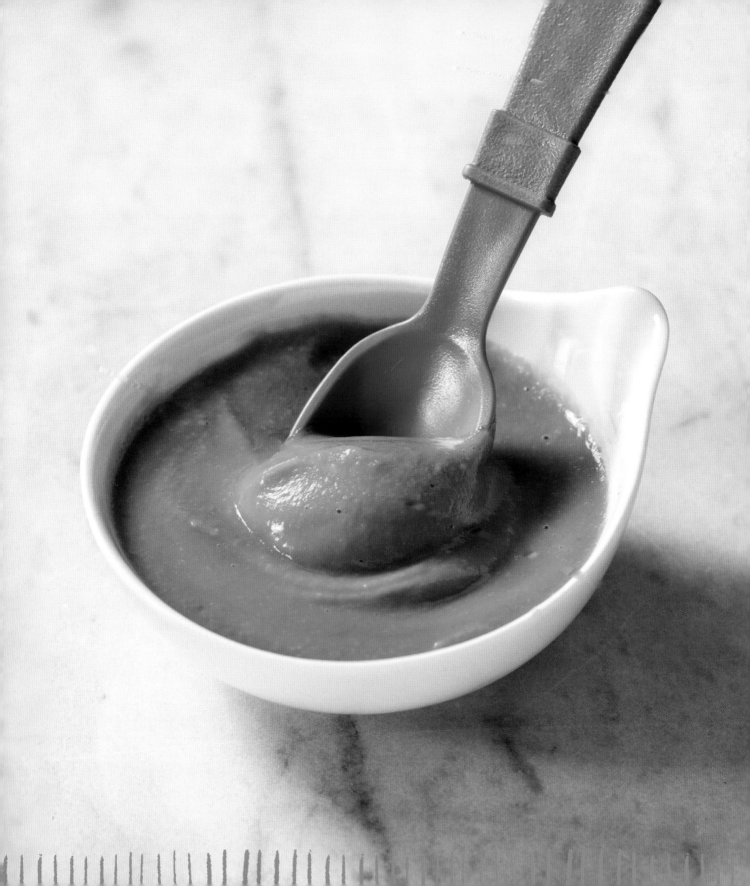

Pea

Makes about 2½ cups
Total Time: 15 minutes

Why This Recipe Works

To make the best green pea puree possible, we turned to the best source for this spring vegetable: the freezer aisle. All we had to do was steam frozen peas until very tender and then process them in a blender with some of their cooking liquid. The resulting puree is springlike and sweet, its color so bright green it almost doesn't look real.

Why Frozen Peas Work Best

Individually frozen soon after shucking from the pod, frozen peas are often sweeter and fresher tasting than the "fresh" peas you have to shuck yourself, which have spent days in storage. This is because the sugars in just-picked peas convert to starches over time. Frozen peas have already been blanched, which stops the process of sugar-to-starch conversion, sets the color of the peas, and cooks them so that they are tender enough to eat.

Don't skip the straining step! Pea skins can add a weird texture, so it's important to pass the puree through a fine-mesh strainer to get a super-smooth finish. You can use a food processor instead of a blender, but the puree will not be quite as smooth.

1½ pounds frozen peas

1. Bring 1 inch water to rolling boil in large saucepan over high heat. Place steamer basket in saucepan and fill basket with peas. Cover and cook until peas are tender, 6 to 8 minutes.

2. Carefully remove steamer basket from saucepan and transfer peas to blender, reserving cooking liquid. Add 1 cup cooking liquid to peas and process on high speed for 1 minute. Scrape down sides of blender jar and continue to process until very smooth, about 1 minute.

3. Strain pea puree through fine-mesh strainer set over bowl, pressing on solids with ladle to extract as much puree as possible; discard solids. Add additional cooking liquid (or breast milk or formula) as needed to thin puree to desired consistency. Let puree cool to room temperature. Serve or store (see page 3 for storage options).

> ### SPICE IT UP
> Add 1 tablespoon finely chopped fresh mint or ¼ teaspoon ground cumin to blender along with peas in step 2.

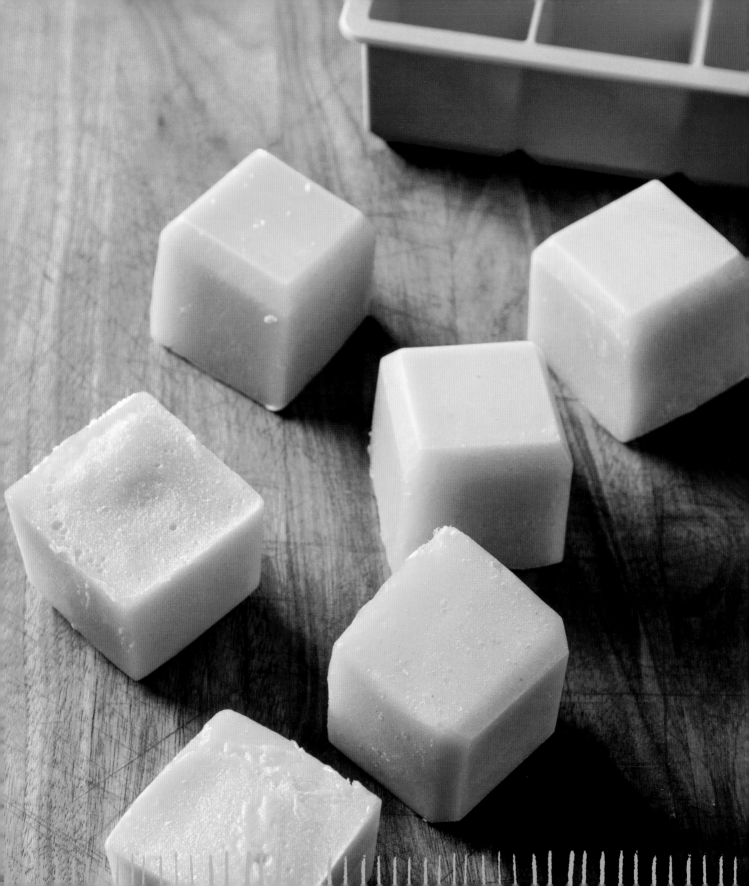

Peach

Makes about 2½ cups
Total Time: 25 minutes

Why This Recipe Works

There are few things better than a freshly picked, super-ripe peach, which is why we first thought raw, ripe peaches would make the freshest tasting puree. But when we pureed them, the raw peaches became oddly...frothy. (Turns out, the fruit's tiny air pockets burst during blending and created that bubbly texture.) Steaming the peaches for just 5 minutes mellowed their flavor and released that trapped air, resulting in a smooth, intensely peachy puree.

A serrated peeler makes quick work of peeling the peaches. You can use 1¼ pounds thawed frozen peach slices in place of the fresh peaches. You can use a food processor instead of a blender, but the puree will not be quite as smooth.

2 pounds peaches, peeled, pitted, and cut into 1-inch pieces

1. Bring 1 inch water to rolling boil in large saucepan over high heat. Place steamer basket in saucepan and fill basket with peaches. Cover and cook until tender, about 5 minutes.

2. Carefully remove steamer basket from saucepan and transfer peaches to blender, reserving cooking liquid. Add ⅓ cup cooking liquid to peaches and process on high speed for 1 minute. Scrape down sides of blender jar and continue to process until very smooth, about 1 minute.

3. Add additional cooking liquid (or breast milk or formula) as needed to thin puree to desired consistency. Let puree cool to room temperature. Serve or store (see page 3 for storage options).

> ### SPICE IT UP
> Add ⅛ teaspoon ground nutmeg or seeds scraped from ½ vanilla bean to blender along with peaches in step 2.

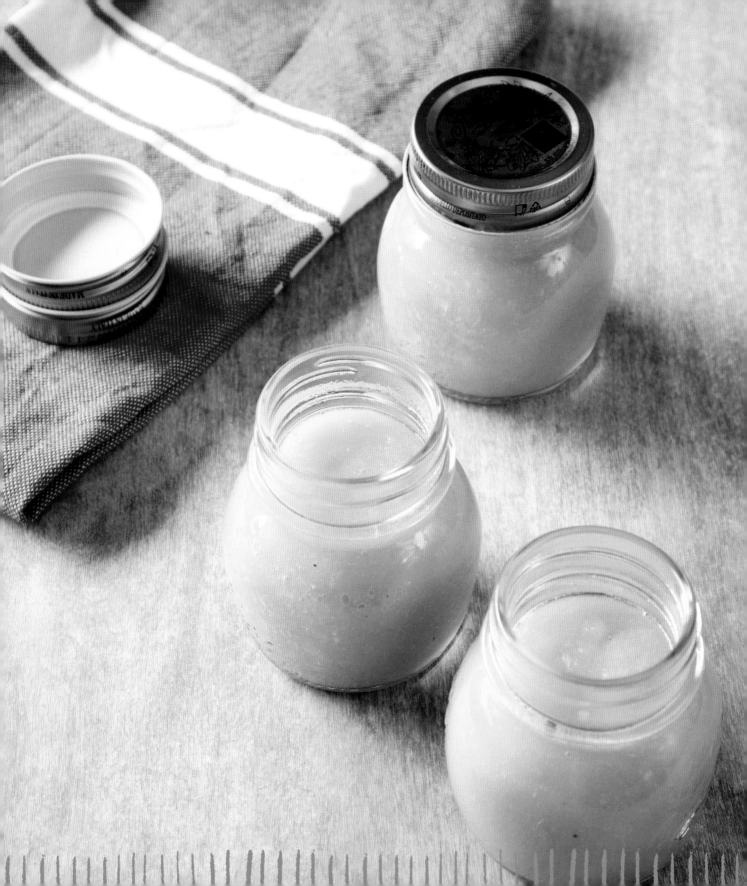

Pear

⚡ ❄ **6+** MONTHS

Makes about 2½ cups
Total Time: 25 minutes

Why This Recipe Works

Pears can cook up grainy, so we knew we had to find a way to ensure a puree with velvety smoothness. First, we tackled the cooking method. Steaming proved the quickest, easiest way to achieve both tenderness and concentrated flavor. Second, we tested the variety and ripeness. Bosc pears are much crisper than other varieties and consistently turned out fibrous purees. Softer varieties such as Anjou and Bartlett yielded smooth, pear-y purees, especially when super ripe.

A ripe Anjou pear will give to slight pressure when pressed at the neck; a Bartlett will turn from light green to yellow when ripe. Do not use Bosc pears in this recipe; they will make the puree grainy. You can use a food processor instead of a blender, but the puree will not be quite as smooth.

2 pounds ripe Bartlett or Anjou pears, peeled, halved, cored, and cut into 1-inch pieces

1 Bring 1 inch water to rolling boil in large saucepan over high heat. Place steamer basket in saucepan and fill basket with pears. Cover and cook until tender, about 10 minutes.

2 Carefully remove steamer basket from saucepan and transfer pears to blender, reserving cooking liquid. Add ⅓ cup cooking liquid to pears and process on high speed for 1 minute. Scrape down sides of blender jar and continue to process until very smooth, about 1 minute.

3 Add additional cooking liquid (or breast milk or formula) as needed to thin puree to desired consistency. Let puree cool to room temperature. Serve or store (see page 3 for storage options).

> SPICE IT UP
> Add ⅛ teaspoon ground ginger or pinch ground cardamom to blender along with pears in step 2.

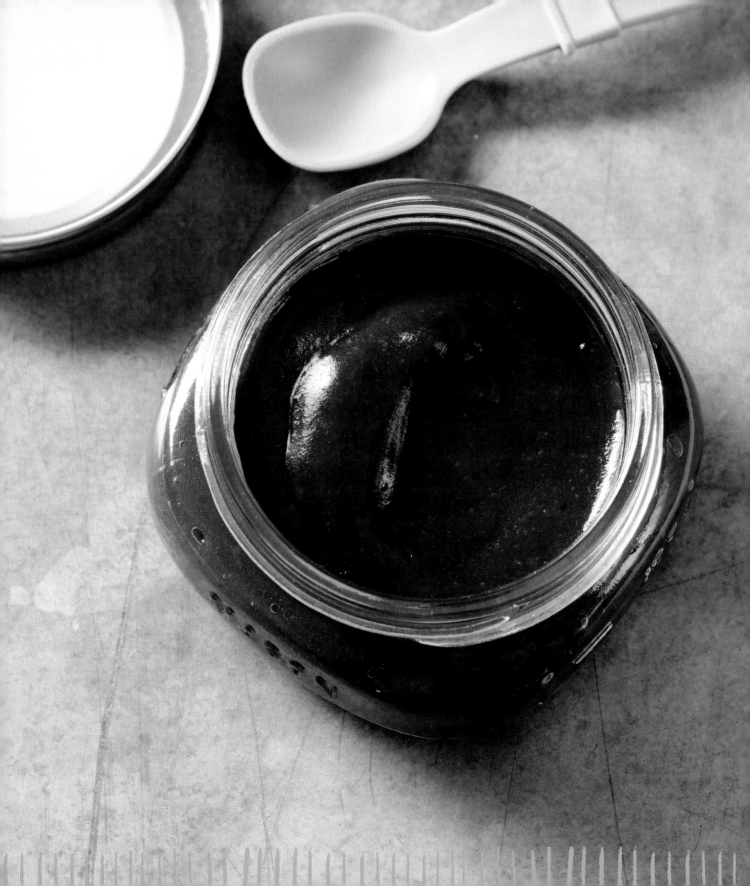

Prune

Makes about ¾ cup
Total Time: 20 minutes

Why This Recipe Works

Digestion and its, ahem, aftereffects are a big part of life with a new baby. As you have most likely found out, introducing solid foods to a baby's diet can cause constipation. Having a way to provide some relief is what we call a parenting win. Prunes (dried plums) are especially high in soluble fiber and can be used as a gentle laxative to keep things regular. Plus, their natural sweetness is very appealing to babies. Making a homemade prune puree turned out to be as simple as rehydrating the dried fruit in hot water and blending it.

✳ APRICOTS WORK, TOO!

Dried apricots are almost as high in soluble fiber as prunes; you can substitute an equal amount of dried apricots for the prunes, if desired. Some babies may be sensitive to the sulfur dioxide that is sometimes used to preserve the color of dried fruit, so we recommend seeking out unsulfured prunes and apricots.

For an accurate measurement of boiling water, bring a full kettle of water to boil, then measure out the desired amount. You can use a food processor instead of a blender, but the puree will not be quite as smooth.

½ cup pitted prunes
¾ cup boiling water

1. Pour boiling water over prunes in medium bowl. Cover and let sit until prunes have softened, about 15 minutes.

2. Transfer prunes and their liquid to blender and process on high speed for 1 minute. Scrape down sides of blender jar and continue to process until very smooth, about 1 minute.

3. Add additional water (or breast milk or formula) as needed to thin puree to desired consistency. Let puree cool to room temperature. Serve or store (see page 3 for storage options).

SPICE IT UP
Add ⅛ teaspoon ground cinnamon or ground allspice to bowl with prunes in step 1.

Portion Size
A little bit of this puree goes a long way for its digestive effect, so we scaled this recipe down to make just a few servings. Portion size ranges from 1 teaspoon twice a day for the youngest solids-eating babies up to 1 tablespoon three times a day for babies around 12 months old, according to our pediatric dietitian.

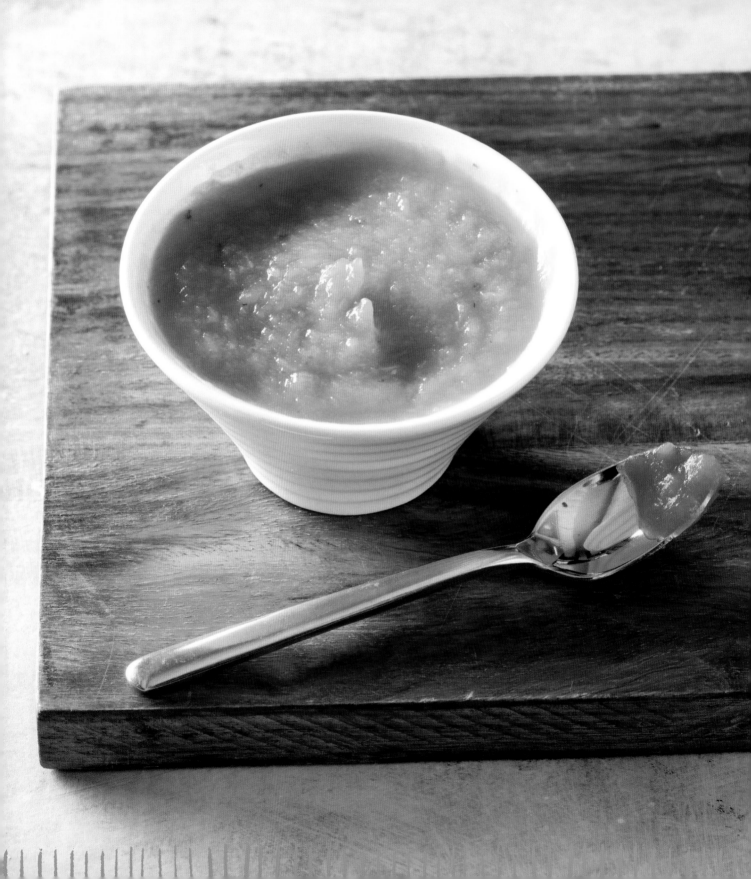

Butternut Squash

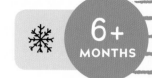

Makes about 2½ cups
Total Time: 1 hour 15 minutes

Why This Recipe Works

Sweet and earthy butternut squash is great pureed, enjoyed by adults (hello, Thanksgiving!) and babies alike. However, when we tasted commercial squash purees, we were dismayed by their sad and even sour flavor. We were excited to find that the squash puree with the best flavor was also the easiest to make. Simply roasting a halved squash on a baking sheet before scooping out the flesh and pureeing it with a little water gave us a smooth puree with concentrated, earthy squash flavor.

If you're in a rush, check out our microwave instructions on page 284. You can use a food processor instead of a blender, but the puree will not be quite as smooth.

1 butternut squash (2½ pounds), halved lengthwise and seeded
1 cup water

1. Adjust oven rack to middle position and heat oven to 425 degrees. Line rimmed baking sheet with parchment paper. Place squash pieces cut side down on prepared sheet and roast until uniformly soft when pressed with tongs, 45 to 60 minutes.

2. Scoop out squash flesh with spoon and transfer to blender; discard skin. Add water to squash and process on high speed for 1 minute. Scrape down sides of blender jar and continue to process until very smooth, about 1 minute.

3. Add additional water (or breast milk or formula) as needed to thin puree to desired consistency. Let puree cool to room temperature. Serve or store (see page 3 for storage options).

> **SPICE IT UP**
> Add ¼ teaspoon ground cumin or ¼ teaspoon ground turmeric to blender along with squash in step 2.

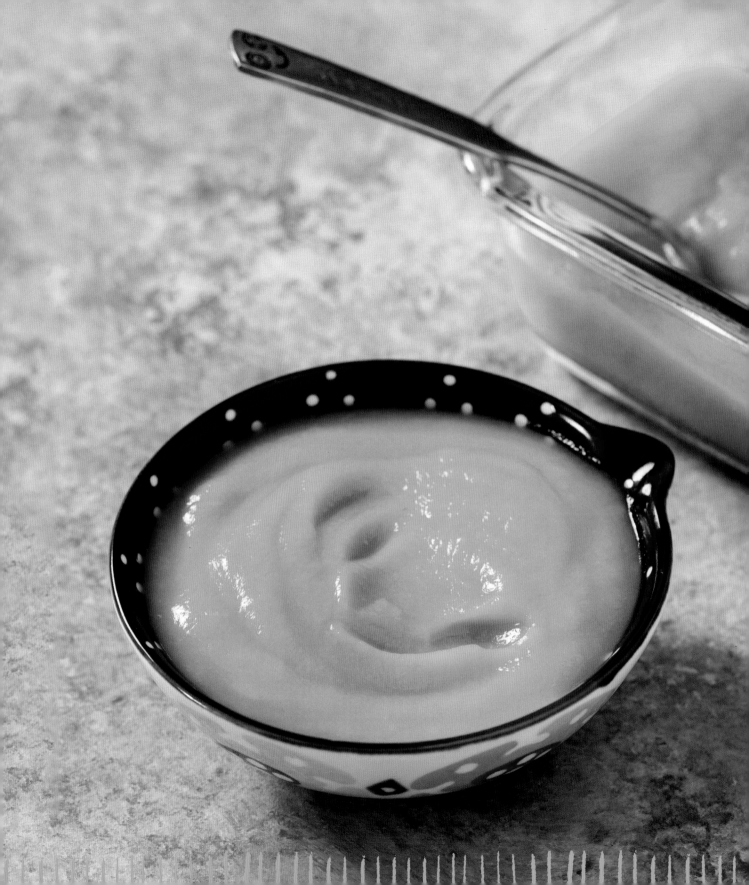

Sweet Potato

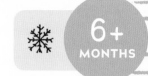

6+ MONTHS

Makes about 2½ cups
Total Time: 1 hour 30 minutes

Why This Recipe Works

Sweet potatoes and common white potatoes are very different. Not only are they different colors, they also come from different botanical families. Most importantly: sweet potatoes contain far less starch and more sugar than white potatoes. This makes sweet potatoes an ideal candidate for a naturally sweet, creamy puree. We found that roasting whole sweet potatoes in the oven for an hour yielded a much sweeter and tastier product, and roasting also increases their vitamin C content. After baking, we blended the sweet potato flesh with water to produce a smooth puree.

SPICE IT UP
Add ¼ teaspoon ground cinnamon or ¼ teaspoon curry powder to blender along with sweet potatoes in step 3.

If you're in a rush, check out our microwave instructions on page 284. You can use a food processor instead of a blender, but the puree will not be quite as smooth.

Vegetable oil spray
3 small sweet potatoes (8 ounces each)
1½ cups water

1   Adjust oven rack to middle position and heat oven to 425 degrees. Set wire rack in aluminum foil–lined rimmed baking sheet and spray with vegetable oil spray.

2   Use fork to prick each sweet potato lightly in 3 places. Place potatoes on prepared rack and bake until potatoes are lightly browned and feel very soft when gently squeezed with tongs, about 1 hour.

3   Cut each potato lengthwise with knife, scoop out flesh with spoon, and transfer to blender; discard skin. Add water and process on high speed for 1 minute. Scrape down sides of blender jar and continue to process until very smooth, about 1 minute.

4   Add additional water (or breast milk or formula) as needed to thin puree to desired consistency. Let puree cool to room temperature. Serve or store (see page 3 for storage options).

Spud Science
Sweet potatoes actually get *sweeter* during cooking thanks to the action of an enzyme that breaks down starch into sugar between 135 and 170 degrees. Baking for a full hour gives the enzymes more time to work. The result? Sweeter sweet potatoes.

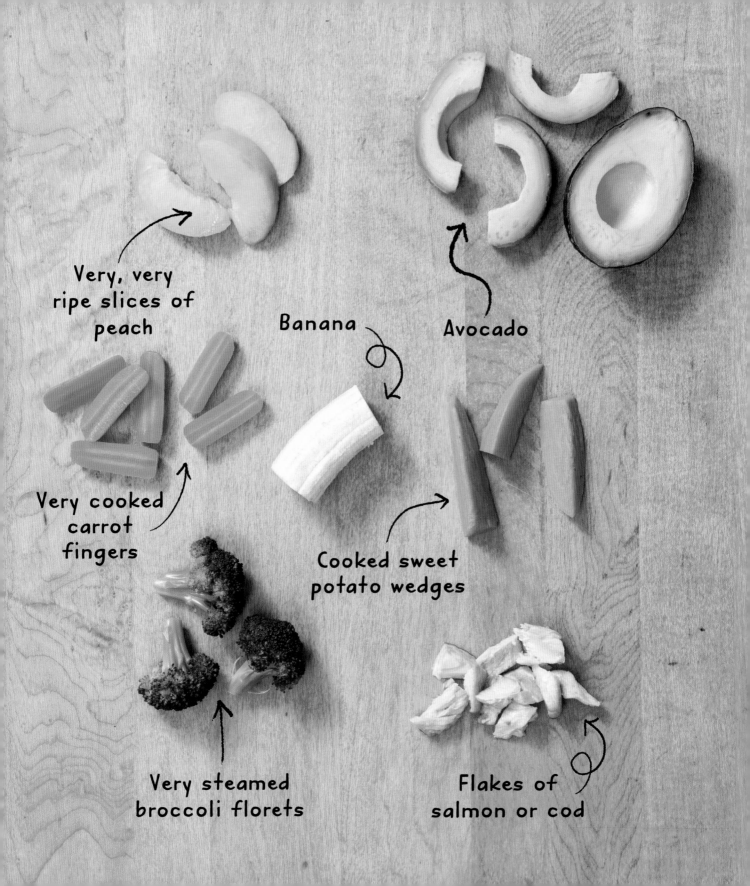

Very, very ripe slices of peach

Banana

Avocado

Very cooked carrot fingers

Cooked sweet potato wedges

Very steamed broccoli florets

Flakes of salmon or cod

FIRST FINGER FOODS

Baby-led weaning, or the practice of skipping purees and introducing solids by letting your baby feed whole foods to him or herself, has become popular in recent years, though in reality has been around for a very long time (purees certainly didn't exist in ancient Rome). This means offering the baby soft, easily graspable finger foods and letting them gnaw, lick, smush, gum, and play with it in whatever manner they choose.

A few things are important when it comes to baby-led weaning: first is to follow your baby's cues for whether he or she is ready to start eating, and then to offer food that is easy and safe to pick up and put in one's mouth. Babies around 6 to 9 months don't have great fine-motor skills, so offering food that is big enough to grasp with the whole hand and long enough to stick out beyond the palm (plus, not too slippery) is key.

In baby-led weaning, babies are encouraged to eat meals with the family, choose how much and what to eat themselves, and eat without expectation on how much to consume. A big part of starting out with solids is playing with food, feeling new textures, and tasting new flavors. Gil Rapley, author of *Baby-Led Weaning*, the 2008 book that brought this old technique back into the spotlight, says that one of the biggest benefits of the technique is bringing the baby into the family eating experience from the very beginning. "Baby meals are particularly rushed because they often happen before the family meal," she says. "The key to baby-led weaning is it's a shared experience. The baby's food and the family food...it looks the same, it is the same. Sharing mealtimes with babies gives them more time to eat food or explore it."

You can try the baby-led weaning experience, offering only whole foods for your baby to feed him or herself, or you can try a combination of letting your baby feed larger pieces of finger food to him or herself along with spoon-feeding him or her purees.

Remember that learning how to feed oneself takes time and practice—and makes a whole lot of mess. To prevent choking or too much gagging (a little gag reflex is normal) avoid hard, round, sticky, or gummy food. Offer foods that are soft enough to mash or gum safely in tiny, toothless mouths.

Here are some of our favorite options (left). Other options include Mini Meatballs (page 103) or slices of veggie burger. For more adventurous finger food ideas, see chapter 3 (page 77).

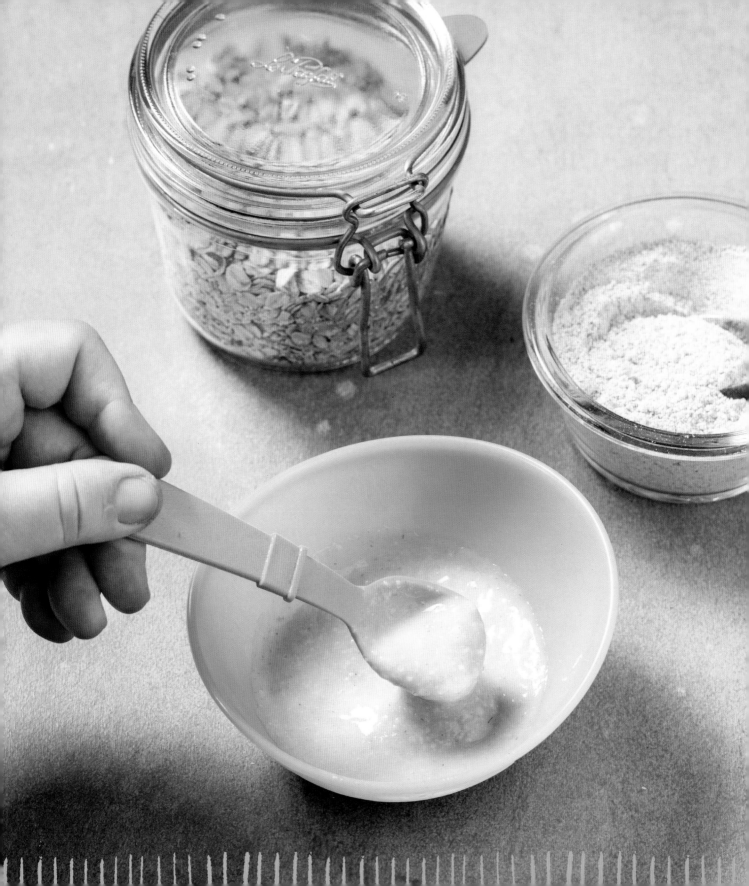

Baby Cereals

Makes 1 to 1⅓ cups dried cereal
Total Time: 5 minutes

Why This Recipe Works

Your first taste of solid food might just have been a grain cereal. Ground into a powder, they are easy to both eat and digest and have been a popular very-first food for decades. Supermarkets sell containers of precooked grain powders to be mixed with water, breast milk, or formula for an easy instant porridge. We wanted to create our own cereal bases from a handful of nutritious whole grains—not only does it save money, these cereals taste better and give you more grain options. See page 34 for how to turn cereal base into porridge.

We had best results grinding the grains in a blender rather than a food processor, as the vortex created during the blending process helped move the grains around in the jar and ensured they were evenly pulverized. If using a food processor, you may need to extend the processing time and pass the ground grains through a fine-mesh strainer to remove any larger pieces.

1 cup white rice, brown rice, millet, rolled oats, or steel-cut oats

1. Process grains in blender on high speed to fine powder, 1 to 3 minutes, scraping down blender jar with rubber spatula as needed. Transfer to airtight container. (See page 34 for cooking directions.)

✳ IMPORTANT TO NOTE!

Our baby cereals, unlike many of the supermarket cereals, need to be cooked after grinding and are meant to be turned into a spoonable porridge (see page 34). Infant cereals should never be added to an infant's bottle for drinking with breast milk or formula unless directed to do so by your pediatrician.

Different Types of Grains

WHITE AND BROWN RICE: A grain of rice is made up of endosperm, germ, bran, and a husk. Brown rice is simply husked, while white rice also has had the germ and bran removed. White rice cooks faster but contains fewer nutrients and flavor.

MILLET: Believed to be the first domesticated cereal grain, this tiny cereal grass seed has a long history. Millet has a mellow corn flavor.

OATS: Rolled oats are made by hulling, cleaning, steaming, and rolling whole oats. Steel-cut oats are partially cooked and then chopped with steel blades.

Turning Dried Baby Cereal into Porridge

Cereal (Ground)	Quantity	Water Amount	Cooking Time/Method	Yield
White Rice	1½ teaspoons	⅓ cup	1½ minutes in microwave	¼ cup
	1 tablespoon	⅔ cup	2½ minutes in microwave	½ cup
	2 tablespoons	1¼ cup	5 to 10 minutes on stovetop	1 cup
Brown Rice	1½ teaspoons	⅓ cup	1½ minutes in microwave	¼ cup
	1 tablespoon	⅔ cup	3 minutes in microwave	½ cup
	2 tablespoons	1¼ cup	5 to 10 minutes on stovetop	1 cup
Millet	1½ teaspoons	¼ cup	1 minute in microwave	¼ cup
	1 tablespoon	½ cup	2 minutes in microwave	½ cup
	2 tablespoons	1 cup	2 to 4 minutes on stovetop	1 cup
Rolled Oats	1½ teaspoons	¼ cup	1½ minutes in microwave	¼ cup
	1 tablespoon	½ cup	3 minutes in microwave	½ cup
	2 tablespoons	1 cup	8 to 10 minutes on stovetop	1 cup
Steel-Cut Oats	1½ teaspoons	¼ cup	1 minute in microwave	¼ cup
	1 tablespoon	½ cup	2 minutes in microwave	½ cup
	2 tablespoons	1 cup	3 to 5 minutes on stovetop	1 cup

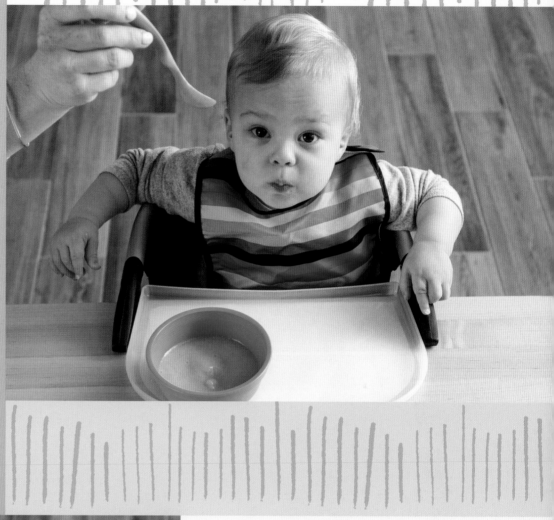

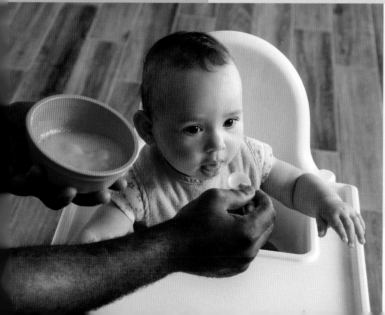

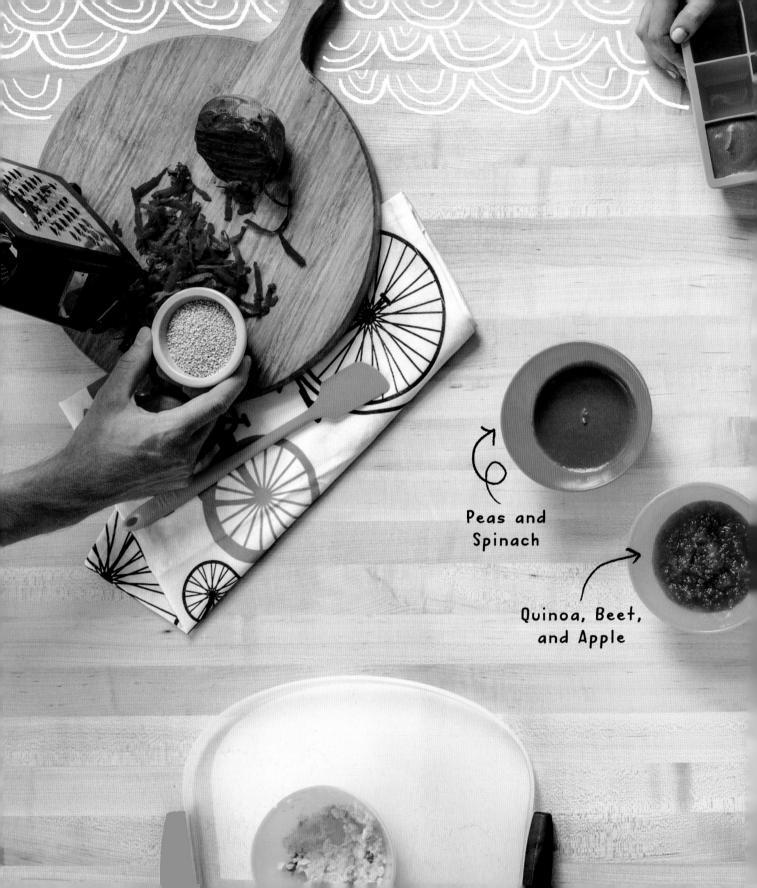

Peas and
Spinach

Quinoa, Beet,
and Apple

ADVENTUROUS COMBINATIONS

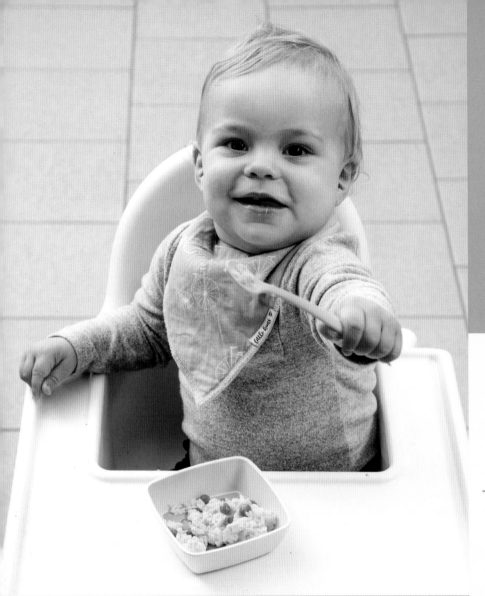

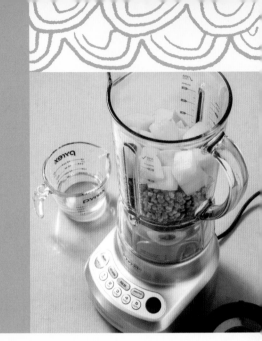

"Great recipe with good ingredients. Love introducing brown rice to my grandbaby."

—Grandparent of 9-month-old, on Chicken, Carrot, and Brown Rice Puree

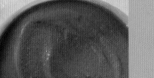

"I did not puree the recipe after cooking since my 12-month-old has a mouthful of teeth! I also used coconut yogurt, as he has a dairy allergy. He loved it!"

—Parent of 12-month-old, on Bulgur, Eggplant, and Yogurt Mash

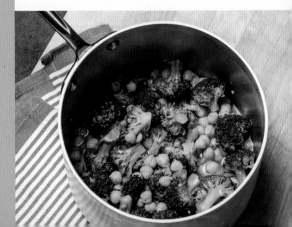

ALL ABOUT
ADVENTUROUS COMBINATIONS

After mastering the basics in chapter 1, you and your baby are ready to move on to more adventurous flavors and textures. For this chapter, our team of test cooks developed a collection of mashes and purees that combine ingredients—everything from fruits and vegetables and grains to dairy, meat, and even fish.

Like for our first chapter, we developed these recipes thinking about nutrition, ease, and flavor. We chose healthy ingredients with the help of our pediatric dietitian. With everything else new parents have going on, dealing with complicated recipes for your babies is not something to add to the list. Note the fast icons ⚡ next to recipes that will take 45 minutes or less.

We wanted each mixture to taste its absolute best, whether that meant roasting the carrots and apples together before pureeing or adding a bit of plain whole milk yogurt to the eggplant barley mash. A big part of the beginning stage of eating is learning about flavor—what flavors exist, how they relate to each other, and if they are good or maybe not so good (yet). Whether or not your baby loves his or her first taste of salmon doesn't really matter; what matters more is that it's being introduced. Each recipe includes options to add *more* flavor to the mix with spices or herbs to help expand your baby's palette. None of the recipes in this chapter include added salt, which is not recommended for babies under 12 months of age. For more on salt, see page vii.

These mixtures range in appropriateness for ages 6 months and up, mainly dependent on texture. Some of the chunkier mashes can be served as finger foods for your baby, straight off a high-chair tray or table. While much of it might end up on clothing, the ground, or even smushed into hair or ears (we've seen it all), remember that eating when under a year old is more about learning *how* to eat than about consuming calories. You're off to a good start.

A NOTE ABOUT STORAGE

We wanted to make sure that if you're making homemade puree, you'll have enough for at least a few meals. Unless otherwise noted, all purees in this chapter can be refrigerated for up to 3 days. Purees that can be frozen are marked with a snowflake icon ❄. To freeze, divide puree evenly into ice cube tray. Once frozen, pop cubes out of tray and transfer to heavy-duty zipper-lock bag. To serve, defrost in refrigerator overnight or microwave 1 cube for 30 to 45 seconds and stir to recombine.

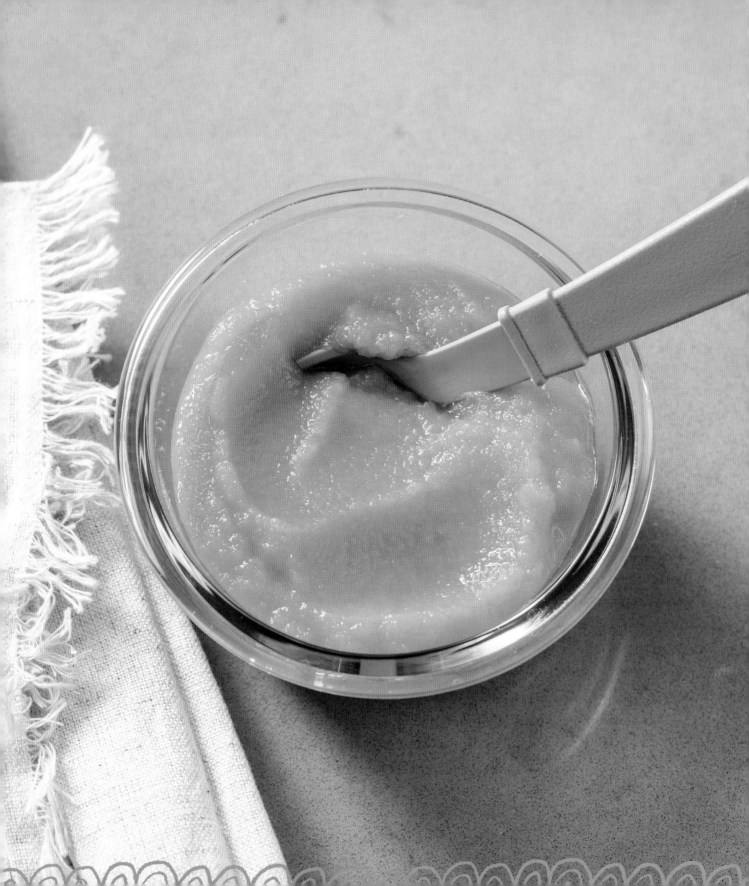

Carrot and Apple

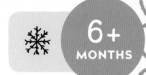

Makes about 2½ cups
Total Time: 50 minutes

Why This Recipe Works

It's like autumn in a bowl of baby food. Roasting carrots and apples brings out a toasty, sweeter flavor that works well in tandem. We jump-started the carrots by using foil to cover them on the baking sheet, causing them to steam as they roasted. After 20 minutes of "steam-roasting," we removed the foil, added the apples to the sheet, and roasted the two together until they were both very tender and lightly browned.

SPICE IT UP

Add pinch ground ginger or pinch nutmeg to blender along with carrots and apples in step 3.

Any variety of apple will work here, but tart apples, like Granny Smith, are more acidic and may not be as appealing to your baby. Do not use frozen carrots in place of fresh carrots. You can use a food processor instead of a blender, but the puree will not be quite as smooth.

4 carrots (10 ounces), peeled and cut into 1-inch pieces
3 Fuji, Gala, or Golden Delicious apples (1¼ pounds), peeled, cored, and cut into 1-inch pieces
¾ cup water

1. Adjust oven rack to middle position and heat oven to 400 degrees. Line rimmed baking sheet with parchment paper. Spread carrots in even layer on prepared sheet and cover tightly with aluminum foil. Roast carrots for 20 minutes.

2. Remove foil, add apples to baking sheet with carrots, and stir to combine. Continue to roast, uncovered, until carrots and apples are tender when pierced with a paring knife and lightly browned, 12 to 14 minutes.

3. Carefully transfer carrots and apples to blender. Add water to blender and process on high speed for 1 minute. Scrape down sides of blender jar and continue to process until very smooth, about 1 minute. Add additional water (or breast milk or formula) as needed to thin puree to desired consistency. Let puree cool to room temperature. Serve or store (see page 39 for storage options).

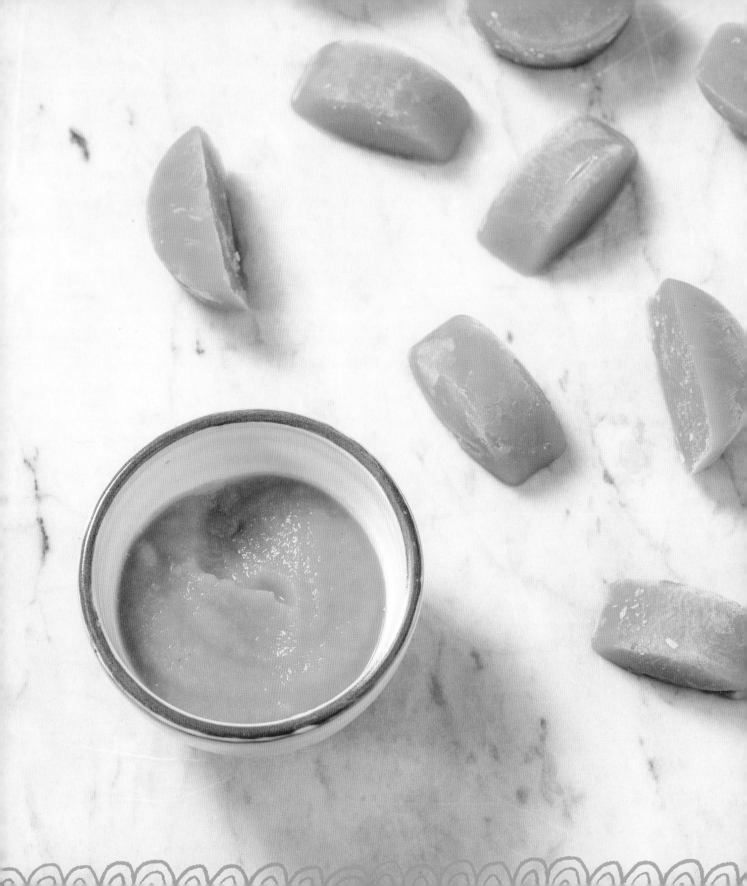

Sweet Potato and Apple

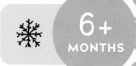

Makes about 2½ cups
Total Time: 50 minutes

Why This Recipe Works

What can we say? Apples and orange vegetables work well together (see Carrot and Apple, page 41). We found that oven roasting gave our mixture of sweet potatoes and apples a deep, earthy flavor and a rich, creamy texture. Peeling and chopping the sweet potato and then giving it a 20-minute head start in the oven, covered with foil, shortened cooking time exponentially. We then added the apples to the baking sheet and roasted them together, uncovered, until they were both super soft and lightly browned.

SPICE IT UP
Add pinch cinnamon or pinch cloves to blender along with sweet potatoes and apples in step 3.

Look for a small or medium sweet potato for this recipe. Any variety of apple will work here, but tart apples, like Granny Smith, are more acidic and may not be as appealing to your baby. You can use a food processor instead of a blender, but the puree will not be quite as smooth.

1 sweet potato (10 ounces), peeled and cut into 1-inch pieces
3 Fuji, Gala, or Golden Delicious apples (1¼ pounds), peeled, cored, and cut into 1-inch pieces
1 cup water

1. Adjust oven rack to middle position and heat oven to 400 degrees. Line rimmed baking sheet with parchment paper. Spread sweet potatoes in even layer on prepared sheet and cover sheet tightly with foil. Roast sweet potatoes for 20 minutes.

2. Remove foil, add apples to baking sheet with sweet potatoes, and stir to combine. Continue to roast, uncovered, until sweet potatoes and apples are very tender when pierced with a paring knife and just beginning to brown, 12 to 14 minutes.

3. Carefully transfer sweet potatoes and apples to blender. Add water to blender and process on high speed for 1 minute. Scrape down sides of blender jar and continue to process until very smooth, about 1 minute.

4. Add additional water (or breast milk or formula) as needed to thin puree to desired consistency. Let puree cool to room temperature. Serve or store (see page 39 for storage options).

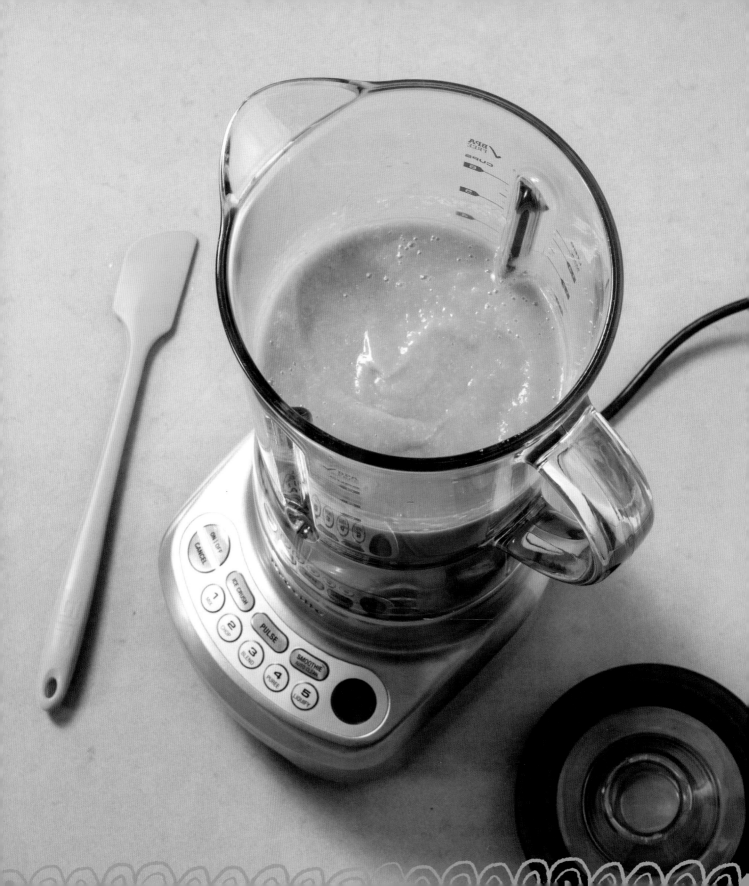

Mango and Pea

Makes about 2½ cups
Total Time: 20 minutes

Why This Recipe Works

Yes, this is a surprising combination. But it turned out to be one of our favorites. The vibrant, tart, fruity flavor of the mango balanced the soft, grassy flavor of the peas. We tested our way through different cooking methods but found that the mango tasted best when we didn't cook it at all.

SPICE IT UP

Add ¼ teaspoon grated lime zest or 2 teaspoons chopped fresh mint to blender along with peas and mangoes in step 2.

You can use 1½ pounds thawed frozen mango chunks in place of the fresh mango. The frozen peas do not need to be thawed before steaming. Be sure to follow the straining step to avoid unappealing texture in the puree. You can use a food processor instead of a blender, but the puree will not be quite as smooth.

1¼ cups frozen peas
2 pounds mangoes, peeled, pitted, and cut into
   1-inch pieces

1. Bring 1 inch water to rolling boil in large saucepan over high heat. Place steamer basket in saucepan and fill basket with peas. Cover and cook until peas are tender, 6 to 8 minutes.

2. Carefully remove steamer basket from saucepan and transfer peas to blender, reserving cooking liquid. Add mangoes and ½ cup cooking liquid to blender and process on high speed for 1 minute. Scrape down sides of blender jar and continue to process until very smooth, about 1 minute.

3. Strain mixture through fine-mesh strainer set over bowl, pressing on solids with ladle to extract as much puree as possible; discard solids. Add additional cooking liquid (or breast milk or formula) as needed to thin puree to desired consistency. Let puree cool to room temperature. Serve or store (see page 39 for storage options).

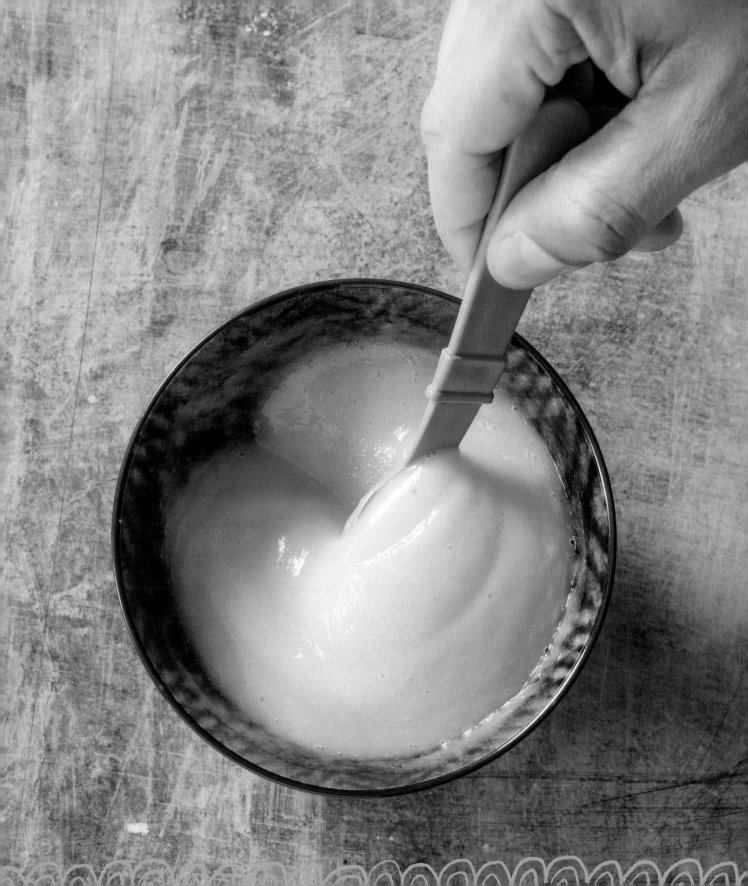

Pear and Zucchini

Makes about 2½ cups
Total Time: 20 minutes

Why This Recipe Works

Steaming zucchini and pears together produces the best flavor in the least amount of steps. Given all of the natural juices contained in both zucchini and pears, we did not need to add any additional cooking liquid to the blender to achieve a consistency we liked. (That said, we do recommend reserving the cooking liquid to thin the puree as desired.)

A ripe Anjou pear will give to slight pressure when pressed at the neck; a Bartlett will turn from light green to yellow when ripe. Do not use Bosc pears in this recipe; they will make the puree grainy. We prefer smaller zucchini, which are more flavorful and less watery than larger ones. You can use a food processor instead of a blender, but the puree will not be quite as smooth.

1½ pounds zucchini, peeled, quartered lengthwise, and cut into 1-inch pieces
1 large ripe Bartlett or Anjou pear (8 ounces), peeled, cored, and cut into 1-inch pieces

1. Bring 1 inch water to rolling boil in large saucepan over high heat. Place steamer basket in saucepan and fill basket with zucchini and pears. Cover and cook until zucchini and pears are tender, 8 to 10 minutes.

2. Carefully remove steamer basket from saucepan and transfer zucchini and pears to blender, reserving cooking liquid. Process on high speed for 1 minute. Scrape down sides of blender jar and continue to process until very smooth, about 1 minute.

3. Add reserved cooking liquid (or breast milk or formula) as needed to thin puree to desired consistency. Let puree cool to room temperature. Serve or store (see page 39 for storage options).

> **SPICE IT UP**
> Add pinch ground nutmeg or 2 teaspoons fresh chopped basil to blender along with zucchini and pears in step 2.

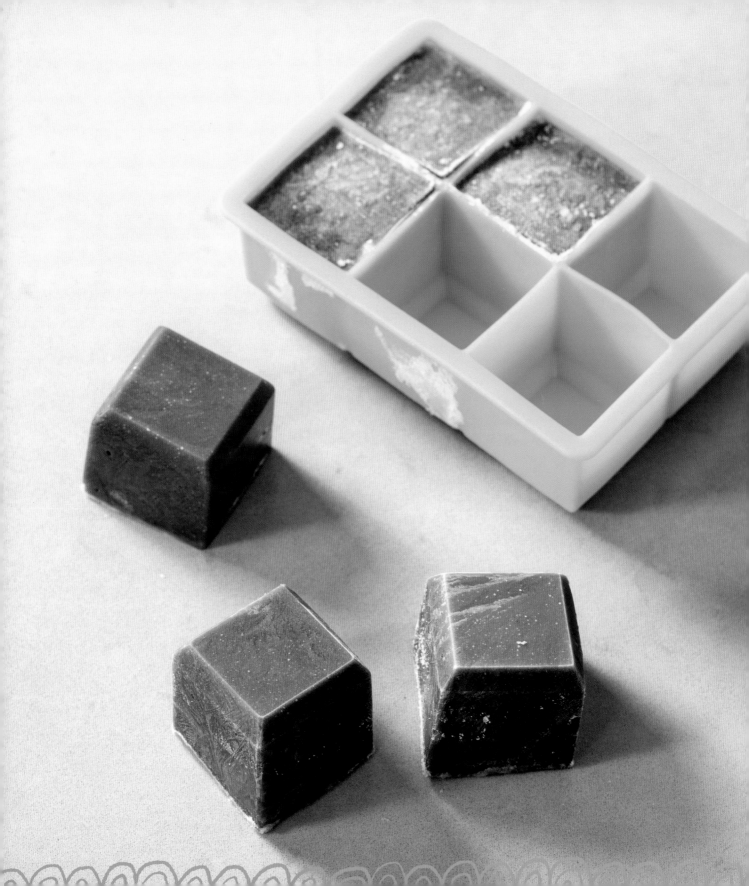

Peas and Spinach

Makes about 2½ cups
Total Time: 20 minutes

Why This Recipe Works

Spinach and peas are the vegetable puree power couple. Their shades of green are bold, and the delicate sweetness of the peas is a nice counterbalance to the earthy spinach. Plus, spinach is a nutritional powerhouse, rich in vitamin A, vitamin C, vitamin K, magnesium, manganese, iron, and folate. We started by steaming the spinach and peas together. To keep the color of this puree bright, we shocked the now-wilted spinach by running the entire steamer basket under cold water just after steaming. Passing the pureed spinach-pea mixture through a fine-mesh strainer creates the best texture.

SPICE IT UP
Add ½ teaspoon curry powder or ground coriander to food processor along with pea mixture in step 2.

Do not substitute frozen spinach for fresh baby spinach, as it will not break down in the blender and it has a different flavor. There is no need to defrost peas before steaming. You can use a food processor instead of a blender, but the puree will not be quite as smooth.

9 ounces (9 cups) baby spinach
2¾ cups frozen peas

1. Bring 1 inch of water to rolling boil in Dutch oven over high heat. Place steamer basket in Dutch oven and fill with spinach and peas. Cover and cook until spinach has wilted, about 6 minutes.

2. Carefully transfer steamer basket to sink, reserving cooking liquid. Run cold water over spinach and peas for 30 seconds. Transfer spinach and peas to blender. Add ½ cup cooking liquid to blender and process on high speed, about 1 minute. Scrape down sides of blender jar and continue to process until smooth, about 1 minute.

3. Strain mixture through fine-mesh strainer set over bowl, pressing on solids with ladle to extract as much puree as possible; discard solids.

4. Add additional cooking liquid (or breast milk or formula) as needed to thin puree to desired consistency. Let puree cool to room temperature. Serve or store (see page 39 for storage options).

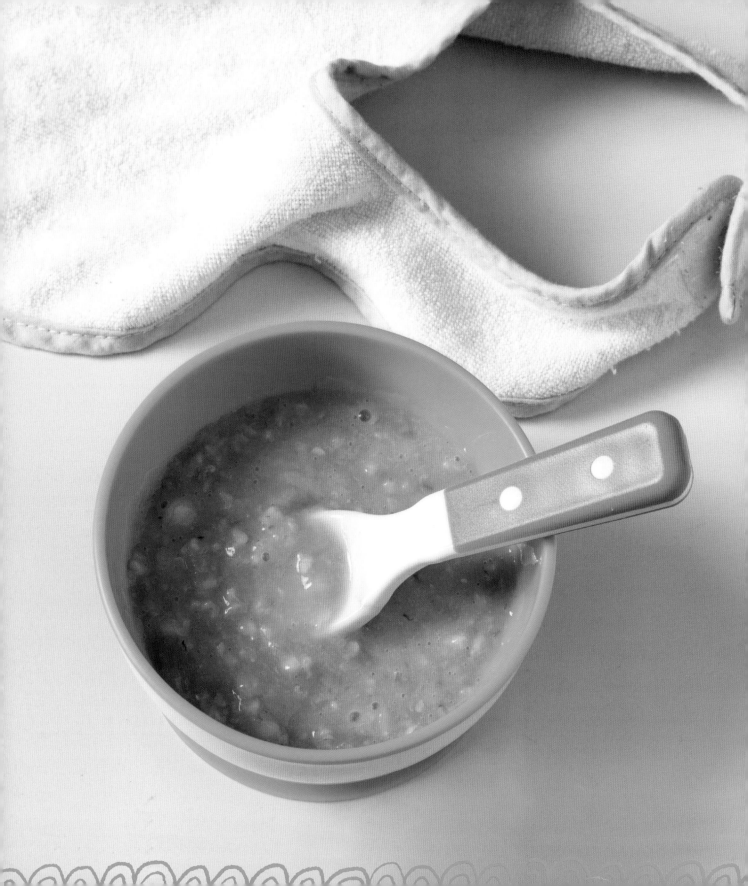

Oatmeal, Peach, and Banana

Makes about 2½ cups
Total Time: 35 minutes

Why This Recipe Works

To tailor the best breakfast ever (oatmeal) to the tastes of a brand-new eater, we made a few changes to the standard recipe. While adults may enjoy a little texture to their oats, we wanted something slightly smoother for a baby. We threw a chopped peach in with the oats while they cooked so it would become soft and easily mashable. Adding a ripe banana gave the mixture a lovely creamy texture and added a sweet balance to the tart stone fruit. No blender necessary: a potato masher brought everything together into a cohesive, new-eater oatmeal.

Oatmeal thickens substantially as it cools, so don't be worried if it looks thin right out of the saucepan. You can substitute 5 ounces frozen sliced peaches, thawed and chopped, for the fresh peach.

3 cups water
⅓ cup old-fashioned rolled oats
1 peach, peeled, halved, pitted, and chopped
1 ripe banana, peeled and chopped

1. Bring water, oats, and peach to boil in large saucepan over medium-high heat. Reduce heat to medium and simmer, stirring occasionally to avoid scorching, until mixture is creamy and peach is very soft, about 20 minutes.

2. Off heat, stir in chopped banana. Use potato masher to mash until mixture has a porridge-like consistency and is uniform in texture. Add additional water (or breast milk or formula) as needed to thin mixture to desired consistency. Let oatmeal mixture cool to room temperature. Serve or store (see page 39 for storage options).

> ### SPICE IT UP
> Add ½ teaspoon ground cinnamon or pinch ground cloves to saucepan along with oats in step 1.

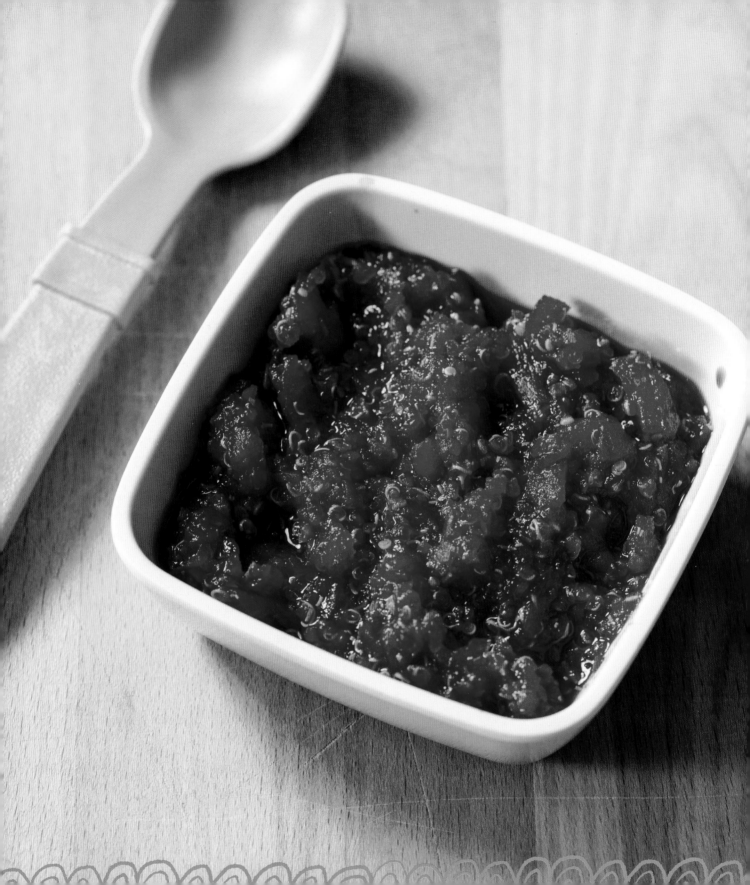

Quinoa, Beet, and Apple

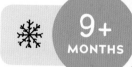

9+ MONTHS

Makes about 2½ cups
Total Time: 50 minutes

Why This Recipe Works

A whole portion of beets might be too intense for a baby palate, but combining earthy, sweet, vibrant beets with apples and quinoa makes a balanced meal with just enough beet flavor. But beets need a long time to become tender while quinoa cooks very fast. Grating beets on the large holes of a box grater solves that problem. Grated beets only needed a 20-minute head start in the saucepan before we added the quinoa and apple.

SPICE IT UP

Add ½ teaspoon ground cardamom to saucepan along with apples and quinoa in step 2.

There are three types of quinoa on the market: white, black, and red. Be sure to buy white quinoa for this recipe, as it has the softest texture of the three quinoas. We like the convenience of prewashed quinoa; rinsing removes the quinoa's bitter protective coating (called saponin). If you buy unwashed quinoa (or if you are unsure if it has been washed), rinse it well before using. Any variety of apple will work here, but tart apples, like Granny Smith, are more acidic and may not be as appealing to your baby. Don't be tempted to use a blender instead of a food processor; it will turn it all into a gluey mess.

2½ cups water
1 beet (4 ounces), peeled and grated
2 Fuji, Gala, or Golden Delicious apples (14 ounces), peeled, cored, and cut into 1-inch pieces
¼ cup prewashed white quinoa

1. Bring 2 cups water and grated beet to boil in large saucepan over medium-high heat. Cover, reduce heat to low, and cook for 20 minutes.

2. Stir in apples and quinoa and continue to cook, covered, until apples and beets are soft and quinoa is tender, about 15 minutes.

3. Carefully transfer beet mixture to food processor. Add remaining ½ cup water and pulse until mixture has a porridge-like consistency and is uniform in texture, about 6 pulses (do not process continuously, as mixture will become bitter and gummy).

4. Add additional water (or breast milk or formula) as needed to thin mixture to desired consistency. Let mixture cool to room temperature. Serve or store (see page 39 for storage options).

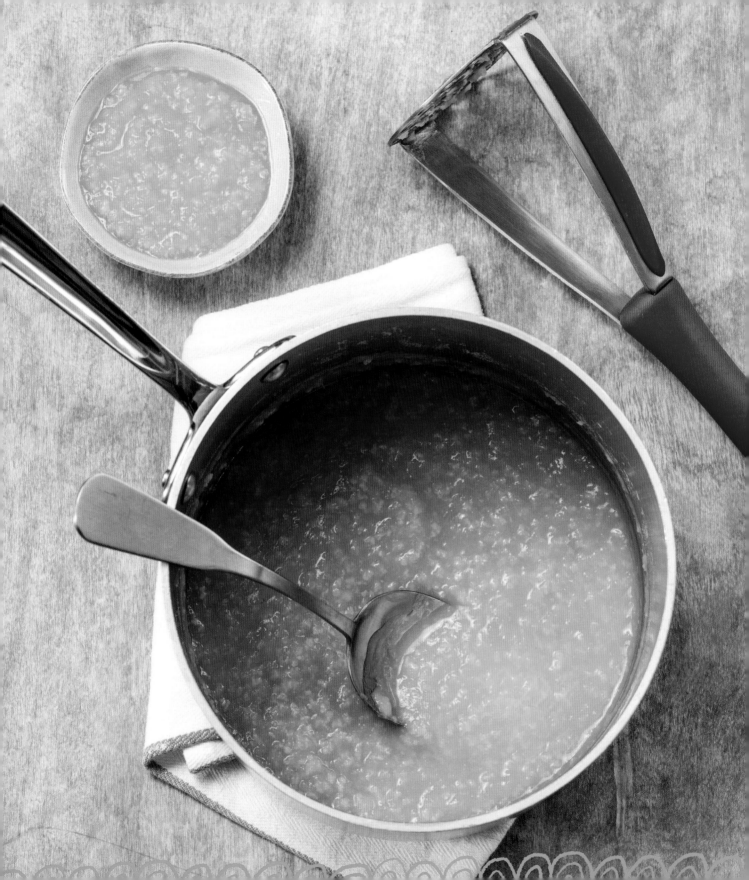

Millet and Squash

Makes about 2½ cups
Total Time: 45 minutes

Why This Recipe Works

For a slightly more adventurous butternut squash–centric meal, we turned to millet, a delicious little grain that cooks quite quickly. We were able to cook the two together in simmering water for just 30 minutes to get a mixture that was soft enough to mash up by hand with a potato masher.

2½ cups water
½ **small butternut squash (10 ounces), peeled, seeded, and cut into ½-inch pieces**
¼ **cup millet, rinsed**

1. Bring water, squash, and millet to boil in large saucepan over medium-high heat. Cover, reduce heat to low, and simmer until squash and millet are very soft, about 30 minutes.

2. Off heat, use potato masher to mash until squash is fully broken down. Add additional water (or breast milk or formula) as needed to thin mixture to desired consistency. Let mixture cool to room temperature. Serve or store (see page 39 for storage options).

> **SPICE IT UP**
> Add ½ teaspoon curry powder or ¼ teaspoon ground nutmeg to saucepan along with squash in step 1.

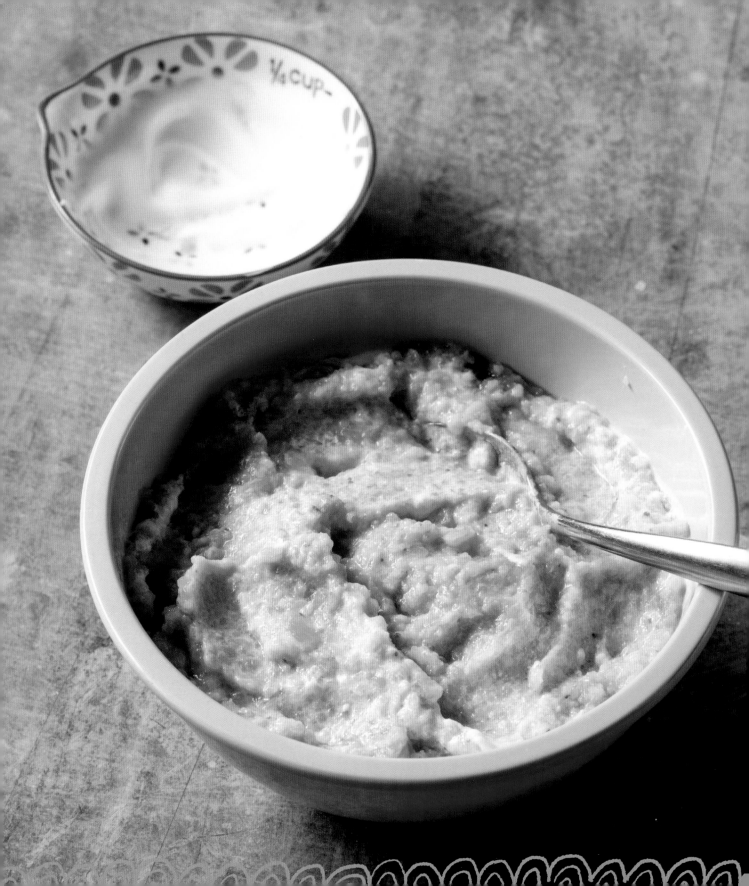

Bulgur, Eggplant, and Yogurt

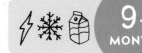

9+ MONTHS

Makes about 2½ cups
Total Time: 25 minutes

Why This Recipe Works

When most people think about baby food, they probably aren't thinking "Eggplant!" But eggplant is an earthy, soft vegetable and is perfect for the new eater—if treated right. We paired it with nutty bulgur and tangy yogurt for a flavorful, lightly textured combination. Eggplant can be bitter, so to make it baby-friendly, we peeled it, thoroughly cooked it, and took care *not* to blend it up. Blending intensifies the bitterness. A bit of plain whole-milk yogurt added creaminess.

Watch for the term "cracked wheat" when purchasing bulgur; while it looks like bulgur, the two are not the same. Cracked wheat is uncooked, whereas bulgur is parcooked, and the two require different cooking methods. Do not use coarse-grind bulgur in this recipe. This recipe calls for one Italian eggplant; half of a larger globe eggplant can be substituted. If freezing this puree, do not add the yogurt in step 3 as directed; instead, stir in the yogurt after thawing.

1¾ cups water
1 Italian eggplant (10 ounces), peeled and cut into
    1-inch pieces
¼ cup fine- or medium-grind bulgur, rinsed
¼ cup plain whole-milk yogurt

1. Bring water, eggplant, and bulgur to boil in large saucepan over medium-high heat. Cover, reduce heat to low, and cook until eggplant is very tender, 10 to 15 minutes.

2. Carefully transfer eggplant mixture to food processor and pulse until mixture has porridge-like consistency and is uniform in texture, about 6 pulses (do not process continuously as mixture will become bitter).

3. Transfer to bowl and stir in yogurt. Let mixture cool to room temperature. Serve or store (see page 39 for storage options).

> ### SPICE IT UP
> Add 1 teaspoon paprika or ground cumin to saucepan along with eggplant in step 1.

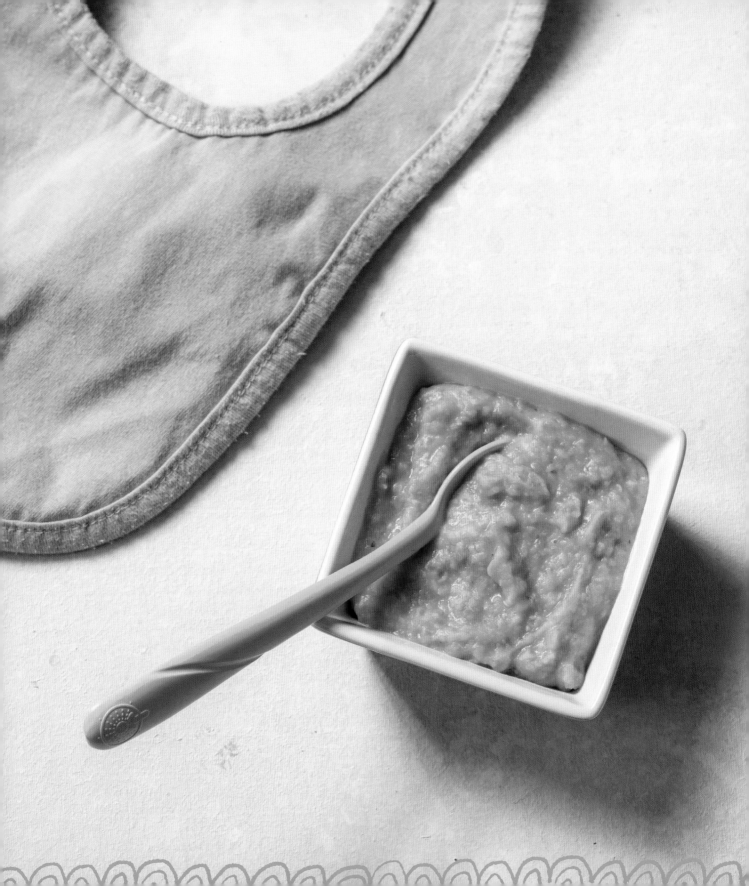

Red Lentil, Carrot, and Coconut Milk

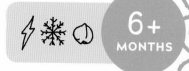

6+ MONTHS

Makes about 2½ cups
Total Time: 35 minutes

Why This Recipe Works

Red lentils are nutrient-dense, tasty little legumes that cook quickly and break down easily into a soft, pulpy mash—perfect for babies who are ready for coarse purees. They have the second-highest ratio of protein per calorie of any legume, after soybeans. We loved the combination of red lentils with carrots; the earthy nuttiness of the lentils was nicely balanced by the mild sweetness of the carrots. To create a pleasantly coarse texture, we used a potato masher after cooking.

For babies not ready for coarse purees, the mixture can be processed in a blender or food processor until it's perfectly smooth.

⅔ cup dried red lentils
3 carrots (8 ounces), peeled and sliced ½ inch thick
1¾ cups water
¼ cup unsweetened canned coconut milk

1. Bring lentils, carrots, water, and coconut milk to boil in large saucepan over high heat. Reduce heat to low, cover, and simmer until lentils and carrots are very tender, 20 to 25 minutes.

2. Off heat, mash lentil mixture with potato masher until it has a porridge-like consistency and is uniform in texture, about 1 minute.

3. Add additional water (or breast milk or formula) as needed to thin mixture to desired consistency. Let mixture cool to room temperature. Serve or store (see page 39 for storage options).

SPICE IT UP
Add ¼ teaspoon ground ginger or ¼ teaspoon ground turmeric to saucepan along with lentils in step 1.

All About *Dal*
For this puree, we took a cue from Indian cuisine, where red lentils are simmered with warm spices and sometimes coconut milk to make a popular dish known as *dal*. Adding a bit of coconut milk gave our simple puree a nice amount of rich, nutty sweetness.

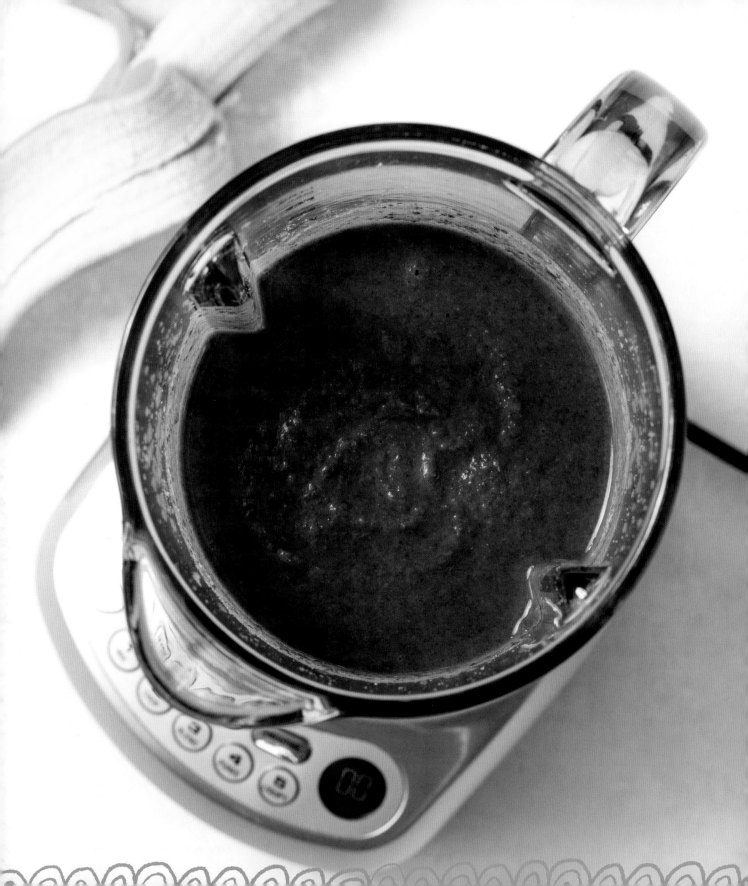

White Bean and Kale

Makes about 2½ cups
Total Time: 25 minutes

9+
MONTHS

Why This Recipe Works

Kale is all the rage in the adult culinary world. Babies, you're next! We started by matching this nutrient-dense green with the creaminess of pureed cannellini beans. And it only took a few tests to find a surprising champion to offset kale's slightly bitter notes: banana. Just half a banana created a creamy, earthy, barely sweet puree.

We developed this recipe with curly kale, which we find nutty and tender once cooked. Avoid red kale and black (or Lacinato) kale as they can be too tough for this application. You can use a food processor instead of a blender, but the puree will not be quite as smooth.

8 ounces curly kale, stemmed and chopped
1 (15-ounce) can no-sodium-added cannellini beans, rinsed
½ ripe banana, peeled and broken into 2 pieces

1 Bring 1 inch water to rolling boil in large saucepan over high heat. Place steamer basket in saucepan and fill basket with kale. Cover and cook until kale is tender, about 10 minutes.

2 Carefully remove steamer basket from saucepan and transfer kale to blender, reserving cooking liquid. Add beans, banana, and 1½ cups cooking liquid to blender and process on high speed for 1 minute. Scrape down sides of blender jar and process until smooth, about 1 minute.

3 Add additional cooking liquid (or breast milk or formula) as needed to thin puree to desired consistency. Let puree cool to room temperature. Serve or store (see page 39 for storage options).

> ### SPICE IT UP
> Add 2 tablespoons chopped fresh basil or 1 teaspoon chopped fresh tarragon to blender along with beans in step 2.

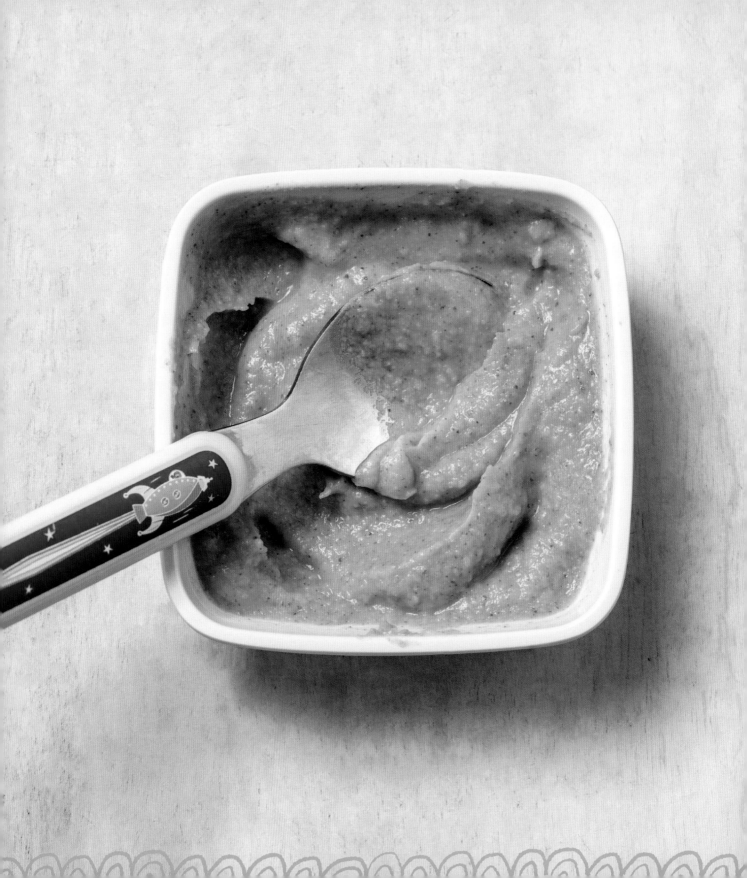

Chickpea and Broccoli

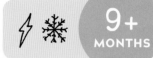

9+ MONTHS

Makes about 2½ cups
Total Time: 20 minutes

Why This Recipe Works

Chickpeas, also known as garbanzo beans, are a staple legume in cuisines around the world. They combine well with countless ingredients, but we loved how their nutty flavor and creamy texture served as a perfect counterpoint to the slightly grassy flavor of broccoli in this velvety puree.

You can substitute 3 cups (8 ounces) thawed frozen broccoli florets for the fresh florets. You can use a food processor instead of a blender, but the puree will not be quite as smooth.

1 teaspoon extra-virgin olive oil
2 garlic cloves, minced
1 (15-ounce) can no-sodium-added chickpeas, rinsed
3 cups broccoli florets (8 ounces), cut into 1-inch pieces
1½ cups water

1   Heat oil in large saucepan over medium heat until shimmering. Add garlic and cook until fragrant, about 30 seconds. Add chickpeas, broccoli, and water and bring to boil. Reduce heat to low, cover, and simmer until chickpeas and broccoli are very tender, about 8 minutes.

2   Carefully transfer chickpea mixture to blender and process on high speed for 1 minute. Scrape down sides of blender jar and continue to process until smooth, about 1 minute.

3   Add additional water (or breast milk or formula) as needed to thin puree to desired consistency. Let mixture cool to room temperature. Serve or store (see page 39 for storage options).

> ### SPICE IT UP
> Add ¼ teaspoon grated lemon zest or ⅛ teaspoon ground ginger to blender along with mixture in step 2.

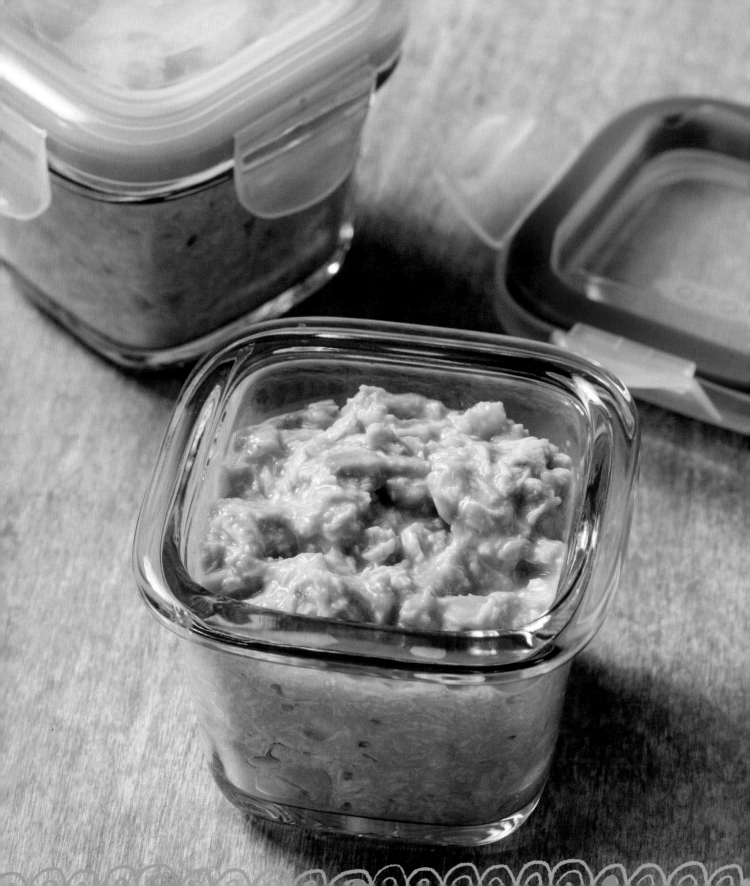

Chicken and Avocado

Makes about 2½ cups
Total Time: 40 minutes

Why This Recipe Works

Baby's first chicken tacos with guacamole! (Minus the taco, plus the blender.) Avocado can go one of two ways when combined with cooked food: it can keep its vibrant green color and delicate, buttery flavor, or it can turn brown and grainy. The latter occurs because of oxidation, an enzymatic reaction that happens when an avocado's broken cells are exposed to oxygen, and it is exacerbated by heat. To avoid this, we tossed the avocado with lime juice (the enzymes don't like acid), and we waited until the chicken was fully cooled before adding the avocado. For an extra limey note, we included a little grated zest in addition to fresh lime juice.

Be sure to use a ripe avocado for this recipe; a ripe avocado will yield slightly to a gentle squeeze when held in the palm of your hand. Underripe avocados will not break down properly in the food processor.

1 avocado, halved, pitted, and cut into 1-inch pieces
½ teaspoon grated lime zest, plus 1 teaspoon juice
¾ cup water
2 (6-ounce) boneless, skinless chicken breasts, trimmed and cut into 1-inch pieces

1. Toss avocado, lime zest, and juice together in small bowl; set aside.

2. Bring water to boil in medium saucepan over medium-high heat. Add chicken, cover, reduce heat to medium-low, and simmer until chicken is opaque and cooked through, about 8 minutes.

3. Carefully transfer chicken and cooking water to food processor. Let chicken cool to room temperature, about 15 minutes.

4. Add avocado mixture to food processor with chicken and pulse until mixture is uniform in texture, 4 to 6 pulses. Add additional water (or breast milk or formula) as needed to thin puree to desired consistency. Serve or store (see page 39 for storage options).

SPICE IT UP

Add 1 teaspoon ground cumin to saucepan along with chicken in step 2. Or, add 1½ teaspoons chopped fresh cilantro to food processor along with avocado in step 4.

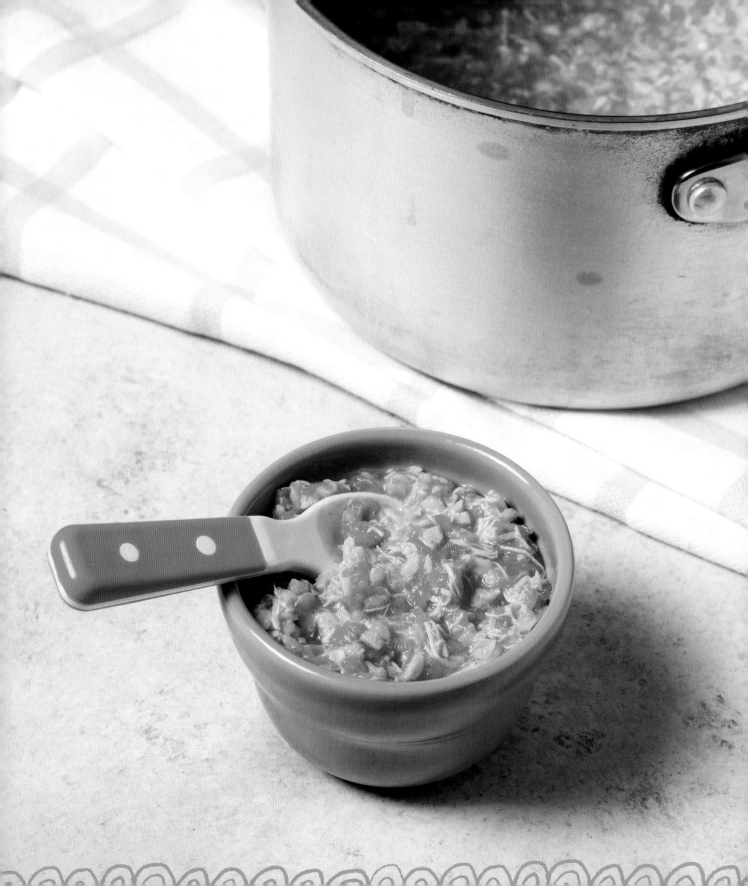

Chicken, Carrot, and Brown Rice

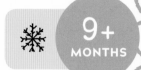

9+ MONTHS

Makes about 2½ cups
Total Time: 55 minutes

Why This Recipe Works

Behold the classic combo of chicken, vegetables, and rice. It's a complete, balanced meal in every bite, especially because we chose to use brown rice. Brown rice is a whole grain and contains more nutrients than its more refined white-rice cousin, but it takes longer to cook. To match the grain's 40-minute cook time, we needed a robust cut of chicken, so we chose chicken thighs, which can withstand longer cooking times.

A potato masher makes quick work of creating the ideal texture for this baby-friendly chicken dinner.

2½ cups water
2 (3-ounce) boneless, skinless chicken thighs, trimmed and cut into 1-inch pieces
3 carrots (8 ounces), peeled and cut into 1-inch pieces
⅓ cup long-grain brown rice

1   Bring water, chicken, carrots, and rice to boil in large saucepan over medium-high heat. Cover, reduce heat to medium-low, and simmer until chicken and carrots are very tender, about 40 minutes.

2   Off heat, mash chicken mixture with potato masher until mixture has a porridge-like consistency and is uniform in texture, about 1 minute.

3   Add additional water (or breast milk or formula) as needed to thin mixture to desired consistency. Let mixture cool to room temperature. Serve or store (see page 39 for storage options).

> **SPICE IT UP**
> Add 1 teaspoon dried thyme to saucepan along with chicken in step 1. Or, add 1 tablespoon chopped fresh parsley to mixture before mashing in step 2.

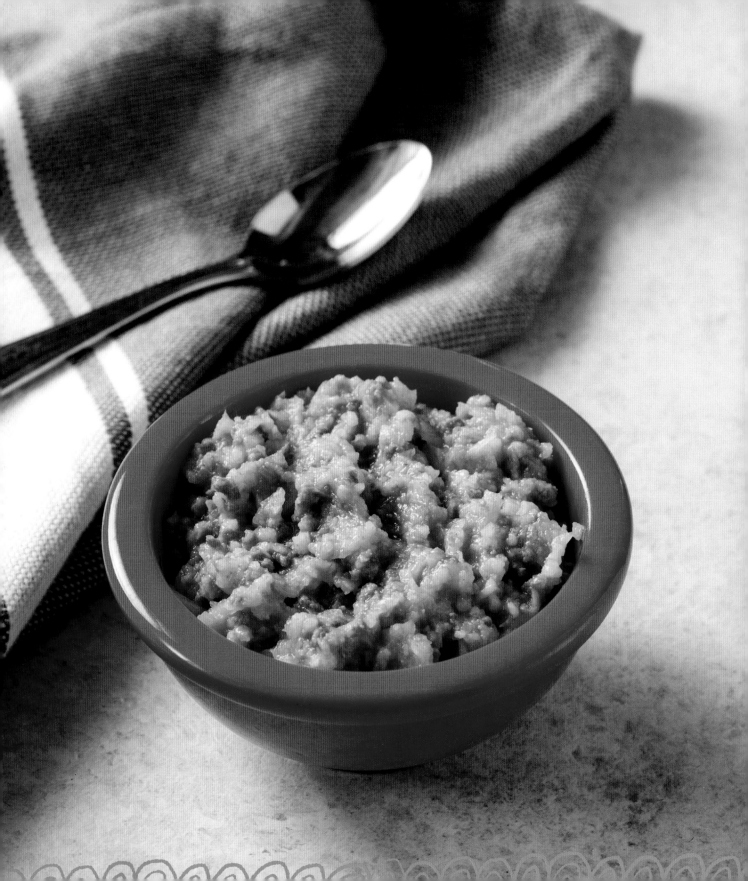

Beef, Parsnip, and Couscous

9+ MONTHS

Makes about 2½ cups
Total Time: 55 minutes

Why This Recipe Works

We know, we know. The combination of "beef" and "puree" isn't necessarily something you've spent your life yearning to cook. But pediatricians often recommend introducing red meat to babies relatively early in their eating careers, and lean ground beef is a quick and easy way to do so. In general, parsnips take much longer to cook than ground beef. But when we tried simmering the parsnips and ground beef together for 40 minutes—a very long time for ground beef!—we found that we loved the flavor. Adding just 2 tablespoons of couscous gave us a cohesive puree.

SPICE IT UP
Add ½ teaspoon ground coriander to saucepan along with beef in step 1. Or, add 1 tablespoon chopped fresh parsley to mixture before mashing in step 4.

This puree is quite thick; thin it to your desired consistency with water (or other liquid of your choice).

1 teaspoon extra-virgin olive oil
6 ounces (85 percent) lean ground beef
1 small shallot, minced
2¼ cups water
2 parsnips (8 ounces), peeled and cut into ½-inch pieces
2 tablespoons couscous

1. Heat oil in large saucepan over medium heat until shimmering. Add beef and shallot and cook, breaking up meat with wooden spoon, until beef is no longer pink, about 2 minutes.

2. Add water and parsnips and bring to boil. Cover, reduce heat to low, and simmer until parsnips are very tender, about 30 minutes.

3. Stir in couscous, cover, and simmer until couscous is tender, about 10 minutes.

4. Off heat, mash beef mixture with potato masher until mixture has a porridge-like consistency and is uniform in texture, about 1 minute.

5. Add additional water (or breast milk or formula) as needed to thin mixture to desired consistency. Let mixture cool to room temperature. Serve or store (see page 39 for storage options).

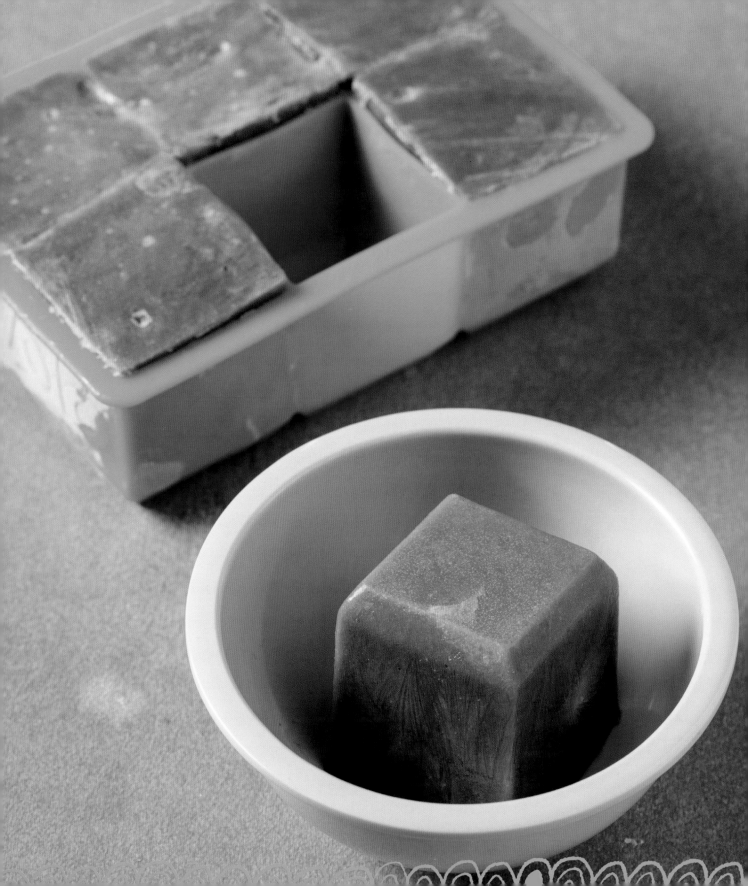

Beef, Sweet Potato, and Carrot

 9+ MONTHS

Makes about 2½ cups
Total Time: 45 minutes

Why This Recipe Works

Again, we know. Making a super-smooth beef puree is not on your life's bucket list. But, again: great for babies and actually pretty delicious. For this beef puree, we paired the beef with sweet potato for its sweet notes and ultracreamy texture. To keep the process as simple as possible, we cooked everything together in a saucepan. Starting with sirloin steak tips guarantees a velvety finish. After about 20 minutes, all the elements were fully cooked and very tender. All that's left is a quick spin in the blender.

You can use a food processor instead of a blender, but the puree will not be quite as smooth.

1 teaspoon extra-virgin olive oil
1 small shallot, chopped
8 ounces sirloin steak tips, trimmed and cut into ½-inch pieces
1 small sweet potato (8 ounces), peeled and cut into ½-inch pieces
1 carrot, peeled and sliced ½ inch thick
1¾ cups water

1 Heat oil in large saucepan over medium heat until shimmering. Add shallot and cook, stirring occasionally, until softened and lightly browned, about 3 minutes.

2 Add steak tips and cook, stirring occasionally, until lightly browned, 3 to 5 minutes. Add sweet potatoes, carrot, and water and bring to boil. Reduce heat to low, cover, and simmer until beef and vegetables are very tender, 20 to 25 minutes.

3 Carefully transfer mixture to blender and process on high speed for 1 minute. Scrape down sides of blender jar and continue to process until smooth, about 1 minute.

4 Add additional water (or breast milk or formula) as needed to thin puree to desired consistency. Let mixture cool to room temperature. Serve or store (see page 39 for storage options).

> ### SPICE IT UP
> Add ¼ teaspoon grated lemon zest or ½ teaspoon paprika to blender along with meat and vegetables in step 3.

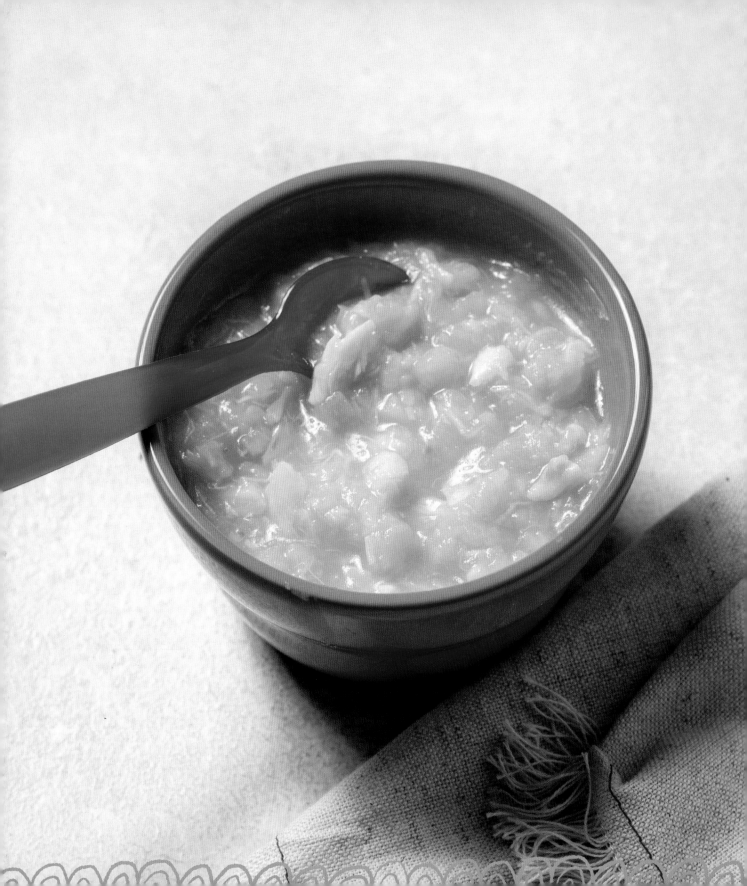

Cod, Potato, and Leek

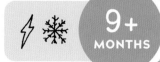

Makes about 2½ cups
Total Time: 45 minutes

Why This Recipe Works

This one's for all you New Englanders out there! The classic combination of cod, potato, and leek in coarse mash form. Mildly sweet and less chewy than poultry or meat, cod is an excellent source of protein that combines well with a range of ingredients. Cooking makes lemon zest bitter, so we added it off the heat. A potato masher transforms the mixture into a creamy yet slightly coarse puree.

SPICE IT UP
Add 1 tablespoon chopped fresh parsley or 1 tablespoon chopped fresh cilantro to saucepan along with lemon zest in step 3.

We preferred Yukon Gold potatoes for their creamy, slightly waxy texture; do not substitute russet potatoes or the puree will be too starchy. We do not recommend processing this mixture in a blender or food processor; the potatoes will become gummy.

2 teaspoons extra-virgin olive oil
1 leek, white and light green parts only, halved lengthwise, sliced thin, and washed thoroughly (about 1½ cups)
1 pound Yukon Gold potatoes (about 2), peeled and cut into ½-inch pieces
1¼ cups water
1 (6-ounce) skinless cod fillet, cut into 1-inch pieces
½ teaspoon grated lemon zest

1. Heat oil in large saucepan over medium heat until shimmering. Add leek, reduce heat to medium-low, and cook, stirring occasionally, until softened, about 3 minutes.

2. Add potatoes and water and bring to boil. Cover, reduce heat to low, and simmer for 10 minutes. Add cod and continue to simmer, covered, until potatoes and cod are very tender, 8 to 10 minutes.

3. Off heat, add lemon zest and mash cod mixture with potato masher until mixture has a porridge-like consistency and is uniform in texture, about 1 minute.

4. Add additional water (or breast milk or formula) as needed to thin mixture to desired consistency. Let mixture cool to room temperature. Serve or store (see page 39 for storage options).

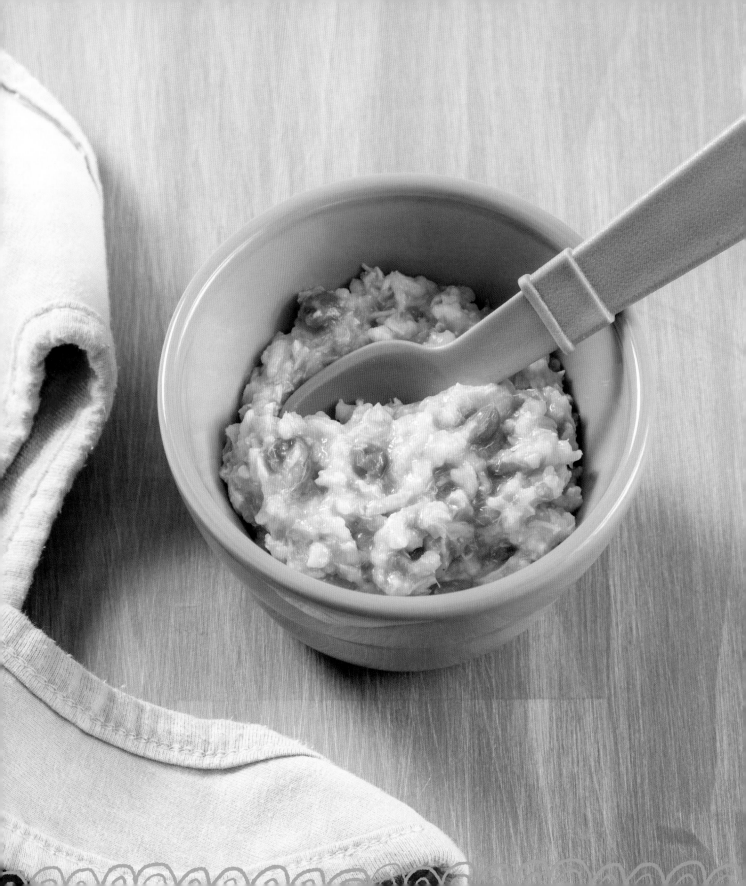

Salmon, Pea, and Rice

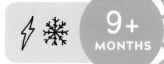

Makes about 2½ cups
Total Time: 30 minutes

Why This Recipe Works

Flecked with pastel pink and green, this is a beautiful mash-up of ingredients. White rice forms an easy-to-digest, creamy base for the nutrient-packed duo of salmon and peas. Salmon is an excellent source of protein and of omega-3 fatty acids, plus its moist texture makes it easy to eat. To make cooking these three main elements as simple as possible, we gave the rice a head start, adding the peas and salmon when the rice was halfway done. A potato masher turned it all into a slightly coarse puree.

We preferred long-grain white rice for its slightly elongated starches, but short-grain white rice can be used as well. We do not recommend processing this mixture in a blender or food processor; the rice will become gummy.

⅓ cup long-grain white rice, rinsed
1¾ cups water
¼ teaspoon grated orange zest plus 2 tablespoons juice
1 (6-ounce) skinless salmon fillet, cut into 1-inch pieces
⅓ cup frozen peas

1. Bring rice, water, and orange juice to boil in large saucepan over high heat. Cover, reduce heat to low, and simmer for 10 minutes. Add salmon and peas and continue to simmer until rice and fish are very tender, 6 to 8 minutes.

2. Off heat, add orange zest and mash salmon mixture with potato masher until mixture has a porridge-like consistency and is uniform in texture, about 1 minute.

3. Add additional water (or breast milk or formula) as needed to thin mixture to desired consistency. Let mixture cool to room temperature. Serve or store (see page 39 for storage options).

> **SPICE IT UP**
> Add 2 teaspoons fresh mint or 1 teaspoon fresh tarragon to mixture along with orange zest in step 2.

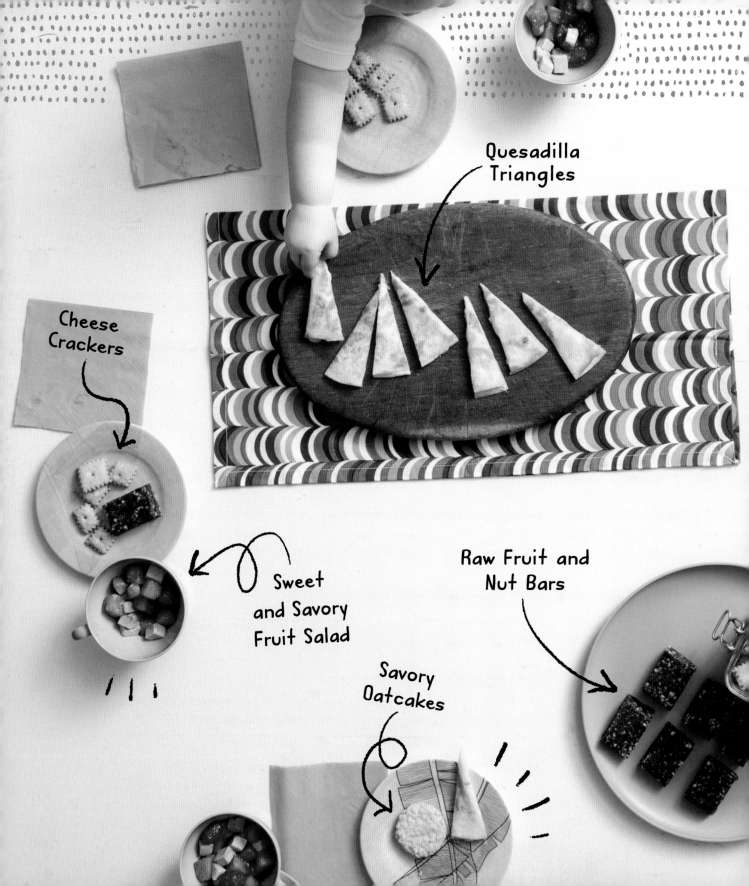

Quesadilla Triangles

Cheese Crackers

Sweet and Savory Fruit Salad

Raw Fruit and Nut Bars

Savory Oatcakes

FINGER FOODS

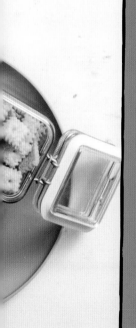

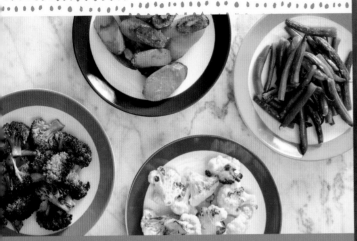

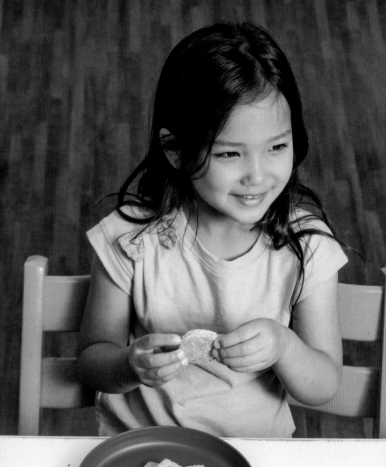

"My 9-month-old dove into this recipe and ate with gusto! (My 3-year-old boycotted all food at this meal, so I'm sorry to say that he didn't have any.) It was pleasant to encounter a recipe that is simple, child-friendly, and relatively quick."

—Parent of 3-year-old and 9-month-old, on Cheesy Rigatoni

"Very easy and very sticky. The older kid loves it; she ate one for a snack and declared it would be her breakfast the next day as well."

—Parent of 6-year-old and 8-month-old, on Raw Fruit and Nut Bars

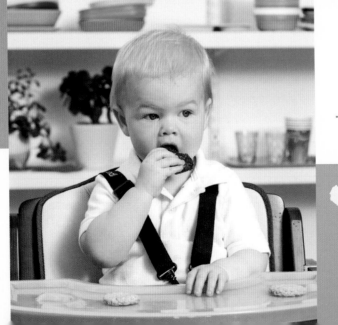

ALL ABOUT FINGER FOODS

Independence. Toddlers want it. Then they don't want it. Then they definitely want it again. As babies become toddlers, the desire for independence is one of the defining factors of their day-to-day life (and yours). One way to express this desire is through food. Toddlers want to feed themselves (until, you know, they suddenly don't). One of the best ways to provide the opportunity? Finger foods.

With that in mind, we set out to create a chapter of fun food easy for toddlers to eat with their hands. Many of these recipes are perfect for snacking. Some are better suited for a small meal. But no matter what, we wanted these recipes to be tasty and easy to make.

Most recipes in this chapter can be completed in 45 minutes or less. Many make a small amount, perfect for a snack to share between a couple of little ones and maybe a nibbly adult, plus or minus, depending on age and appetite. Others create larger batches and freeze well. (See page 285 for more on toddler serving sizes.)

You'll find a range of flavors and textures in this chapter to continue the introduction to new food experiences. We kept an eye on nutrition (hello, Tiny Carrot Muffins, page 107) and flavor (our Cheesy Rigatoni, page 101, is better than anything that comes in a box).

Remember that it's fun not only for toddlers to eat with their hands, but for grown-ups, too!

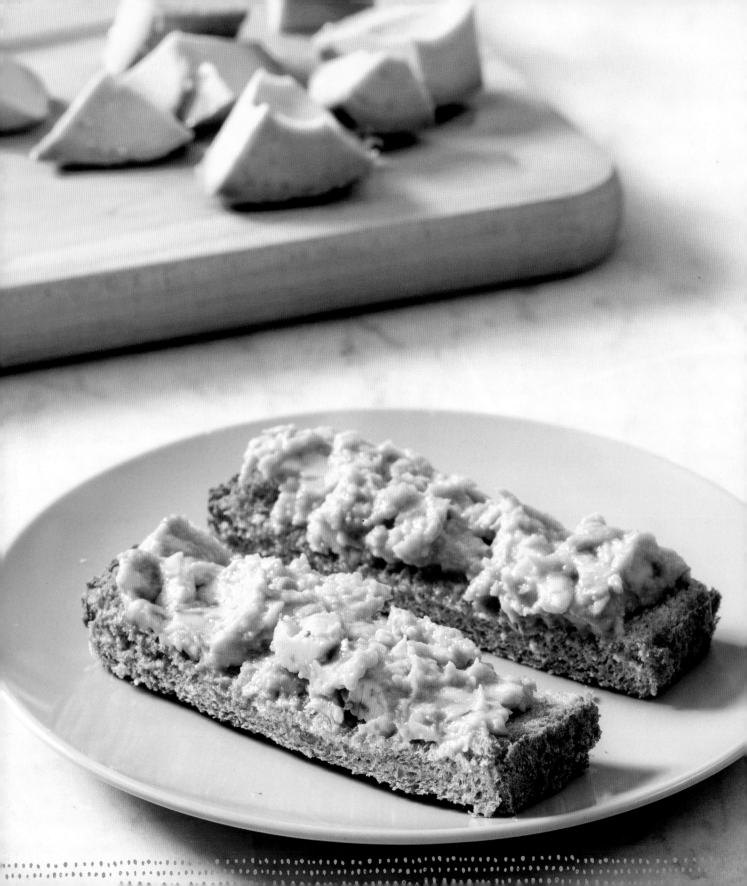

Avocado Toast Sticks

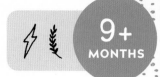
9+ MONTHS

Makes 4 toast sticks
Total Time: 10 minutes

Why This Recipe Works

Avocado toast is a trendy meal for adults. (See every hip café menu everywhere.) But it's also great for kids of all ages. It's simple yet flavorful, and avocado is packed with healthy fats and potassium. The creamy avocado contrasts with the crisp, toasty bread beneath it. To tailor this snack to toddlers, we used half an avocado and sliced one piece of toast into four easy-to-grasp sticks. Lime juice provided a nice pop of acidity and prevented the avocado from oxidizing and turning brown (though brown avocados are still safe to eat).

We like to add a pinch of salt, but feel free to omit the seasoning, particularly if your child is under 12 months—avocado and lime make a flavorful couple without any enhancement.

½ ripe avocado, pitted and cut into 1-inch pieces
1 teaspoon lime juice
Pinch salt (optional)
1 slice hearty whole-wheat sandwich bread

1　Combine avocado, lime juice, and salt, if using, in bowl. Use fork to mash mixture together until mostly smooth.

2　Toast bread until golden brown on both sides, 1 to 2 minutes.

3　Spread avocado mixture evenly on toast. Cut avocado toast crosswise into 4 sticks. Serve.

SPICE IT UP
Add ¼ teaspoon ground coriander or 1 teaspoon minced fresh cilantro or mint to avocado mixture in step 1.

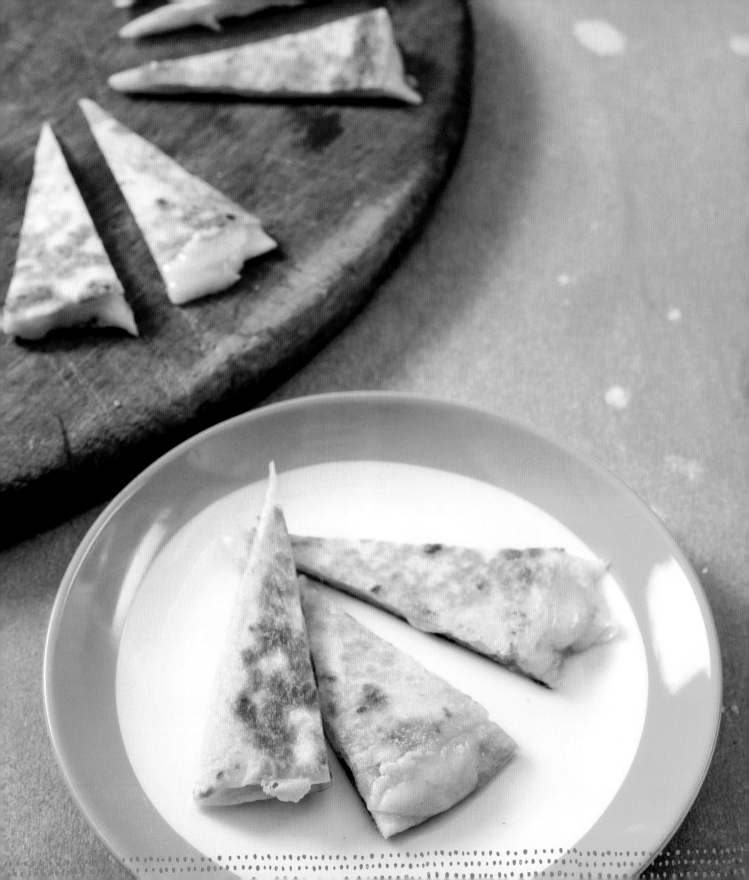

Quesadilla Triangles

12+ MONTHS

Makes 8 triangles
Total Time: 10 minutes

Why This Recipe Works

It's just you and a hungry, hungry toddler. Call in the quesadilla! Quesadillas are fast and easy, suitable for a snack or simple meal. You only need three ingredients—a tortilla, shredded cheese, and some vegetable oil—and the recipe comes together in minutes. Brushing the exterior of the tortilla with oil and starting our quesadilla in a cold skillet, which we then heated gently, gave us golden-brown results.

HAM AND CHEESE QUESADILLA TRIANGLES

Sprinkle 1 tablespoon finely chopped deli ham onto cheese before folding tortilla in half in step 1.

TOMATO AND CHEESE QUESADILLA TRIANGLES

Sprinkle 1 tablespoon finely chopped tomatoes onto cheese before folding tortilla in half in step 1.

It's important to cool your quesadilla before cutting it, or the hot cheese will ooze out. You can double this recipe and cook two quesadillas in the same skillet (just arrange the straight, folded edges of the two quesadillas next to each other in the center of the skillet). Serve these plain, or let your child have fun dipping them into sour cream, mild salsa, yogurt, or even Mashed Avocado (page 7).

1 (8-inch) flour tortilla
1 ounce cheddar or Monterey Jack cheese, shredded (¼ cup)
2 teaspoons canola oil

1. Lay tortilla on cutting board and sprinkle cheese over half of tortilla. Fold tortilla in half over cheese, forming half-moon shape, and press to flatten.

2. Brush top of quesadilla with 1 teaspoon oil. Place quesadilla, oiled side down, in 10-inch nonstick skillet. Brush second side of quesadilla with remaining 1 teaspoon oil.

3. Cook quesadilla over medium heat until bottom is crisp and lightly browned, 1 to 2 minutes. Flip quesadilla and cook until second side is crisp and lightly browned, 1 to 2 minutes.

4. Slide quesadilla out of skillet onto cutting board and let cool for 3 minutes. Slice into 8 wedges and serve.

Omelet Rolls

Makes 1 omelet
Total Time: 10 minutes

Why This Recipe Works

We wanted to develop a simple, fast method for preparing a single egg that would be fun to eat. And all you need to create this crepe-like omelet roll is one beaten egg and a 10-inch nonstick skillet. (Not needed: a ton of skill.) We simply heated some olive oil, added the egg, swirled it into a single layer, and then lowered the heat and quickly covered the pan. After about 1 minute, the egg was set and easily released onto the cutting board, where we could roll the omelet into a log and slice it into playful pinwheels.

You will need a 10-inch nonstick skillet with a tight-fitting lid for this recipe. We like to add a pinch of salt, but feel free to omit the seasoning, particularly if your child is under 12 months.

1 large egg
Pinch salt (optional)
1 teaspoon extra-virgin olive oil

1 Whisk egg and salt, if using, in bowl until well combined and uniform yellow color. Heat oil in 10-inch nonstick skillet over medium-low heat until shimmering, swirling pan to coat with oil. Add egg mixture and swirl skillet to coat bottom with egg mixture in even layer.

2 Reduce heat to low, cover, and cook until egg is set, about 1 minute. Uncover and carefully slide omelet onto cutting board (see "Rolling an Omelet," right). Roll omelet into tight log, then slice crosswise into 1-inch pieces. Serve.

OMELET ROLLS WITH CHEESE
Sprinkle 2 tablespoons shredded cheddar or Monterey Jack cheese or 1 tablespoon crumbled feta cheese over egg mixture before covering skillet in step 2.

OMELET ROLLS WITH SPINACH
Sprinkle 2 tablespoons finely chopped baby spinach over egg mixture before covering skillet in step 2.

OMELET ROLLS WITH HERBS
Add ¼ teaspoon minced fresh dill or 1 teaspoon minced fresh parsley or cilantro to bowl with egg in step 1.

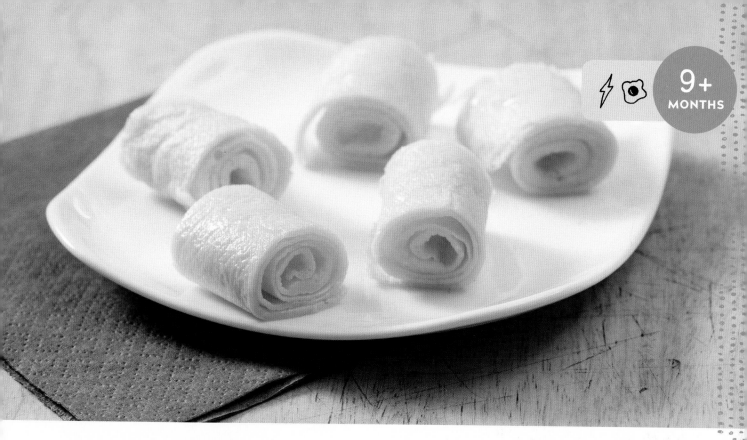

ROLLING AN OMELET

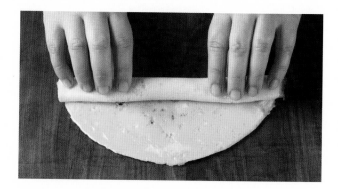

1. Slide omelet onto cutting board, then roll omelet into tight log.

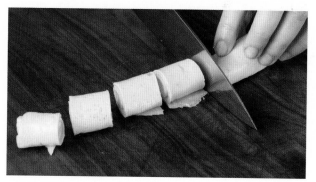

2. Slice omelet roll crosswise into 1-inch pieces.

Frittata Bites

Makes 6 mini frittatas
Total Time: 45 minutes

Why This Recipe Works

To make frittatas in small, graspable portions, we turned to the muffin tin. For an easy (and appealing) flavor combo, we sautéed some potatoes and shallots and then added a little Parmesan cheese. We divided this mixture evenly among the muffin cups and then topped each portion with a simple egg-dairy mixture. Half-and-half, with its slightly higher fat content than milk, helped the frittatas release from the pan (rather than getting stuck). You can serve whole or cut into pieces, whatever your toddler prefers.

✳ STORAGE INFORMATION

Leftovers can be refrigerated in airtight container for up to 24 hours.

You will need a 10-inch nonstick skillet with a tight-fitting lid and a 6-cup nonstick muffin tin (or you can fill half of the cups of a nonstick 12-cup muffin tin) for this recipe. Make sure to spray the tin well with vegetable oil spray to further help the eggs release. This recipe can easily be doubled.

4 large eggs
2 tablespoons half-and-half
Salt
2 teaspoons extra-virgin olive oil

1 small Yukon Gold potato (6 ounces), peeled, quartered lengthwise, and sliced thin
1 shallot, chopped
2 tablespoons grated Parmesan cheese

1. Adjust oven rack to lower-middle position and heat oven to 425 degrees. Generously spray 6-cup nonstick muffin tin with vegetable oil spray. Whisk eggs, half-and-half, and pinch salt together in bowl; set aside.

2. Heat oil in 10-inch nonstick skillet over medium heat until shimmering. Add potato, shallot, and pinch salt and cover. Reduce heat to medium-low and cook, stirring occasionally, until potato is tender, 10 to 12 minutes. Transfer to separate bowl and let cool slightly, about 2 minutes. Stir in cheese.

3. Divide potato mixture evenly among 6 muffin cups. Using ladle, evenly distribute egg mixture over filling in muffin cups.

4. Bake until frittatas are lightly puffed and just set in center, 8 to 10 minutes. Transfer muffin tin to wire rack and let cool for 10 minutes. Run butter knife around edges of frittatas to loosen, then gently remove frittatas. Serve.

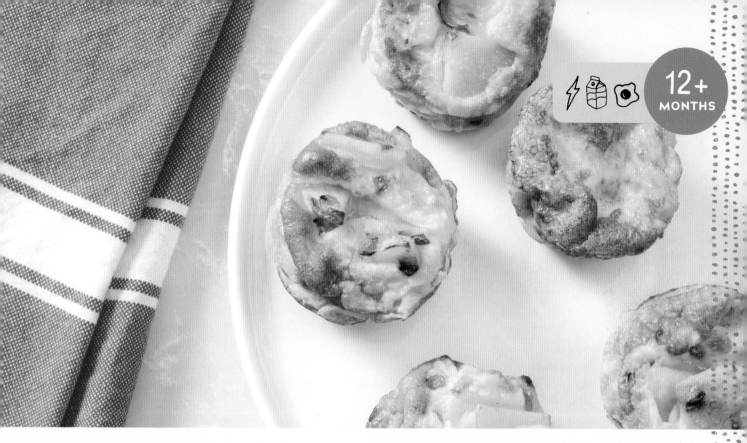

BROCCOLI-CHEDDAR FRITTATA BITES

Omit potato. In step 2, after heating oil, add shallot to skillet and cook, stirring occasionally, until softened, about 3 minutes. Add 2¼ cups broccoli florets, chopped into ½-inch pieces, to skillet, cover, reduce heat to medium-low, and cook until broccoli is bright green and tender, about 5 minutes. Substitute ¼ cup shredded cheddar cheese for Parmesan.

ASPARAGUS-FETA FRITTATA BITES

Omit potato. In step 2, after heating oil, add shallot to skillet and cook, stirring occasionally, until softened, about 3 minutes. Add 8 ounces (about ½ bunch) asparagus, trimmed and sliced thin, to skillet, cover, reduce heat to medium-low, and cook, stirring occasionally, until asparagus is bright green and tender, about 3 minutes. Substitute 2 tablespoons crumbled feta cheese for Parmesan.

Zucchini-Carrot Fritters

Makes 6 fritters
Total Time: 35 minutes

Why This Recipe Works

In the Venn diagram of vegetables and foods most toddlers will eat, veggie fritters sit right in the center. We set out to create a recipe for a fritter that would be light, moist, and easy for small humans to handle. We started with the simple combination of zucchini with carrots. Shredding and lightly salting the vegetables, letting them drain, and then squeezing them in a clean dish towel eliminated excess moisture and kept the fritters from becoming soggy. We bound the mixture together with just a bit of flour and an egg, and then we pan-fried the patties in a nonstick skillet to get crispy results.

Use the large holes of a box grater or the shredding disk of a food processor to shred the vegetables. Make sure to squeeze the shredded vegetables until they are quite dry or the fritters might fall apart in the skillet. This recipe can be doubled to make 12 fritters but will need to be cooked in two batches; wipe the skillet clean between batches. Serve the fritters with yogurt for dipping, if desired.

1 small zucchini, shredded (1 cup)
2 small carrots, peeled and shredded (1 cup)
¼ teaspoon salt

1 large egg, lightly beaten
2 tablespoons all-purpose flour
1 tablespoon extra-virgin olive oil

1. Toss zucchini and carrots with salt and let drain in fine-mesh strainer set over medium bowl for 10 minutes.

2. Wrap zucchini and carrots in clean dish towel and thoroughly squeeze out as much liquid as possible. Wipe bowl clean and transfer zucchini and carrots to bowl. Stir in beaten egg until well combined. Sprinkle flour over mixture and stir to combine.

3. Line large plate with paper towels. Heat oil in 12-inch nonstick skillet over medium heat until shimmering. Drop 2-tablespoon-size portions of batter into skillet and use back of spoon to press batter into 2-inch fritters (you should have 6 fritters total). Cook until golden brown on both sides, about 3 minutes per side.

4. Transfer fritters to prepared plate to drain. Serve (making sure they've cooled enough for young eaters).

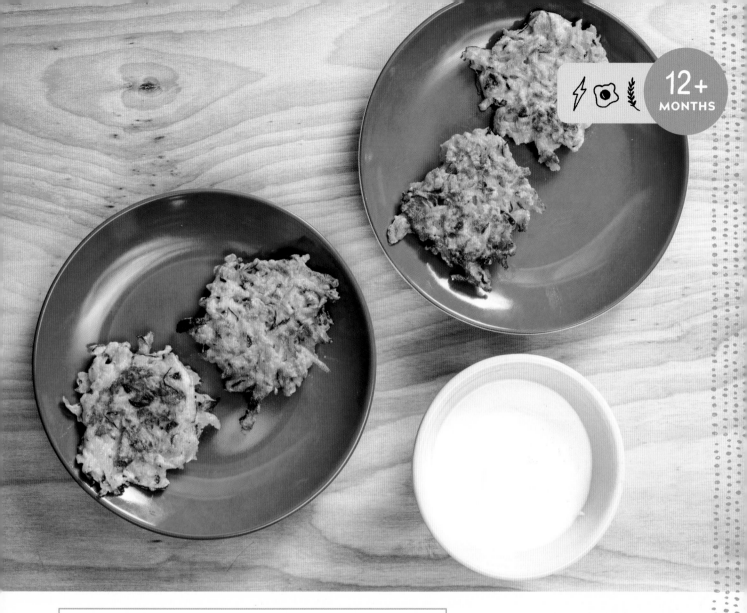

ZUCCHINI-CARROT FRITTERS WITH FETA AND DILL

Add ¼ cup crumbled feta cheese and ½ teaspoon minced fresh dill to vegetable mixture along with egg in step 2.

ZUCCHINI-CARROT FRITTERS WITH PARMESAN AND BASIL

Add ¼ cup grated Parmesan cheese and 1 tablespoon minced fresh basil to vegetable mixture along with egg in step 2.

✳ STORAGE INFORMATION

Leftovers can be refrigerated in airtight container for up to 24 hours.

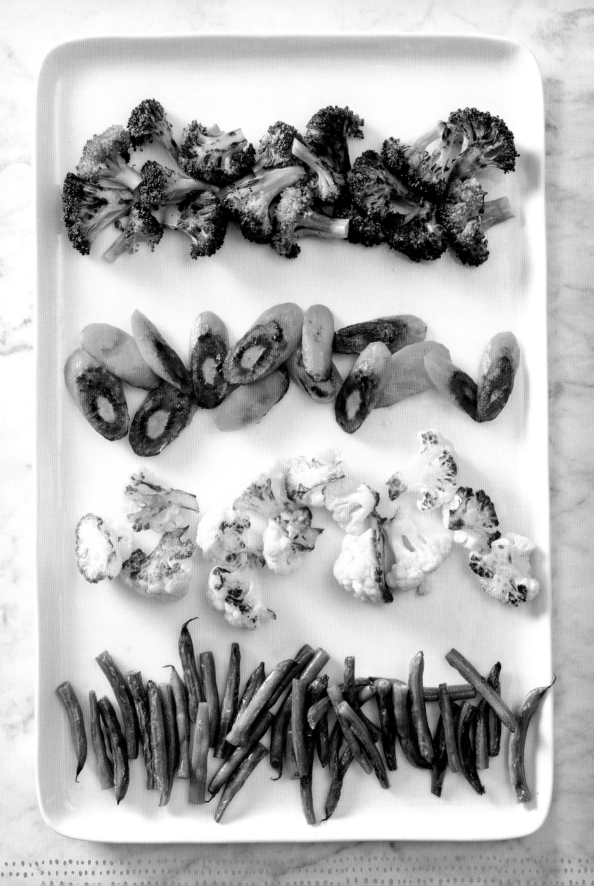

Skillet-Roasted Broccoli

12+ MONTHS

Makes about 1½ cups
Total Time: 20 minutes

Why This Recipe Works

This quick and easy method for skillet-roasting a small portion of broccoli also works for a variety of other vegetables, including cauliflower, green beans, and carrots. A single batch yields just the right amount of roasty, tender veggies for a couple of healthy snacks, or as part of a meal. For a streamlined approach, we simultaneously browned and steamed the broccoli—by cooking the florets covered in a nonstick skillet. The resulting veggies were lightly browned on all sides and perfectly tender. Look for florets that are similarly sized to ensure even cooking.

✳ STORAGE INFORMATION

Leftovers can be refrigerated in airtight container for up to 2 days.

You will need a 10-inch nonstick skillet with a tight-fitting lid for this recipe.

2 teaspoons extra-virgin olive oil
1½ cups broccoli florets (4 ounces), halved lengthwise
Pinch salt
Lemon wedges (optional)

1. Heat oil in 10-inch nonstick skillet over medium heat until shimmering. Add broccoli to skillet and arrange in single layer, cut sides down. Sprinkle with salt, cover skillet, and cook until bottoms of florets are evenly browned, about 2 minutes.

2. Stir broccoli and reduce heat to low. Cover and continue to cook, stirring occasionally, until florets are tender and lightly browned on all sides, 7 to 9 minutes.

3. Transfer broccoli to plate. Serve with lemon wedges, if using.

SKILLET-ROASTED CAULIFLOWER

Substitute 1½ cups cauliflower florets, halved lengthwise, for broccoli florets. In step 2, increase cooking time to 8 to 10 minutes.

SKILLET-ROASTED CARROTS

Substitute 2 carrots, peeled and sliced ½ inch thick on bias, for broccoli florets. In step 2, increase cooking time to 8 to 10 minutes.

SKILLET-ROASTED GREEN BEANS

Substitute 4 ounces green beans, trimmed and cut into 2-inch lengths (2 cups), for broccoli florets.

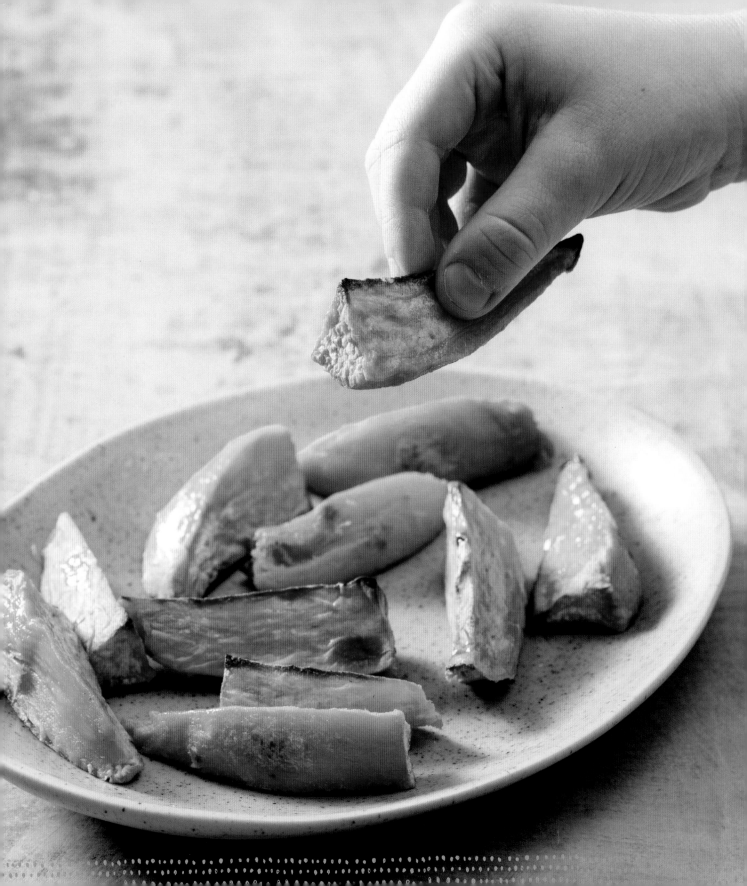

Roasted Sweet Potato Wedges

Makes 12 small wedges
Total Time: 45 minutes

Why This Recipe Works

Sweet potatoes are a nutritional win. Luckily, their candy-like natural sweetness makes them an easy sell. Leaving the potato skins on while roasting protected the bottoms of the sweet potato wedges from scorching in the oven, allowing us to bake them long enough to become soft and buttery inside. You can easily peel the skins off before serving, especially for younger babies and toddlers.

✳ STORAGE INFORMATION

Leftovers can be refrigerated in airtight container for up to 2 days.

We like to add a pinch of salt, but feel free to omit the seasoning, particularly if your child is under 12 months.

1 small sweet potato (8 ounces), unpeeled
1 teaspoon extra-virgin olive oil
Pinch salt (optional)

1. Adjust oven rack to middle position and heat oven to 425 degrees. Line rimmed baking sheet with parchment paper.

2. Cut sweet potato in half crosswise. Then cut each half in half lengthwise to create 4 quarters. Cut each quarter lengthwise into 3 wedges (you should have 12 small wedges).

3. Combine sweet potato wedges, oil, and salt, if using, in bowl and toss to coat. Arrange sweet potato wedges, skin side down, on prepared sheet. Bake until soft and lightly browned, about 25 minutes.

4. Transfer sheet to wire rack. Carefully peel off and discard skins, if desired. Serve (making sure they've cooled enough for young eaters).

SPICED SWEET POTATO WEDGES
Add ¼ teaspoon ground cumin and ¼ teaspoon chili powder to bowl with sweet potato wedges in step 3.

GARLIC AND THYME SWEET POTATO WEDGES
Add ½ teaspoon minced fresh thyme and ½ teaspoon garlic powder to bowl with sweet potato wedges in step 3.

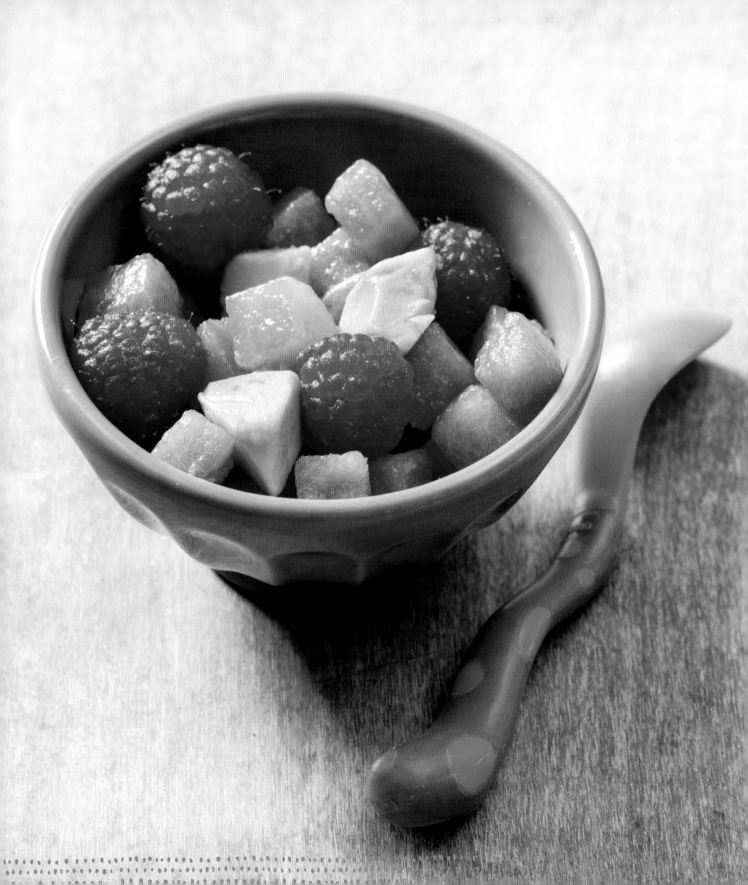

Sweet and Savory Fruit Salad

Makes about 1 cup
Total Time: 10 minutes

Why This Recipe Works

To create a fruit salad suitable for eaters 9 months and up, we auditioned different combinations of soft, graspable fruits until we settled on our two favorites: watermelon and raspberries. Avocado made a soft, savory addition. Since fruit salad doesn't taste as good after a few days in the refrigerator, we decided to make a relatively small batch (which is easily doubled or even tripled if you're feeding a crowd). A lime, olive oil, and sugar dressing brought the salad together.

We like to add a pinch of salt, but feel free to omit the seasoning, particularly if your child is under 12 months.

1 teaspoon extra-virgin olive oil
½ teaspoon lime juice
½ teaspoon sugar
Pinch salt (optional)

½ cup seedless watermelon, cut into ½-inch pieces
¼ avocado, cut into ½-inch pieces
¼ cup raspberries

1. Whisk oil, lime juice, sugar, and salt, if using, together in medium bowl.

2. Add watermelon, avocado, and raspberries to bowl and toss gently to coat with dressing. Serve.

Glazed Tofu Sticks

Makes 6 sticks
Total Time: 40 minutes

Why This Recipe Works

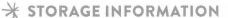

These tasty tofu sticks are crispy on the outside, moist on the inside, and burnished with a light glaze that balances sweet, savory, and tangy flavors. Plus, they're simple to make. After draining the prepared tofu sticks on paper towels, we crisped them up in a bit of oil in a nonstick skillet. We then turned off the heat and poured in a mixture of soy sauce, maple syrup, lemon juice, and ginger; the residual heat was enough to reduce the mixture to a light glaze that coated the tofu.

This recipe can be doubled to make 12 tofu sticks; wipe the skillet clean between batches. You can store unused tofu covered with water and refrigerated in a covered container, changing the water daily, and make the recipe throughout the week.

2 (1-inch-thick) slabs firm tofu, sliced crosswise from 14-ounce block
1½ teaspoons low-sodium soy sauce
1½ teaspoons maple syrup
1 teaspoon lemon juice
⅛ teaspoon ground ginger
1 teaspoon canola oil

1. Lay tofu slabs flat on cutting board and slice each slab lengthwise into three ½-inch-thick sticks (you should have 6 sticks) (see "Cutting Tofu into Sticks," right). Arrange tofu sticks on paper-towel-lined plate, let drain for 20 minutes, then press dry with paper towels.

2. While tofu drains, combine soy sauce, maple syrup, lemon juice, and ginger in small bowl; set aside.

3. Heat oil in 8-inch nonstick skillet over medium-high heat until shimmering. Cook tofu until golden brown and crisp on all 4 sides, about 2 minutes per side.

4. Off heat, add soy sauce mixture to skillet and gently toss tofu sticks to coat evenly. Serve.

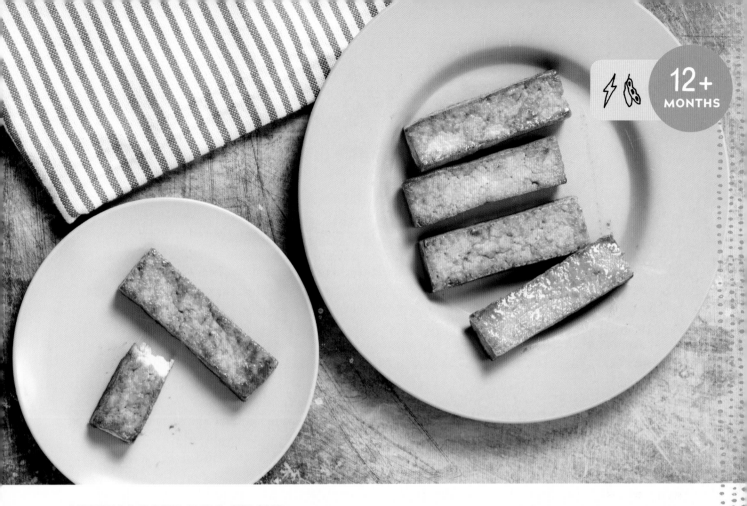

CUTTING TOFU INTO STICKS

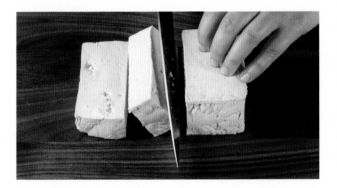

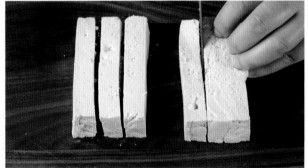

(1) Remove 14-ounce block of tofu from package and discard liquid. Slice two 1-inch-thick slabs crosswise from block of tofu. (Reserve remaining tofu for another use.)

(2) Slice each slab lengthwise into three ½-inch-thick sticks (you should have 6 sticks).

Brown Rice Balls with Spinach and Edamame

Makes 12 balls
Total Time: 1 hour

Why This Recipe Works

Onigiri are a perennially popular Japanese lunch box staple. Traditional onigiri are adorable little bundles of white sushi rice stuffed with morsels of ingredients like fish, pickled plums, or sea vegetables. For our own take on this tasty snack, we first swapped out white rice for short-grain brown rice to boost the nutritional content. And instead of stuffing tidbits of ingredients *into* the balls of rice, we pulsed our add-ins—spinach, edamame, nori, scallion, and ginger—right into the rice mixture using a food processor. You don't have to be an expert onigiri maker to form the rice balls when the ingredients are pulsed together. But you still get the fun of eating these adorable snacks.

You can substitute ¼ teaspoon ground ginger for the fresh ginger. You can serve these with low-sodium soy sauce for dipping or a squeeze of fresh lemon or lime juice.

1 cup water
½ cup short-grain brown rice
½ cup baby spinach
⅓ cup frozen shelled edamame beans, thawed and patted dry
1 scallion, sliced thin
1 (8-by-7½-inch) sheet nori, crumbled (optional)
2 teaspoons toasted sesame oil
½ teaspoon grated fresh ginger
⅛ teaspoon salt

1 Bring water and rice to boil in medium saucepan over high heat. Reduce heat to low, cover, and simmer until rice is tender and water is absorbed, 30 to 35 minutes. Remove saucepan from heat, lay clean folded dish towel underneath lid, and let sit for 10 minutes. Uncover and fluff rice with fork.

2 Pulse spinach, edamame, scallion, nori, if using, sesame oil, ginger, and salt in food processor until mixture is finely ground (mixture should not be smooth), about 12 pulses. Add rice and pulse until rice is coarsely chopped and mixture is well combined, about 8 pulses.

3 Divide rice mixture into 12 portions (about 1½ tablespoons each). Using lightly moistened hands, roll each portion into ball. Serve.

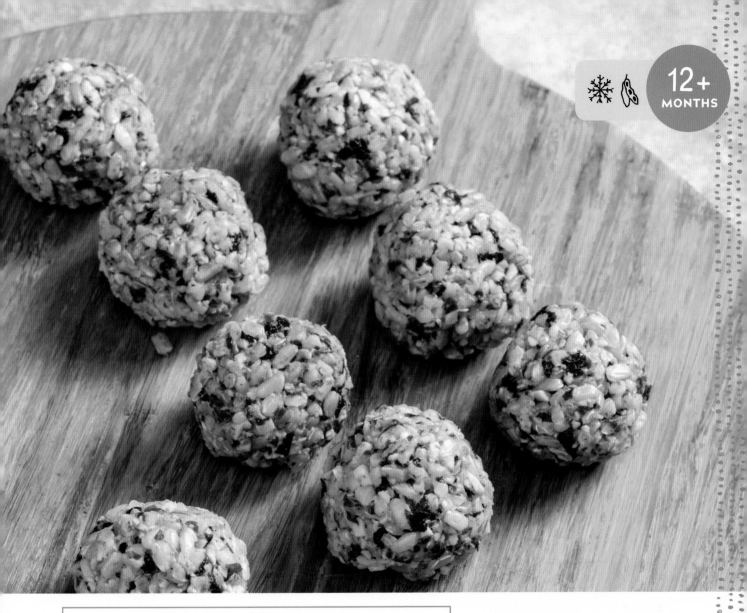

CURRIED BROWN RICE BALLS WITH SPINACH AND CHICKPEAS

Omit nori and ginger. Add ¼ teaspoon curry powder to water and rice in step 1. Substitute ⅓ cup rinsed canned chickpeas for edamame, extra-virgin olive oil for sesame oil, and 1 tablespoon chopped fresh cilantro for scallion.

✳ STORAGE INFORMATION

Brown Rice Balls can be refrigerated up to 3 days or frozen up to 1 month. To freeze, arrange rice balls in single layer on plate and freeze. Once frozen, transfer to a heavy-duty zipper-lock bag. To serve if frozen, fully thaw rice ball in refrigerator. Microwave until heated through, about 15 seconds.

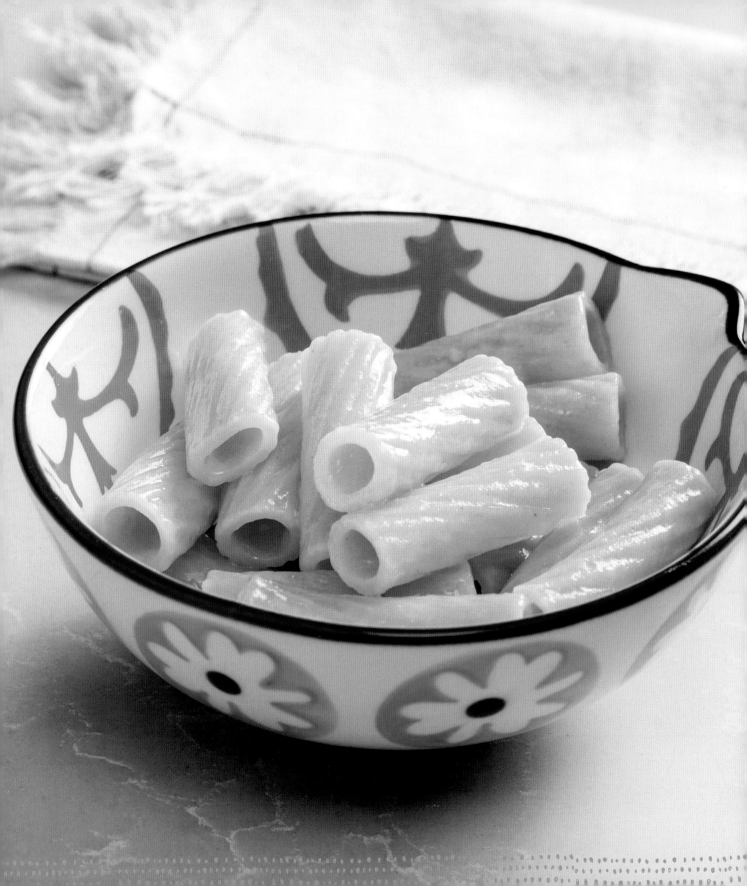

Cheesy Rigatoni

12+
MONTHS

Makes about 1½ cups
Total Time: 30 minutes

Why This Recipe Works

Even the most basic boxed macaroni and cheese requires a few steps: boil water, cook and strain pasta, stir together sauce ingredients, return noodles to the pot. We wanted to make a snack-size batch of simple, from-scratch, cheesy pasta that would be even easier to prepare than the kind from a box. Our first improvement? Eliminate the need to drain the pasta. We spent some time experimenting with the ratios of pasta to butter and water. In the end, we added just enough water to the skillet so that the pasta cooked up tender and almost all the remaining water evaporated—the buttery, starch-infused liquid left made our creamy sauce.

It's important to add the Parmesan at the very end, off the heat. This allows the aged cheese to melt gently and slowly. If it is subjected to too much heat too quickly, it will clump. You will need a 10-inch skillet with a lid for this recipe. The sauce ratio will not work in other size skillets. Avoid preshredded Parmesan products that contain additives, as they are generally stiff and fibrous compared with the fluffy strands of freshly grated cheese, and thus they measure and melt differently. For the best results, grate the cheese on a rasp-style grater or the small holes of a box grater.

2¼ cups water
1 cup rigatoni
1 tablespoon unsalted butter
⅛ teaspoon salt
¼ cup grated Parmesan cheese

1. Bring water, rigatoni, butter, and salt to vigorous simmer in 10-inch skillet over medium-high heat. Cook, stirring frequently, until pasta is tender and almost all liquid has evaporated and a thin layer of milky-white liquid coats bottom of skillet, 14 to 16 minutes.

2. Off heat, sprinkle Parmesan over pasta. Cover skillet and let pasta sit for 5 minutes. Uncover and stir to thoroughly combine and emulsify. Serve.

CHEESY RIGATONI WITH LEMON AND BASIL
Add 1 teaspoon lemon juice and 1 teaspoon minced fresh basil to pasta along with Parmesan in step 2.

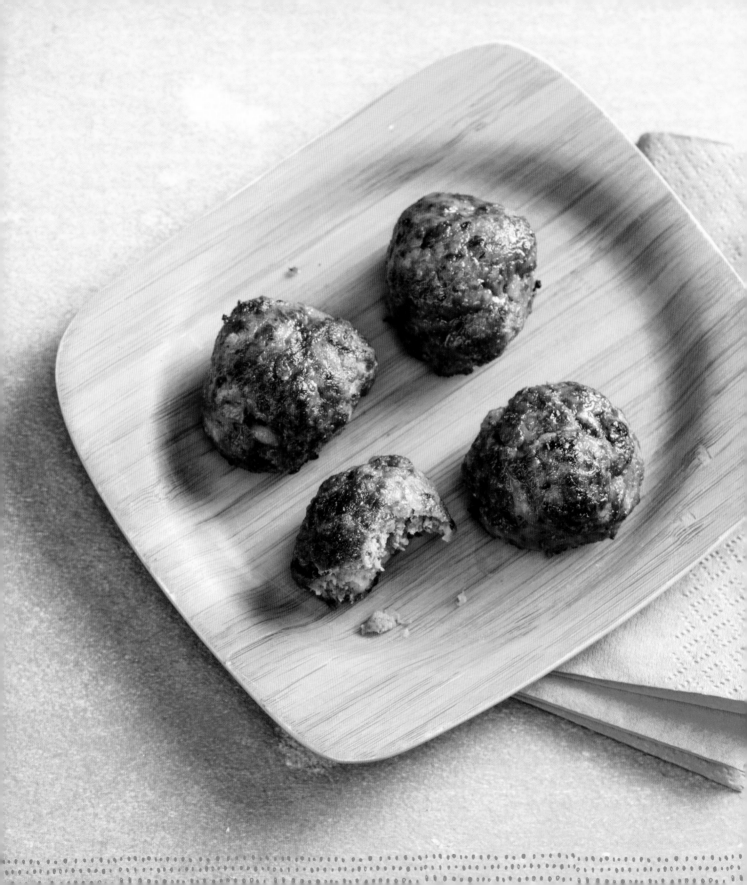

Mini Meatballs

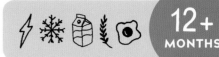

12+
MONTHS

Makes 24 meatballs
Total Time: 45 minutes

Why This Recipe Works

There are so many ways to make meatballs (we know, we've made them all)—from simple to all-day affairs. For the purpose of finger food, we wanted a quick, hands-off method that would allow us to make a big batch that didn't rely on sauce and wouldn't make a big mess. We decided to turn to the oven. For these baked meatballs, we use a simple panade, or a mixture of bread and milk, which helps to keep meatballs moist and tender. They bake for about 20 minutes—more than enough time to clean up!

✳ STORAGE INFORMATION

Meatballs can be refrigerated for up to 3 days or frozen up to 1 month. To freeze, place cooked, cooled meatballs in single layer on plate and freeze. Once frozen, transfer to heavy-duty zipper-lock bag. To serve, place meatballs on foil-lined rimmed baking sheet and reheat in 400-degree oven until sizzling, about 15 minutes.

These meatballs are delicious on their own or dipped into our Hand-Squished Roasted Tomato Sauce (page 213).

2 slices hearty white sandwich bread, crusts removed, torn into 1-inch pieces
¼ cup whole milk
1 tablespoon extra-virgin olive oil
1 small onion, chopped fine
½ teaspoon salt

2 garlic cloves, minced
1 teaspoon dried oregano
1 ounce Parmesan cheese, grated (½ cup)
1 large egg, lightly beaten
2 tablespoons minced fresh parsley
1 pound (85 percent) lean ground beef

1 Adjust oven rack to upper-middle position and heat oven to 450 degrees. Line rimmed baking sheet with aluminum foil and spray foil with vegetable oil spray. Mash bread and milk together with fork in large bowl until mixture forms smooth paste; set aside.

2 Heat oil in 10-inch skillet over medium heat until shimmering. Add onion and salt and cook until softened and lightly browned, 5 to 7 minutes. Stir in garlic and oregano and cook until fragrant, about 30 seconds. Transfer onion mixture to bowl with bread mixture. Stir in Parmesan, egg, and parsley until well combined.

3 Add beef and gently mix with your hands until well combined. Divide meat mixture into 24 portions (about 1½ tablespoons each) and roll each portion into ball. Arrange meatballs evenly on prepared sheet.

4 Bake meatballs until well browned and cooked through, 18 to 20 minutes, rotating sheet halfway through baking. Serve.

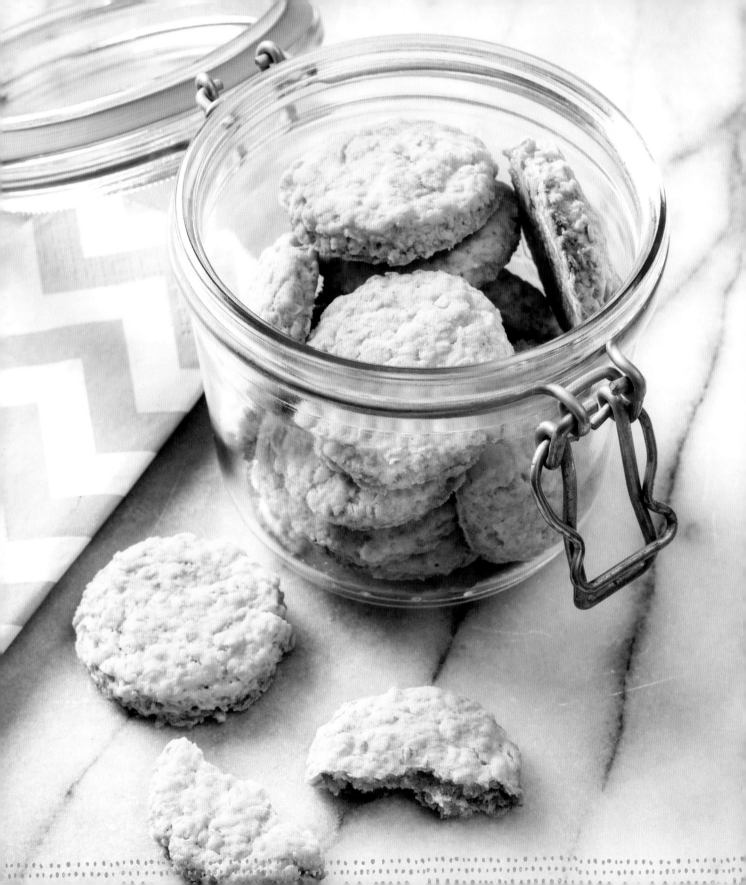

Savory Oatcakes

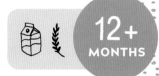

Makes 12 small oatcakes
Total Time: 45 minutes, plus cooling time

Why This Recipe Works

Oatcakes are a traditional Scottish biscuit, packed with oats and more savory than sweet. The type and treatment of the oats determine the success of these little biscuits. Old-fashioned oats are oat kernels that have been rolled flat and need a lot of water in order to fully rehydrate. To account for this, you often have to break them down by pulsing them in a food processor. Sure this method works, but it seemed like a laborious step for a simple snack. Instead, we opted for quick-cooking oats since they have already been broken down into smaller flakes and thus need no further processing before being added to the dough.

✳ STORAGE INFORMATION

Oatcakes can be stored at room temperature for up to 1 week.

It's important to rest the dough for 10 minutes after mixing. This short rest time allows the oats to hydrate, making the dough more pliable. No need for a rolling pin: you can use your hands to pat the dough into an even layer before cutting out the biscuits. If you don't have a biscuit cutter, you can use a round cookie cutter or a small glass. Do not substitute steel-cut, old-fashioned rolled, or instant oats in this recipe.

⅓ cup water
3 tablespoons unsalted butter, melted and cooled
1 cup (3 ounces) quick oats
⅓ cup (1⅔ ounces) all-purpose flour
2 teaspoons sugar
¾ teaspoon baking powder
½ teaspoon salt

1 Adjust oven rack to middle position and heat oven to 350 degrees. Line rimmed baking sheet with parchment paper.

2 Whisk water and butter together in small bowl. Whisk oats, flour, sugar, baking powder, and salt together in large bowl. Add water mixture to oat mixture and use rubber spatula to stir until well combined (dough will be sticky). Let dough sit at room temperature for 10 minutes.

3 Scrape dough out onto floured counter and use floured hands to pat dough into 8-inch circle (dough should be ¼ inch thick).

4 Use 2-inch biscuit cutter to cut out 12 rounds of dough (gather and press scraps together to cut the last few rounds). Use metal offset spatula to transfer rounds to prepared sheet.

5 Bake until oatcakes are golden brown, about 25 minutes, rotating sheet halfway through baking. Transfer sheet to wire rack and let oatcakes cool on sheet, about 30 minutes. Serve.

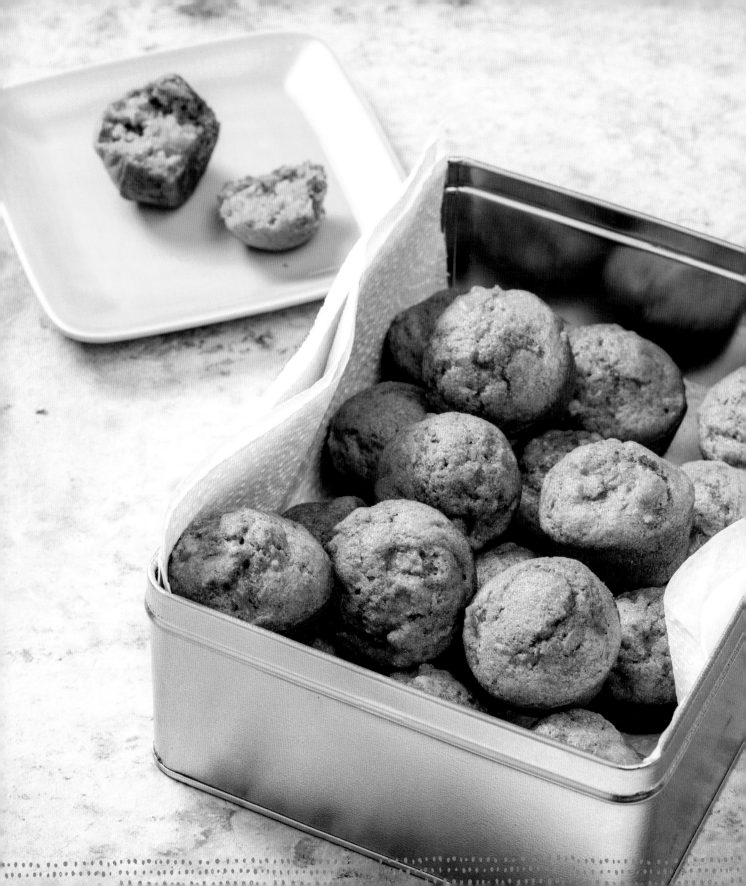

Tiny Carrot Muffins

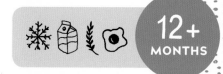

Makes 24 mini muffins
Total Time: 40 minutes, plus cooling time

Why This Recipe Works

Yes, carrots are healthy, but the best part about adding them to these muffins? They're 88 percent water. This means that as they cook in the batter, some of this water becomes steam, giving the muffins an airy, fluffy texture. To make these muffins even healthier, we opted for whole-wheat flour and yogurt in place of the usual white flour and butter. Warm spices like cinnamon and ginger give these muffins a signature carrot-cake flavor.

✳ STORAGE INFORMATION

Muffins can be stored at room temperature for up to 3 days or frozen for up to 1 month. To freeze, place muffins in single layer in heavy-duty zipper-lock bag. To serve, thaw muffins at room temperature. To serve warm, heat thawed muffins in 300-degree oven for 8 to 10 minutes.

You can use either light or dark brown sugar in this recipe. If you don't have a mini muffin tin, you can use a standard muffin tin. Divide batter evenly among 12 muffin cups and bake for about 15 minutes.

1 cup (5½ ounces) whole-wheat flour
¾ teaspoon baking powder
½ teaspoon baking soda
½ teaspoon ground cinnamon
½ teaspoon ground ginger
¼ teaspoon salt
½ cup plain whole-milk yogurt
⅓ cup packed (2⅓ ounces) brown sugar
¼ cup canola oil
2 large eggs
½ teaspoon vanilla extract
1 cup shredded carrots (2 small carrots)

1. Adjust oven rack to middle position and heat oven to 375 degrees. Grease one 24-cup mini muffin tin.

2. Whisk flour, baking powder, baking soda, cinnamon, ginger, and salt together in medium bowl. Whisk yogurt, sugar, oil, eggs, and vanilla together in large bowl. Using rubber spatula, stir in carrots until fully incorporated. Add flour mixture and stir until just combined.

3. Divide batter evenly among mini-muffin cups (about 1 heaping tablespoon per cup). Bake until toothpick inserted in center of muffin comes out clean, 10 to 12 minutes. Let muffins cool in muffin tin on wire rack for 10 minutes. Remove muffins from muffin tin and let cool completely on rack, about 30 minutes. Serve.

TINY CARROT MUFFINS WITH RAISINS
Add ⅓ cup golden raisins to flour mixture in step 2.

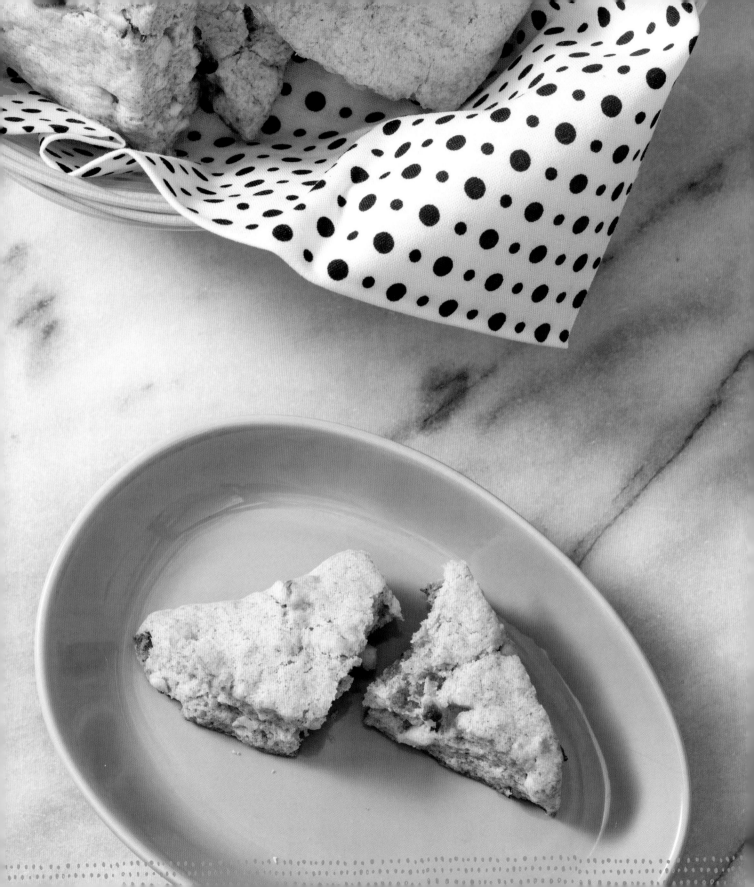

Baby Apple Scones

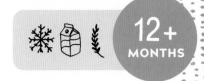

12+ MONTHS

Makes 10 small scones
Total Time: 45 minutes, plus cooling time

Why This Recipe Works

We set out to create a slightly healthier version of the classic coffeehouse treat—and make it a good fit for tiny hands. Scones are often flaky little sugar bombs, so to start, we reduced the amount of sugar and went for a combination of whole-wheat and all-purpose flours. To avoid adding excess moisture, we stirred dried apples into the dough. Heavy cream provides richness and just enough liquid to pull the dough together without making it gummy or tough. The result? Tender, lightly sweetened mini scone snacks.

✳ STORAGE INFORMATION

Scones can be stored at room temperature for up to 3 days or frozen for up to 1 month. To freeze, place cooled scones in single layer in heavy-duty zipper-lock bag. To serve, thaw scones at room temperature. To serve warm, refresh thawed scones in 300-degree oven for 8 to 10 minutes.

½ cup (2½ ounces) all-purpose flour
½ cup (2¾ ounces) whole-wheat flour
1½ teaspoons baking powder
2 tablespoons sugar
¼ teaspoon salt

3 tablespoons unsalted butter, chilled and cut into ¼-inch pieces
½ cup heavy cream
½ cup dried apples, chopped fine

1 Adjust oven rack to middle position and heat oven to 425 degrees. Line rimmed baking sheet with parchment paper.

2 Process all-purpose flour, whole-wheat flour, baking powder, sugar, and salt in food processor until combined, about 10 seconds.

3 Add butter and pulse until mixture resembles coarse meal, about 6 pulses. Add cream and pulse until dough forms large clumps, 6 to 8 pulses. Add apples and pulse until evenly incorporated, about 4 pulses.

4 Transfer dough to lightly floured counter and knead dough by hand until it just comes together, 5 to 10 seconds. Pat dough into 12½-by-2½-inch rectangle. Cut rectangle into 5 even squares, then cut each square diagonally to form 10 triangles.

5 Transfer scones to prepared sheet. Refrigerate until dough is chilled, 10 to 15 minutes.

6 Bake scones until lightly browned, 10 to 12 minutes, rotating sheet halfway through baking. Transfer scones to wire rack and let cool for at least 10 minutes before serving.

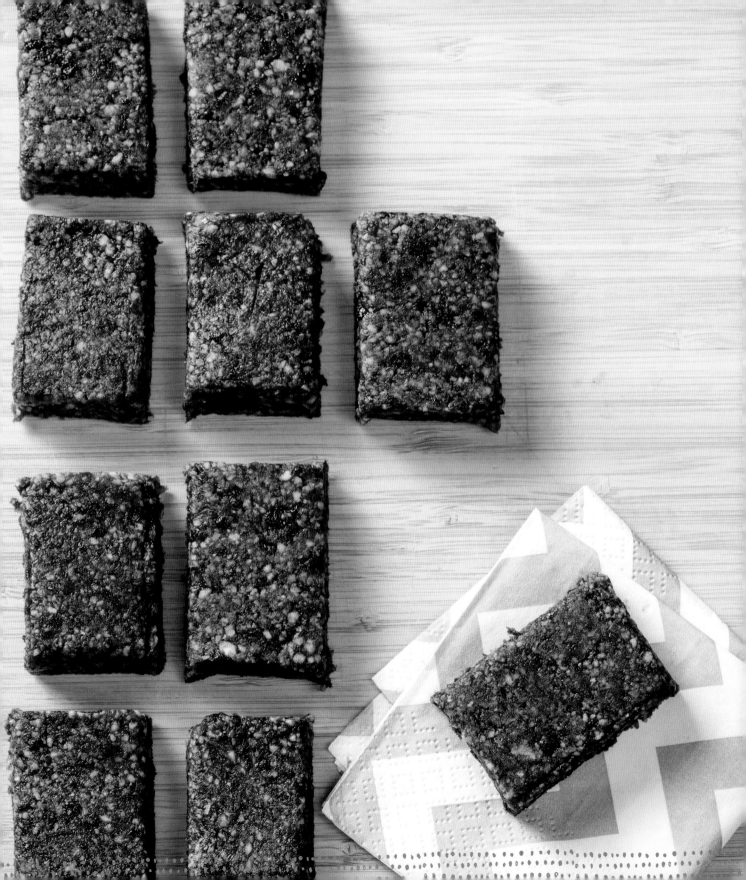

Raw Fruit and Nut Bars

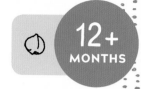

12+ MONTHS

Makes 12 small bars
Total Time: 15 minutes, plus chilling time

Why This Recipe Works

You might be familiar with various raw fruit and nut bars, packaged in bright colors and sold at the supermarket for...not a tiny amount of money. We wanted to create our own homemade version that, with a bit of bulk buying, would reduce the cost and allow you to customize and make a portable, compact, and protein-packed snack—no baking required. The basic ingredient list for these commercial bars is simple: dried fruit (often dates), nuts (often almonds), spices, and salt. Dates are naturally moist and therefore excellent for holding all the ingredients together. We wanted to reduce the amount of dates (they're very sweet!) and found that rehydrating other dried fruits worked as well. All you need is a food processor to finely chop the ingredients, press the mixture into a pan, chill it, and slice it into bars.

✳ **STORAGE INFORMATION**

Bars can be refrigerated for up to 1 week.

The test kitchen's preferred loaf pan measures 8½ by 4½ inches; if you use a 9-by-5-inch loaf pan, the bars will be slightly thinner but will still work.

1 cup hot water
¾ cup dried cherries, dried apricots, or dried cranberries (or a mixture of two or three)
3 ounces pitted dates, chopped (½ cup)
1 cup raw whole almonds
¼ teaspoon ground cinnamon
¼ teaspoon salt

1. Line 8½-by-4½-inch loaf pan with plastic wrap, letting excess hang over sides of pan.

2. Combine water, cherries, and dates in bowl. Let sit until fruit has softened, 5 to 10 minutes. Drain well and pat fruit dry with paper towels.

3. Process almonds, cinnamon, and salt in food processor until finely ground, about 20 seconds. Add drained fruit and pulse until fruit is very finely chopped and mixture starts to clump together, 15 to 20 pulses.

4. Transfer mixture to prepared pan and spread into even layer with rubber spatula. Fold excess plastic wrap over top and, using hands, press to flatten. Refrigerate until firm, about 1 hour.

5. Transfer chilled fruit and nut mixture to cutting board and discard plastic wrap. Slice in half lengthwise, then cut each half crosswise into 6 pieces (you should have 12 bars). Serve.

Cheese Crackers

Makes 64 small crackers
Total Time: 1 hour, plus cooling time

Why This Recipe Works

While we love eating store-bought cheese crackers (who doesn't?), we wanted a more homemade option—with real cheese and no preservatives. The dough for these crackers proved to be surprisingly simple. We mixed cheese, flour, butter, a little cornstarch, a touch of salt, and a spoonful of water in the food processor. The butter warmed up during mixing, making it difficult to create crackers, but after a stint in the refrigerator, the dough was easy to roll out and cut into perfectly shaped individual crackers. To re-create the look of the classic supermarket cheese cracker, we used yellow cheddar cheese for the classic neon-orange color (though white cheddar worked just as well), and we poked a small hole in the center of each cracker using the blunt side of a wooden skewer.

This recipe is easy to scale up: double all the ingredients, divide the crackers between two rimmed baking sheets, and bake one sheet at a time.

3 ounces sharp yellow cheddar cheese, shredded (¾ cup)
½ cup (2½ ounces) all-purpose flour
1 teaspoon cornstarch
⅛ teaspoon salt
3 tablespoons unsalted butter, cut into 3 pieces and chilled
1 tablespoon water

1   Process cheddar, flour, cornstarch, and salt in food processor until combined, about 30 seconds. Add butter and process until mixture resembles wet sand, about 20 seconds. Add water and pulse until dough forms large clumps, about 5 pulses.

2   Transfer dough to counter and pat dough into 6-inch square. Wrap dough in plastic wrap and refrigerate until firm, about 30 minutes.

3   Meanwhile, adjust oven rack to middle position and heat oven to 350 degrees. Line rimmed baking sheet with parchment paper.

4   Discard plastic wrap and transfer dough to lightly floured counter. Roll dough into rough 9-inch square, about ⅛ inch thick. Use fluted pastry wheel, pizza wheel, or paring knife to trim dough into neat 8-inch square. Slice square into 8 strips, each 1 inch wide, then make 8 perpendicular slices, each 1 inch wide, to form 64 squares.

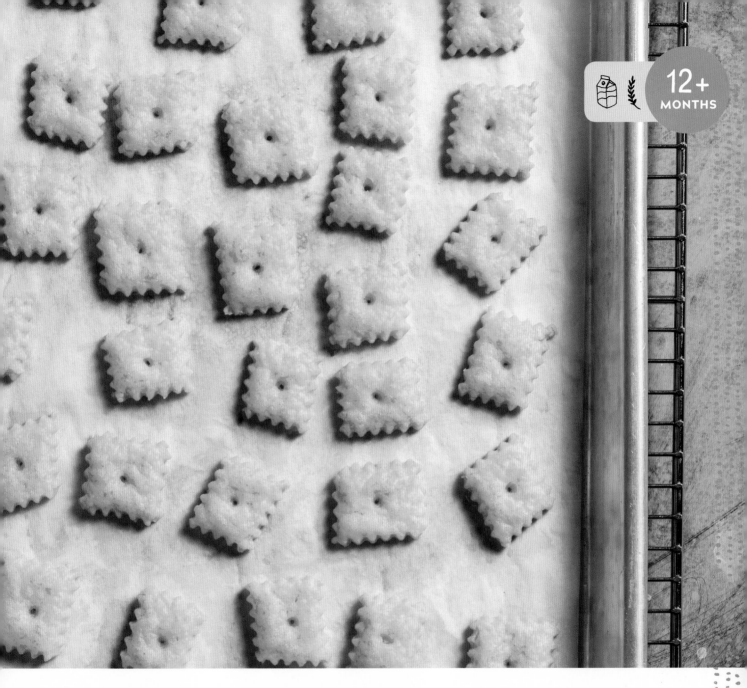

5 Place squares on prepared sheet (they can be close together, but not touching). Use blunt end of skewer to poke hole through center of each square. Bake until golden around edges, 16 to 18 minutes, rotating each sheet halfway through baking. Let crackers cool completely on sheet, about 15 minutes. Serve.

* STORAGE INFORMATION

Crackers can be stored at room temperature for up to 1 week.

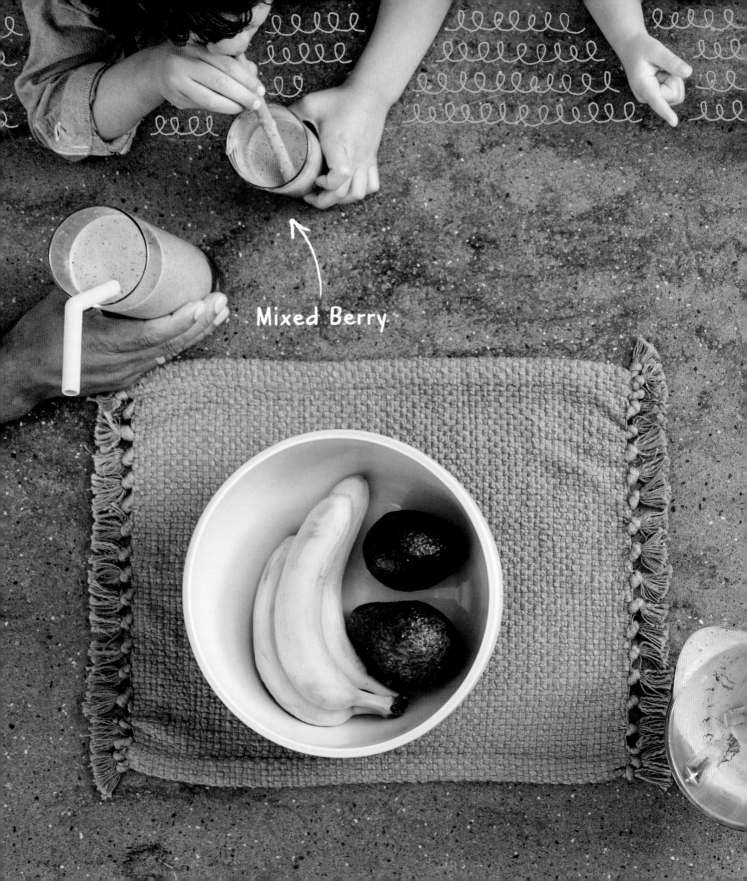

Mixed Berry

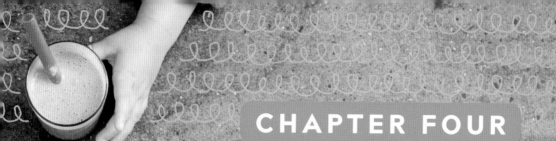

18+
MONTHS

SMOOTHIES

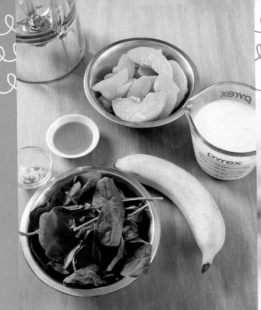

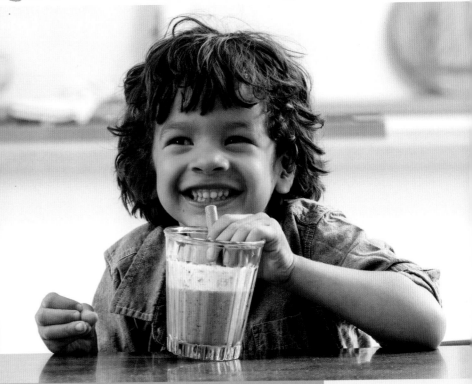

"Our whole family had this as a snack. Our toddler wanted more!"

—Parent of 18-month-old, on Blueberry Avocado Smoothie

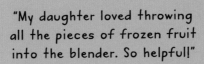

"My daughter loved throwing all the pieces of frozen fruit into the blender. So helpful!"

—Parent of 3-year-old, on Strawberry Mango Smoothie

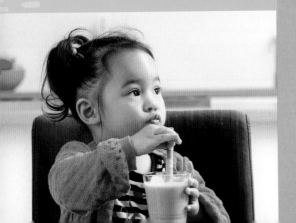

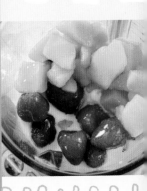

ALL ABOUT SMOOTHIES

Smoothies are simple recipes with high reward. They're refreshingly cold; they're naturally sweet; they're full of healthy fruits, vegetables, and (sometimes) nut butters or dairy for a nice protein boost. Plus, making smoothies at home guarantees that they are wholesome and nutritious (premade supermarket smoothies can contain unnecessary added salt, sugar, preservatives, additives, and thickeners).

When developing these smoothie recipes, we worked hard to include nutritional-powerhouse ingredients—think kale, spinach, carrots, avocado—while taking care to never let any of the resulting smoothies taste like a salad. We often started each recipe by blending up a banana with a pinch of salt for the creamiest base. We used frozen fruit whenever possible—in part because it's convenient, but also because it eliminates the need for flavor-diluting ice. Each recipe makes 3 cups, enough for a snack for at least one toddler (or two) and a grown-up. Our pediatric dietitian recommends a serving size of 2 to 4 ounces for snacks for toddlers.

We've found that toddlers not only love to drink smoothies, but they also love to participate in their creation: start by having your child break a banana into pieces and toss it into the blender jar. Note that many of these recipes contain salt and/or honey, which are not recommended for babies under 12 months.

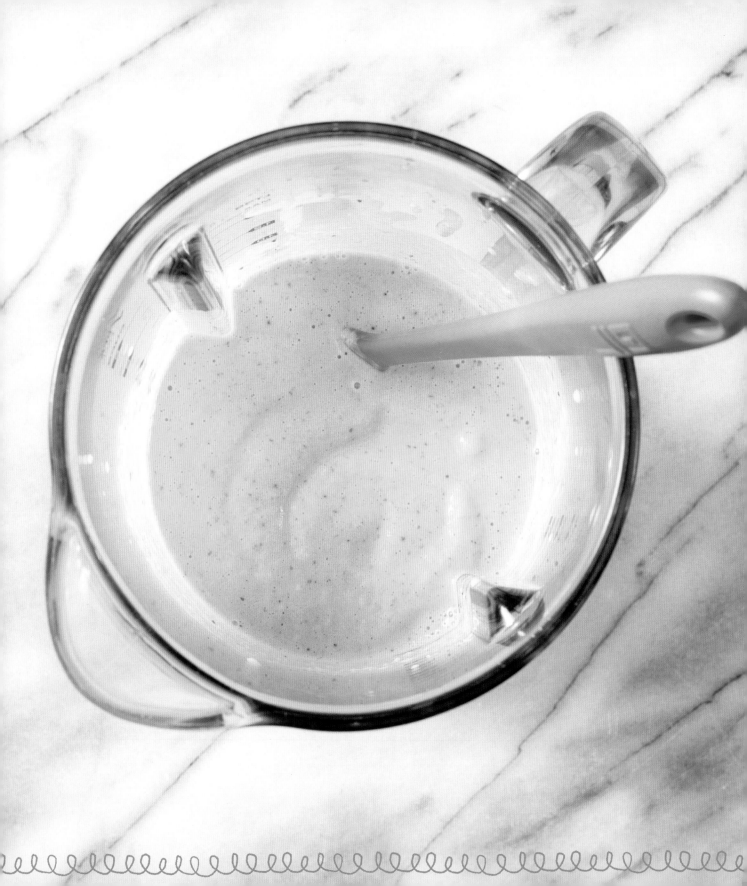

Strawberry Mango

18+ MONTHS

Makes about 3 cups
Total Time: 10 minutes

Why This Recipe Works

Strawberry banana is a classic, delicious flavor combination...but a little predictable. We wanted something bright to add to the mix. Pineapple made the mixture too acidic. Mango, however, brought a floral sweetness that complemented the strawberry and also lent just a bit of tartness. A tablespoon of honey and a pinch of salt balanced the pucker. (Salt actually brings out the sweetness in the fruit.)

You can substitute whole-milk Greek yogurt for the whole-milk yogurt, but your smoothies will be thicker; thin with additional milk as needed.

1 ripe banana, peeled and broken into 4 pieces
1 tablespoon honey
Pinch salt
1 cup frozen strawberries
1 cup frozen mango chunks
1 cup plain whole-milk yogurt
¼ cup whole milk

1. Process banana, honey, and salt in blender on high speed until smooth, about 10 seconds.

2. Add strawberries, mango, yogurt, and milk and continue to process until smooth, about 1 minute, scraping down sides of blender jar as needed. Serve.

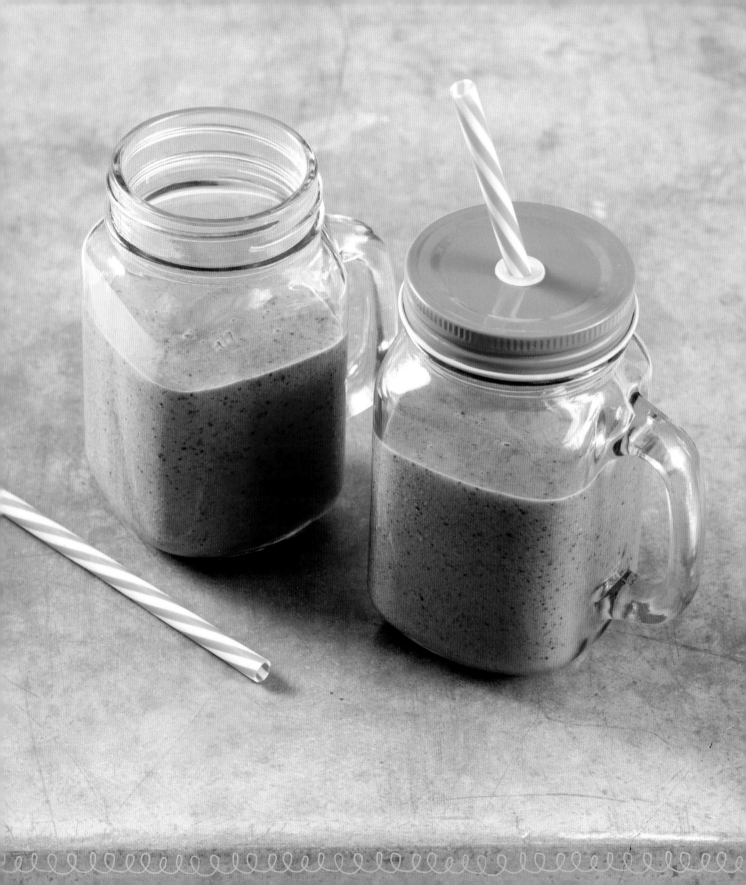

Mixed Berry

Makes about 3 cups
Total Time: 10 minutes

Why This Recipe Works

The combination of strawberries, blackberries, blueberries, and raspberries can deliver bright, summery sweetness, even in the middle of winter. Using frozen berries made this a year-round smoothie (see "Why We Use Frozen Fruit," below).

You can substitute whole-milk Greek yogurt for the whole-milk yogurt, but your smoothies will be thicker; thin with additional milk as needed.

1 ripe banana, peeled and broken into 4 pieces
1 tablespoon honey
Pinch salt

2 cups frozen mixed berries
1 cup plain whole-milk yogurt
¼ cup whole milk

1. Process banana, honey, and salt in blender on high speed until smooth, about 10 seconds.

2. Add berries, yogurt, and milk and continue to process until smooth, about 1 minute, scraping down sides of blender jar as needed. Serve.

Why We Use Frozen Fruit

When it comes to smoothies, we almost always choose frozen fruit over fresh. This is because frozen fruit (everything from berries to mangoes) is flash-frozen at the peak of ripeness, preserving the nutrients and giving us consistent results at a fraction of the cost of fresh fruit. Using frozen fruit also keeps the smoothie cold without needing to add any ice to the mix.

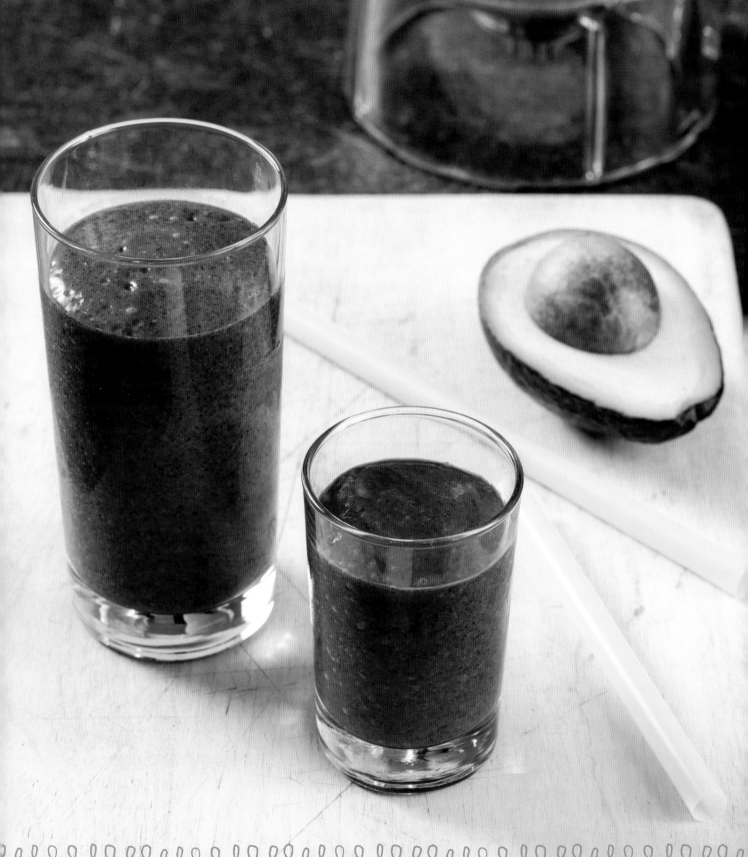

Blueberry Avocado

Makes about 3 cups
Total Time: 10 minutes

Why This Recipe Works

An avocado in a smoothie is not as strange as it sounds. Avocados are soft and creamy and therefore blend beautifully, plus their natural richness provides body and healthy fat. We decided to pair our avocado with tangy frozen blueberries (see page 121 for more on why we use frozen fruit). Almond milk was a great neutral, calcium-packed liquid to bring the smoothie together. (Bonus: vegan! But you can also substitute cow's milk.) A couple tablespoons of lemon juice and a pinch of salt brought the flavors into focus.

1 ripe banana, peeled and broken into 4 pieces
Pinch salt
1½ cups unsweetened almond milk
1½ cups frozen blueberries
½ avocado, pitted and cut into 1-inch pieces
2 tablespoons lemon juice

1. Process banana and salt in blender on high speed until smooth, about 10 seconds.

2. Add almond milk, blueberries, avocado, and lemon juice and continue to process until smooth, about 1 minute, scraping down sides of blender jar as needed. Serve.

Avocado Magic
Avocados not only add a beautiful creaminess to smoothies like this one, they are also packed with nutrients. Avocados are one of the only fruits that have an abundance of heart-healthy monounsaturated fat and are a great source of fiber; vitamins C, E, and K; riboflavin; copper; and potassium.

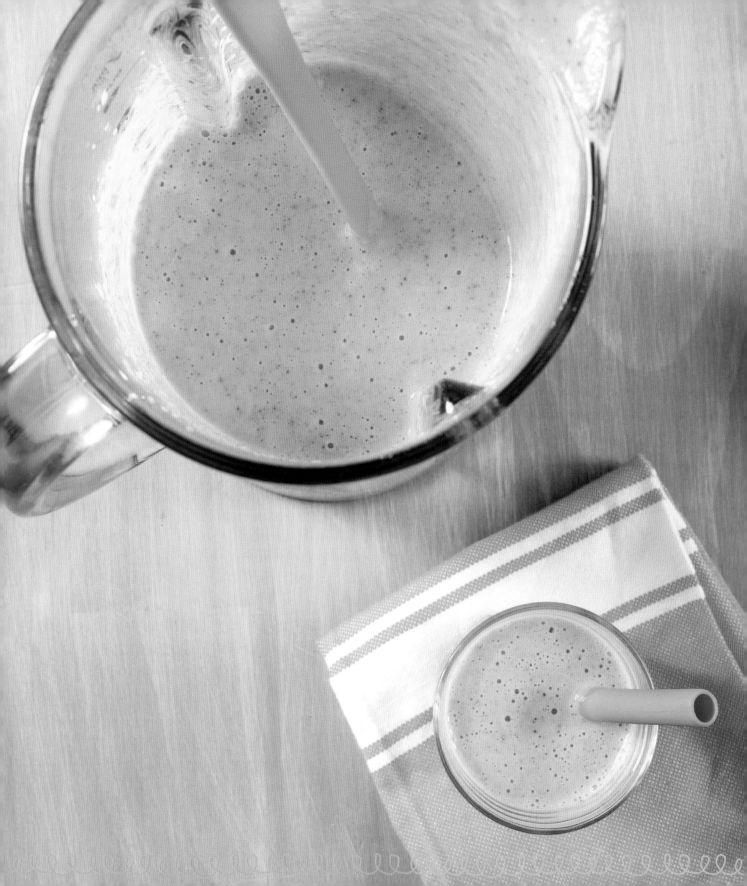

Peach Spinach

Makes about 3 cups
Total Time: 10 minutes

Why This Recipe Works

Fresh summer peaches are delicious, but in most parts of the country the availability of good peaches is fleeting. That's why we love frozen sliced peaches: they are available year-round, they are picked and processed at the peak of ripeness, and there's no pitting or peeling required (see page 121 for more on why we use frozen fruit). Adding a handful of nutrient-dense baby spinach turned our smoothie a beautiful light green. A tablespoon of honey kept things sweet alongside the more savory spinach.

You can substitute whole-milk Greek yogurt for the whole-milk yogurt, but your smoothies will be thicker; thin with additional milk as needed.

1 ripe banana, peeled and broken into 4 pieces
1 tablespoon honey
Pinch salt
2 cups frozen peaches
1 ounce (1 cup) baby spinach
1 cup plain whole-milk yogurt
¼ cup whole milk

1 Process banana, honey, and salt in blender on high speed until smooth, about 10 seconds.

2 Add peaches, spinach, yogurt, and milk and continue to process until smooth, about 1 minute, scraping down sides of blender jar as needed. Serve.

Green Power

Dark leafy greens—a group that includes spinach, kale, collards, and Swiss chard—are some of the most nutrient-dense foods out there. They're packed with chlorophyll; fiber; calcium; antioxidants; vitamins A, C, E, and K; and some B vitamins like folate. Among dark greens, spinach is one of the most accessible for its mild flavor and tender texture. Plus, it gives your smoothie a nice springlike hue.

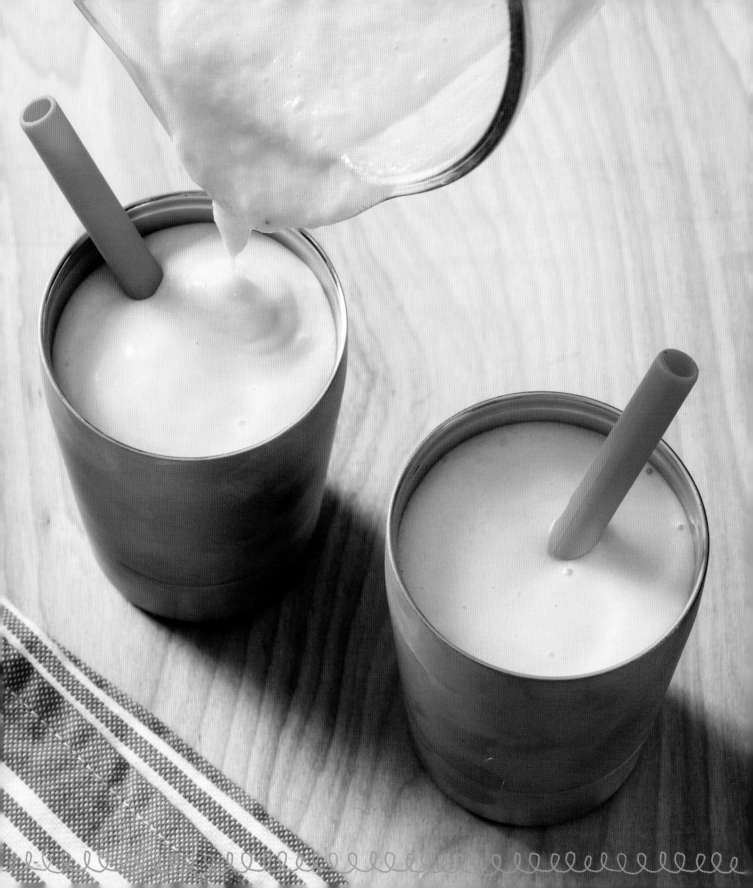

Pineapple Coconut

⚡ 🥥 **18+ MONTHS**

Makes about 3 cups
Total Time: 10 minutes

Why This Recipe Works

With the image of a tropical vacation in our mind's eye, we set out to create a bright, pineapple-y smoothie to bring summer even to the darkest winter months. Frozen pineapple was the obvious choice for our smoothie base (see page 121 for more on why we use frozen fruit). A banana added creaminess. Canned coconut milk added an ultracreamy, tropical flourish. (No, *you're* thinking about piña coladas.) We thinned out this dense smoothie with a bit of water to keep it dairy free.

1 ripe banana, peeled and broken into 4 pieces
1 tablespoon honey
Pinch salt
2 cups frozen pineapple chunks
½ cup unsweetened canned coconut milk
½ cup water

1 Process banana, honey, and salt in blender on high speed until smooth, about 10 seconds.

2 Add pineapple, coconut milk, and water and continue to process until smooth, about 1 minute, scraping down sides of blender jar as needed. Serve.

The World of Canned Coconut

Coconut milk is not the thin liquid found inside the coconut itself—that is called coconut water. Coconut milk is a product made by steeping equal parts shredded coconut meat and either warm milk or water. The meat is pressed or mashed to release as much liquid as possible, the mixture is strained, and the result is coconut milk! The same method is used to make coconut cream, but the ratio of coconut meat to liquid is higher, about 4 to 1. (The cream that rises to the top of coconut milk after it sits a while is also referred to as coconut cream.) Finally, cream of coconut—not to be confused with coconut cream—is a sweetened product based on coconut milk that also contains thickeners and emulsifiers.

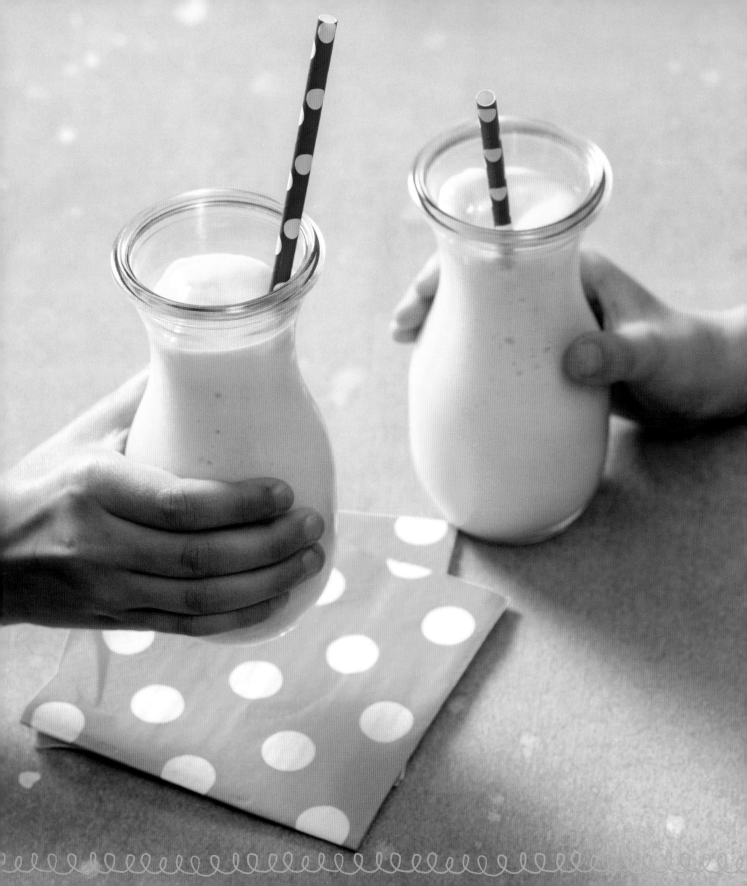

Mango Yogurt

Makes about 3 cups
Total Time: 15 minutes

Why This Recipe Works

A standard offering in Indian cuisine, a lassi is a chilled yogurt drink meant to cool you down when eating spicy food or during the hottest days of summer. Lassis can be savory, seasoned with salt and spices, or sweet, made with fruit, sugar or honey, and sometimes essences like rose water. The sweet mango lassi is by far the most popular, and we decided to make our own. A touch of honey brought out the mango's floral notes, and a squeeze of lime gave the drink a nice tang.

While in most smoothies we prefer frozen fruit, this mango-centric recipe tasted best with fresh, very ripe mangoes. (But frozen mangoes can be substituted.) If your fresh mangoes are not very sweet, you may need to add additional honey. You can substitute whole-milk Greek yogurt for the whole-milk yogurt, but your smoothies will be thicker; thin with additional water as needed.

2 mangoes, peeled, pitted, and chopped (2½ cups)
1 cup plain whole-milk yogurt
1 cup ice cubes
2 teaspoons honey
1 teaspoon lime juice
Pinch salt

1. Process mango, yogurt, ice, honey, lime juice, and salt in blender on high speed until smooth, about 1 minute, scraping down sides of blender jar as needed. Serve.

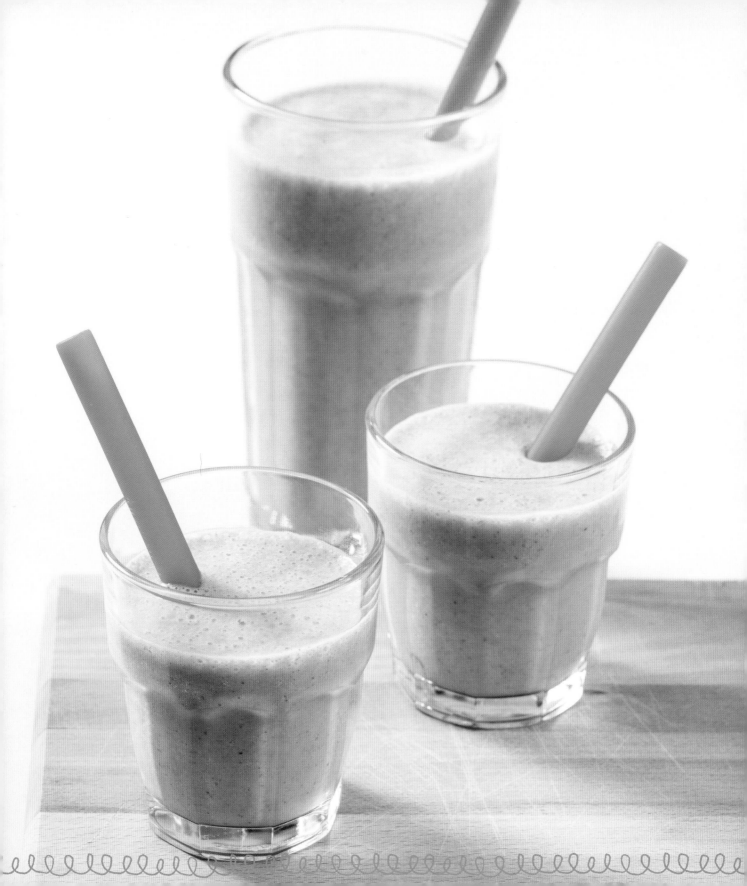

Kale Pineapple

Makes about 3 cups
Total Time: 10 minutes

Why This Recipe Works

Green smoothies can be a tough sell for some vegetable-averse adults but are a great way of adding some kale to your toddler's snack routine. It's all about the balance. For this recipe, we used sweet and tangy pineapple to counter kale's bitter notes, as well as a touch of honey and a banana for sweetness and a smooth texture. Blending the mixture with yogurt and a little water ensures that the fibrous kale gets fully broken down.

You can substitute frozen chopped kale for fresh kale. You can substitute whole-milk Greek yogurt for the whole-milk yogurt, but your smoothies will be thicker; thin with additional water as needed.

1 ripe banana, peeled and broken into 4 pieces
1 tablespoon honey
Pinch salt
1 cup frozen pineapple chunks

1 cup chopped kale leaves
1 cup plain whole-milk yogurt
½ cup water

1 Process banana, honey, and salt in blender on high speed until smooth, about 10 seconds.

2 Add pineapple, kale, yogurt, and water and continue to process until smooth, about 1 minute, scraping down sides of blender jar as needed. Serve.

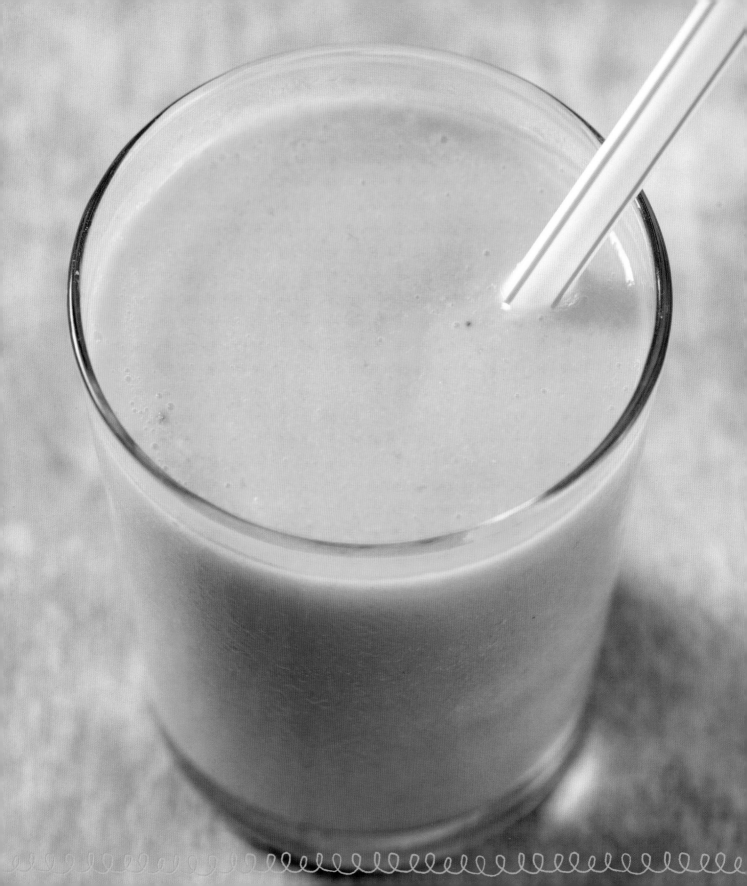

Gingery Carrot Mango

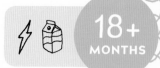

18+ MONTHS

Makes about 3 cups
Total Time: 10 minutes

Why This Recipe Works

This smoothie is a bright-orange billboard for the delicious combination of carrots, mango, and ginger. We chose carrots for their natural sweetness but didn't want to cook them (if nothing else, smoothies should be quick and easy). Happily, we found that we could leave the carrots raw; we just needed to give them extra time in the blender to break down before adding the other ingredients. A ripe banana along with some yogurt provided a creamy base. Frozen mango gave us a pretty orange-on-orange color palette. To balance the flavors, we added a bit of honey and salt. For a little kick, we added some grated fresh ginger.

3 carrots, peeled and chopped
1 cup ice cubes
½ cup water
1½ cups frozen mango chunks
1 ripe banana, peeled and broken into 4 pieces
½ cup plain whole-milk yogurt
1 tablespoon honey
¼ teaspoon grated ginger
Pinch salt

1   Process carrots, ice, and water in blender on high speed until smooth, about 2 minutes, scraping down sides of blender as needed.

2   Add mango, banana, yogurt, honey, ginger, and salt and continue to process until smooth, about 1 minute. Serve.

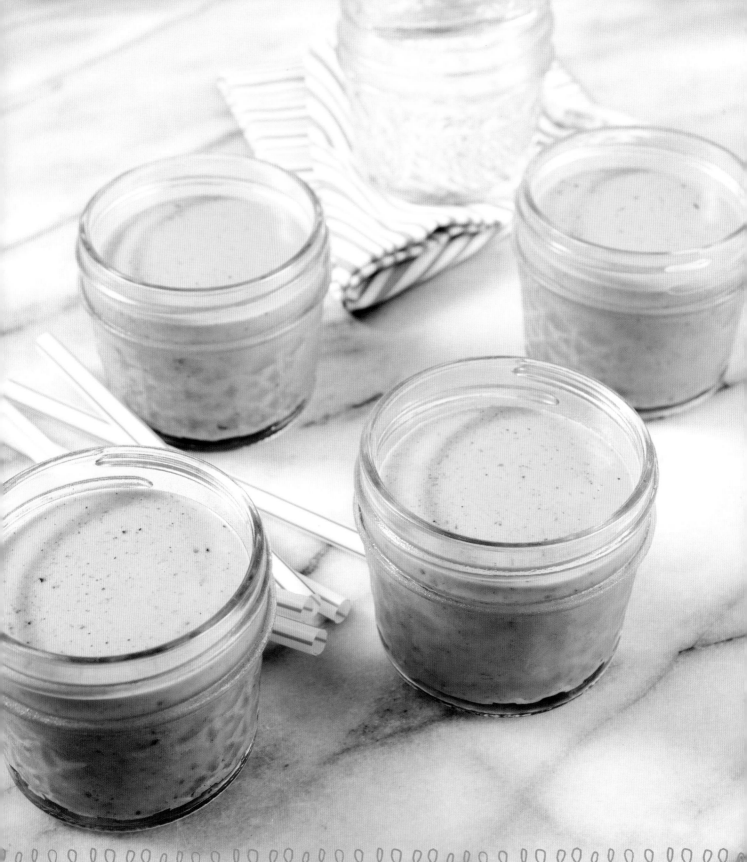

Cherry Almond

Makes about 3 cups
Total Time: 10 minutes

18+
MONTHS

Why This Recipe Works

Think of this smoothie as a sippable PB&J. Using frozen fruit removed the time-consuming task of pitting cherries, and it also meant we didn't have to dilute the flavor of the smoothie with ice to keep the smoothie cold. A scoop of rich almond butter complemented the brightness of the cherries, while a banana provided background sweetness and a smooth, creamy texture. Yogurt and a pinch of salt rounded things out with savory tang.

You can substitute whole-milk Greek yogurt for the whole-milk yogurt, but your smoothies will be thicker; thin with additional milk as needed.

1 ripe banana, peeled and broken into 4 pieces
¼ cup almond butter
Pinch salt

2 cups frozen sweet cherries
1 cup plain whole-milk yogurt
¼ cup whole milk

1 Process banana, almond butter, and salt in blender on high speed until smooth, about 10 seconds.

2 Add cherries, yogurt, and milk and continue to process until smooth, about 1 minute, scraping down sides of blender jar as needed. Serve.

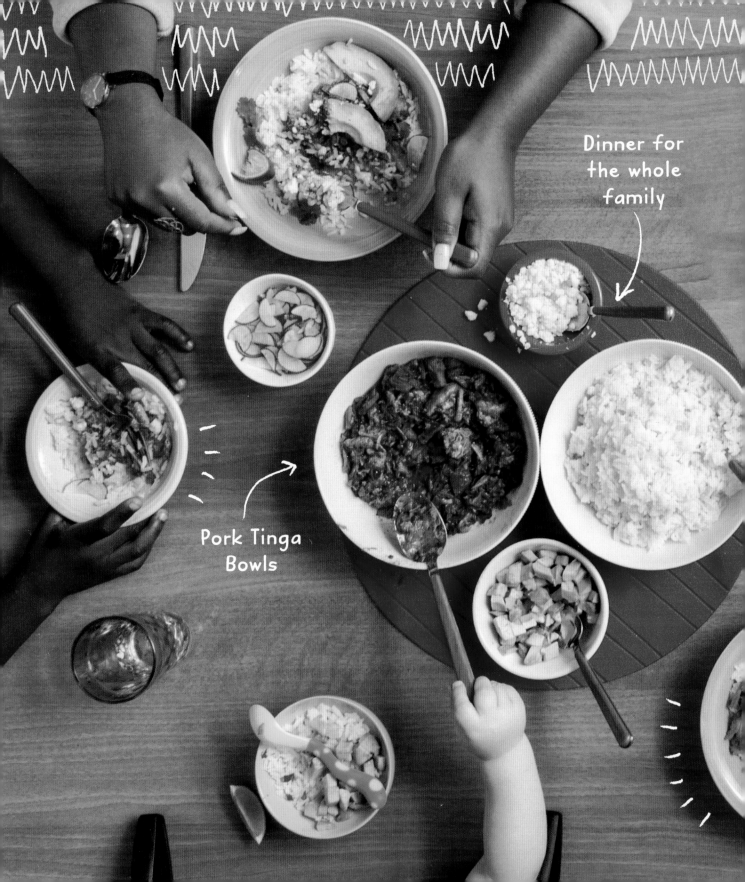

Dinner for the whole family

Pork Tinga Bowls

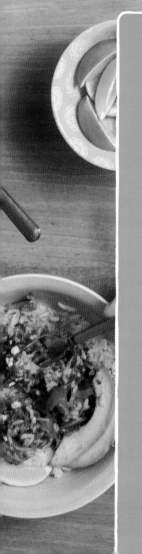

FAMILY MEALS

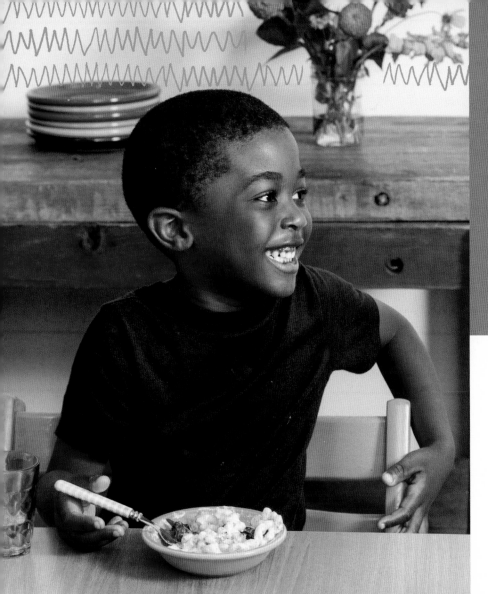

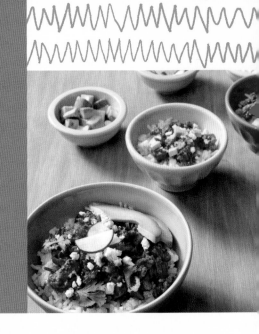

"Our kids loved the chicken and the sweet potatoes. Have never attempted kale with them and all were reluctant at first, but everyone ate it. 'I liked the whole thing,' said my 5-year-old."

—Parent of 5-year-old, 3-year-old, and 16-month-old, on One-Pan Chicken with Kale and Sweet Potatoes

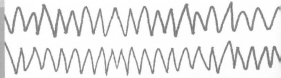

"Children ate it right up and didn't even mention the 'hidden' vegetables. The 7-year-old says that they were great, and the 3-year-old actually sat and ate it without complaint, which is success enough!"

—Parent of 7-year-old and 3-year-old, on Turkey-Veggie Burgers with Roasted Fingerling Potatoes

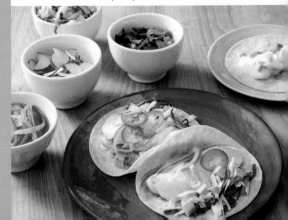

ALL ABOUT FAMILY MEALS

Yes, it might sound crazy. The whole family sitting down to dinner. Together. With just one meal—for everyone—cooked and served. No separate baby food. No separate toddler food. No separate adult food. And on a weeknight no less. It might not be every-night possible. But, it *is* possible.

At America's Test Kitchen, we believe that healthy eating starts with cooking at home and eating together. We also know how hard this is to accomplish when life is already so busy and your family contains people of all ages, each with their own food preferences. With that in mind, we set out to create a chapter full of recipes that are easy to make, attractive to a wide range of ages, and, most important, flexible.

Flexibility is important for family meals for a few reasons. Preferences are fickle and ever changing, and families come in every possible configuration. Flexibility in terms of flavor came first on our priority list. Although we did not create mild recipes for this chapter, we do provide tips for how to leave out more potent ingredients and tone things down for your more particular eaters if that's what you want to do. We created recipes that invite kids (and grown-ups) to add their own toppings whenever possible.

Second, we went for flexibility in terms of serving size. Do you have one kid? Five kids? Are you a family of one adult? Two or three or five adults? Unlike most traditional recipes, we built serving-size flexibility into many of the recipes in this chapter. When possible, we note the amount of food a recipe makes rather than the number of people it serves. Most serve enough for two to four adults, but the proteins (like chicken breasts or fish fillets) can be easily scaled up or down to accommodate your particular situation. Kids of different ages and appetites need different amounts of food. (See page 285 for more on serving sizes for toddlers.)

In this chapter, there are a handful of recipes that work not only for adults and kids, but also for babies under 12 months old who are still eating purees or are in the beginning stages of feeding themselves (One-Pan Chicken with Kale and Sweet Potatoes, page 140; Oven-Roasted Chicken Breasts with Chickpeas, Swiss Chard, and Chermoula, page 142; Cumin-Crusted Chicken Thighs with Cauliflower Rice, page 146; Garlicky Chicken and Brown Rice Soup, page 148; and Red Lentil Soup with Arugula and Fennel Salad, page 184). In these recipes, you'll see notes ⬦ for creating purees or fine mashes or chopping into small pieces for easy pickup. Added salt is not recommended for babies under 12 months (a tiny amount is fine), so in these recipes we call for no-sodium-added products and only add minimal salt until a portion for the baby has been reserved. (For more on this, see page vii.) The remaining recipes in this chapter are meant for adults and kids over 12 months old.

Most importantly, we want you to sit down together and enjoy being a family over a table of good food.

One-Pan Chicken with Kale and Sweet Potatoes

Makes 3 to 4 bone-in chicken breasts, plus sides
Total Time: 1 hour

Why This Recipe Works

Sheet-pan meals are great for busy weeknights. All the ingredients can roast alongside one another in one pan, emerging from the oven ready to serve all at the same time. (Bonus: minimal cleanup!) The trick is making sure all the components—often different sizes and shapes—cook at the same rate. The solution for this tasty mix of ingredients is just some simple geometry: sweet potatoes go on the perimeter of the baking sheet, the kale goes in the center, and the chicken goes on top of the kale to protect the delicate greens from burning. Massaging the kale before cooking helped it to become nice and tender.

Note that three chicken breasts will serve two adults plus one to two kids. This recipe will not work with just one or two chicken breasts (the vegetables will burn), but you can scale up, if desired, adding an additional chicken breast to the same sheet pan. We developed this recipe with curly kale. Avoid red kale and black (or Lacinato) kale, as they have a tendency to burn in this recipe. It's important to season with salt and pepper to taste after removing the portion for babies, since otherwise it will be underseasoned for adults.

¼ cup extra-virgin olive oil
2 garlic cloves, minced
2 teaspoons grated lemon zest
½ teaspoon minced fresh thyme
Salt and pepper
½ cup plain whole-milk yogurt
1 tablespoon water

8 ounces curly kale, stemmed and cut into 2-inch pieces
1½ pounds sweet potatoes, peeled and cut into 1-inch pieces
1 teaspoon paprika
3 to 4 (10- to 12-ounce) bone-in split chicken breasts, trimmed and halved crosswise

1. Adjust oven rack to upper-middle position and heat oven to 450 degrees. Whisk oil, garlic, lemon zest, thyme, ⅛ teaspoon salt, and ⅛ teaspoon pepper together in small bowl until combined. In separate bowl whisk together yogurt, water, 1 tablespoon oil mixture, and ¼ teaspoon salt; set aside.

2. Vigorously squeeze and massage kale with hands in large bowl until leaves are uniformly darkened and slightly wilted, about 1 minute. Arrange kale in pile in center of rimmed baking sheet.

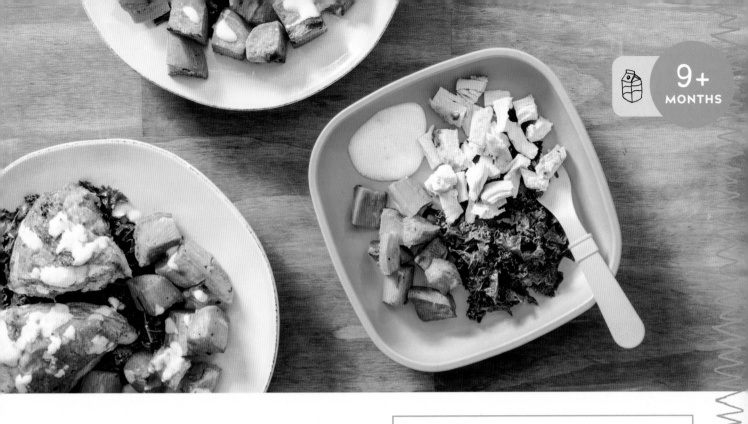

3 Add sweet potatoes and 1 tablespoon oil mixture to now-empty bowl and toss to coat. Arrange sweet potatoes in single layer around edges of sheet. Whisk paprika into remaining oil mixture and add to now-empty bowl along with chicken. Toss until chicken is well coated. Place chicken, skin side up, on top of kale in center of sheet.

4 Transfer sheet to oven and roast until chicken registers 165 degrees, 25 to 35 minutes, rotating sheet halfway through roasting. Transfer chicken to serving platter, tent with aluminum foil, and let rest for 5 to 10 minutes.

5 Toss vegetables with any accumulated pan juices and transfer to platter with chicken. Season with salt and pepper to taste. Drizzle ¼ cup yogurt sauce over chicken and vegetables and serve, passing remaining yogurt sauce separately.

TIPS FOR BABIES

For babies (9 to 12 months): In step 5, don't season with salt and pepper. Make a fine mash by transferring small portion of vegetable mixture to food processor. Remove the skin from 1 piece of chicken, pull off as much meat as desired, and add it to the processor with the vegetables. Pulse to desired consistency, scraping down the sides of the bowl as needed.

TIPS FOR TODDLERS

Simply chop chicken, sweet potatoes, and kale into smaller pieces as needed and serve with yogurt sauce, if desired.

Oven-Roasted Chicken Breasts with Chickpeas, Swiss Chard, and Chermoula

Makes 2 to 4 bone-in chicken breasts, plus sides
Total Time: 1 hour and 10 minutes

Why This Recipe Works

To bring exciting flavor to lean chicken breasts, we turned to chermoula, a bold Moroccan green sauce. Our version is made with cilantro, lemon, and a good dose of garlic and spices. Not only is it a tasty topping to drizzle over the chicken, it seasons a side of chickpeas and Swiss chard. The best thing about this punchy sauce? You can add as much (or as little) as you like.

You will need a 12-inch skillet with a tight-fitting lid for this recipe. The pan will be very full when you add the Swiss chard leaves in step 5, but they will wilt. We use unsalted chickpeas and broth to make this recipe appropriate for babies under 12 months old; families without babies can use regular chickpeas and broth and omit salt in step 6. It's important to season with salt and pepper to taste after removing the portion for babies, since otherwise it will be underseasoned for adults. Note that two chicken breasts will serve one adult plus one to two kids. Cook the number of chicken breasts that feed your family.

¾ cup fresh cilantro leaves
¼ cup plus 1 teaspoon extra-virgin olive oil
2 tablespoons lemon juice, plus lemon wedges for serving
4 garlic cloves, minced
½ teaspoon ground cumin
½ teaspoon paprika
⅛ teaspoon cayenne pepper
Salt and pepper

2 to 4 (10- to 12-ounce) bone-in split chicken breasts, trimmed and halved crosswise
12 ounces Swiss chard, stems chopped, leaves cut into 2-inch pieces
2 (15-ounce) cans unsalted chickpeas, drained and rinsed
1 cup unsalted chicken broth

1. Adjust oven rack to middle position and heat oven to 450 degrees. Process cilantro, ¼ cup oil, lemon juice, garlic, cumin, paprika, cayenne, and ¼ teaspoon salt in food processor until combined, about 1 minute, scraping down sides of bowl as needed; set aside.

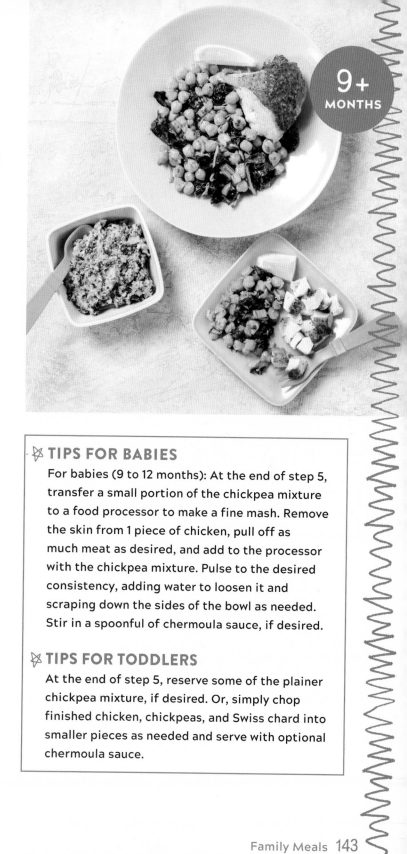

2. Pat chicken dry with paper towels and season with salt and pepper. Heat remaining 1 teaspoon oil in 12-inch skillet over medium-high heat until just smoking. Place chicken, skin side down, in skillet and cook until well browned, 6 to 8 minutes.

3. Transfer browned chicken pieces, skin side up, to rimmed baking sheet (do not wipe out skillet). Transfer sheet to oven and roast until chicken registers 165 degrees, about 20 minutes, rotating sheet halfway through cooking.

4. Meanwhile, heat fat remaining in skillet over medium heat until shimmering. Add Swiss chard stems and cook, stirring occasionally, until softened and lightly browned, about 3 minutes.

5. Stir in chickpeas and broth and bring to simmer. Add Swiss chard leaves, cover, reduce heat to medium-low, and cook until chickpeas are warmed through and Swiss chard has wilted, about 4 minutes. Uncover, increase heat to high, and cook until nearly all liquid has evaporated, 2 to 3 minutes.

6. Off heat, stir 2 tablespoons chermoula sauce and ¼ teaspoon salt into chickpeas; transfer to serving dish. Drizzle chicken with remaining chermoula sauce and serve with chickpeas and lemon wedges.

⊰ TIPS FOR BABIES

For babies (9 to 12 months): At the end of step 5, transfer a small portion of the chickpea mixture to a food processor to make a fine mash. Remove the skin from 1 piece of chicken, pull off as much meat as desired, and add to the processor with the chickpea mixture. Pulse to the desired consistency, adding water to loosen it and scraping down the sides of the bowl as needed. Stir in a spoonful of chermoula sauce, if desired.

⊰ TIPS FOR TODDLERS

At the end of step 5, reserve some of the plainer chickpea mixture, if desired. Or, simply chop finished chicken, chickpeas, and Swiss chard into smaller pieces as needed and serve with optional chermoula sauce.

Parmesan Chicken Cutlets with Warm Bulgur Salad

Makes 3 to 6 chicken cutlets, plus side
Total Time: 45 minutes

Why This Recipe Works

Think of this dish as the best chicken fingers you'll ever eat. Plus, it's easily done on a weeknight! We gave these chicken cutlets a crispy, crunchy coating using a combination of panko bread crumbs and Parmesan cheese. Bulgur is made from parboiled or steamed wheat kernels that are then dried, partially stripped of their outer bran layer, and coarsely ground. There are four grind sizes, from fine to extra coarse. We chose the smallest, finest grind, which is couscous-like in appearance and, happily, the most readily available in most stores, because it becomes cooked and fluffy in just 5 (!) minutes.

You can make your own chicken cutlets from 8-ounce boneless, skinless chicken breasts: pop them in the freezer for 15 minutes to firm up, then halve them horizontally, and pound them to an even ½-inch thickness. Use the large holes of a box grater to shred the Parmesan. Do not use coarse- or medium-grind bulgur in this recipe. Note that three chicken cutlets will serve two adults plus one to two kids. Cook the number of chicken cutlets that feed your family. To serve a larger family, double the flour, egg, Parmesan, panko, and chicken cutlets, and cook the chicken in two batches, wiping out the skillet and adding 3 additional tablespoons oil for the second batch.

1½ cups water
1 cup fine-grind bulgur
Salt and pepper
¼ cup all-purpose flour
1 large egg
1½ ounces Parmesan cheese, shredded (½ cup)
½ cup panko bread crumbs
3 to 6 (4-ounce) chicken cutlets, ½ inch thick, trimmed
¼ cup extra-virgin olive oil
1 tablespoon lemon juice, plus lemon wedges for serving
6 ounces cherry tomatoes, quartered
4 ounces fresh mozzarella cheese, cut into ½-inch pieces (1 cup)
¼ cup chopped fresh basil
½ cup pitted kalamata olives, halved (optional)

1 Bring water to boil in large saucepan over medium-high heat. Stir in bulgur and ½ teaspoon salt. Cover, remove from heat, and let sit until liquid is absorbed and bulgur is tender, about 5 minutes.

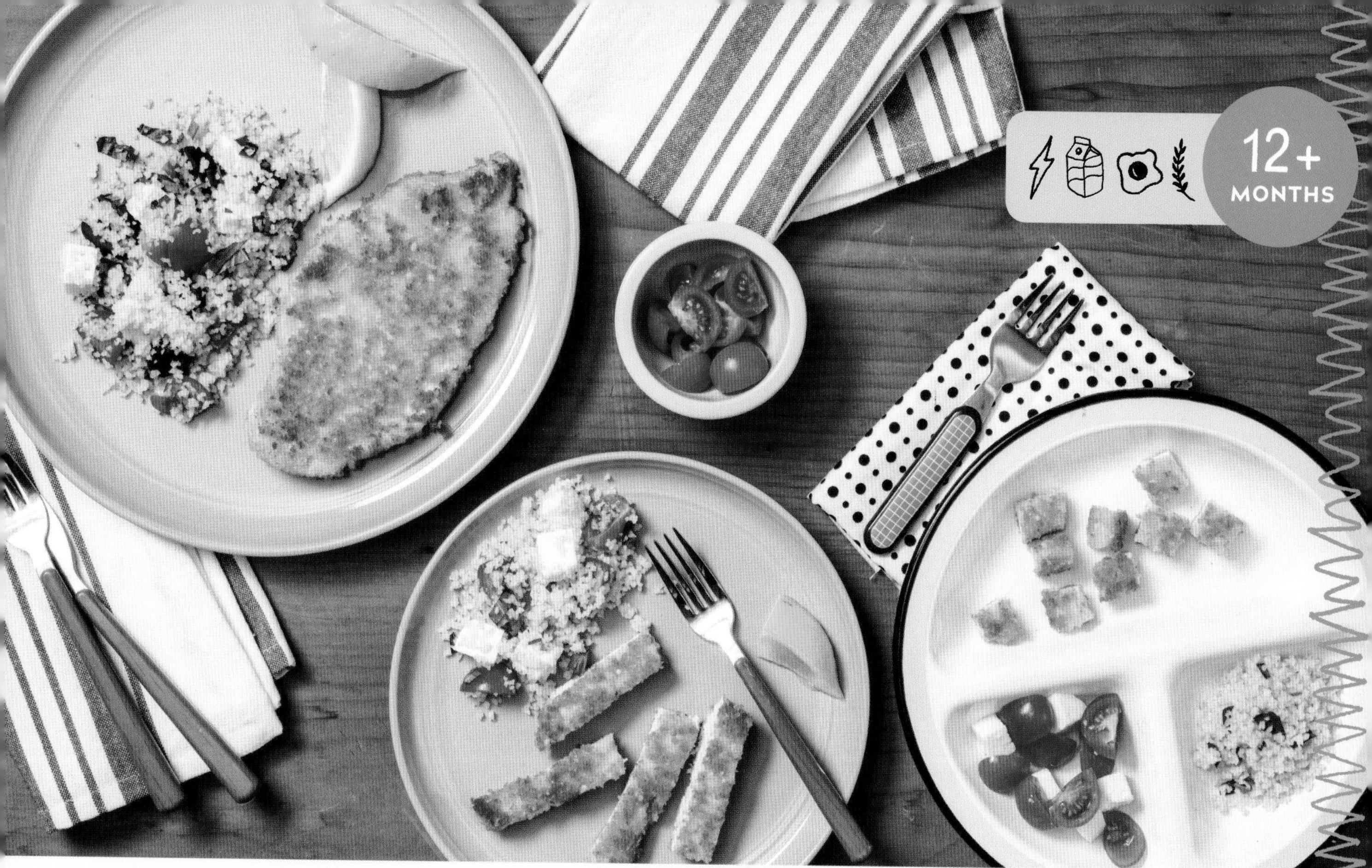

2. Meanwhile, spread flour in shallow dish. Beat egg in second shallow dish. Combine Parmesan and panko in third shallow dish. Pat cutlets dry with paper towels and season with salt and pepper. Working with 1 cutlet at a time, dredge cutlets in flour, dip in egg, then coat with panko mixture, pressing gently to adhere; transfer to large plate.

3. Heat 3 tablespoons oil in 12-inch nonstick skillet over medium heat until shimmering. Add cutlets and cook until chicken is golden brown and crisp on both sides, 3 to 4 minutes per side. Transfer cutlets to paper-towel-lined serving platter.

4. Fluff bulgur with fork, then stir in lemon juice and remaining 1 tablespoon oil. Add tomatoes, mozzarella, basil, and olives, if using, and gently stir to combine. Season with salt and pepper to taste. Serve chicken with bulgur salad and lemon wedges.

TIPS FOR TODDLERS

In step 4, transfer a small portion of bulgur to a bowl and stir in a little tomato, mozzarella, basil, and/or olives (or let them choose!). Cut a cutlet into smaller pieces as needed and serve with the bulgur.

Cumin-Crusted Chicken Thighs with Cauliflower Rice

Makes 4 to 8 bone-in chicken thighs, plus side
Total Time: 55 minutes

Why This Recipe Works

Chicken and rice is a classic combination. We gave it a twist by using arroz con pollo as our inspiration. And we made it deliciously healthy with cauliflower rice, a fresh and satisfying substitute that's easy to make in the food processor. (Just blitz to small pieces and you're done!) This dish is easy to turn into baby-friendly food since the food processor is already out to make the cauliflower rice.

Be sure to keep the rendered chicken fat in the skillet after step 2; this schmaltz adds flavor and richness to the cauliflower. It's important to season with salt and pepper to taste after removing the portion for babies, since otherwise it will be underseasoned for adults. Note that four chicken thighs will serve one adult plus one to two kids. Scale chicken up to fit the size of your family.

4 to 8 (5- to 7-ounce) bone-in chicken thighs
Salt and pepper
1 tablespoon canola oil
1½ teaspoons cumin seeds
1 head cauliflower (2 pounds), cored and chopped coarse
4 garlic cloves, minced
1 teaspoon paprika
½ teaspoon ground coriander
1 red bell pepper, stemmed, seeded, and chopped
⅓ cup frozen peas
¼ cup chopped fresh cilantro
1½ teaspoons grated lime zest plus 1 tablespoon juice, plus lime wedges for serving

1. Adjust oven rack to upper-middle position and heat oven to 375 degrees. Pat chicken dry with paper towels and season with salt and pepper. Heat oil in 12-inch nonstick skillet over medium-high heat until just smoking. Place chicken, skin side down, in skillet and cook until well browned, 6 to 8 minutes.

2. Transfer browned chicken pieces, skin side up, to rimmed baking sheet and sprinkle cumin seeds over top (do not wipe out skillet). Transfer sheet to oven and roast until chicken registers 175 degrees, 15 to 20 minutes, rotating sheet halfway through roasting. Tent with aluminum foil and let rest 5 to 10 minutes.

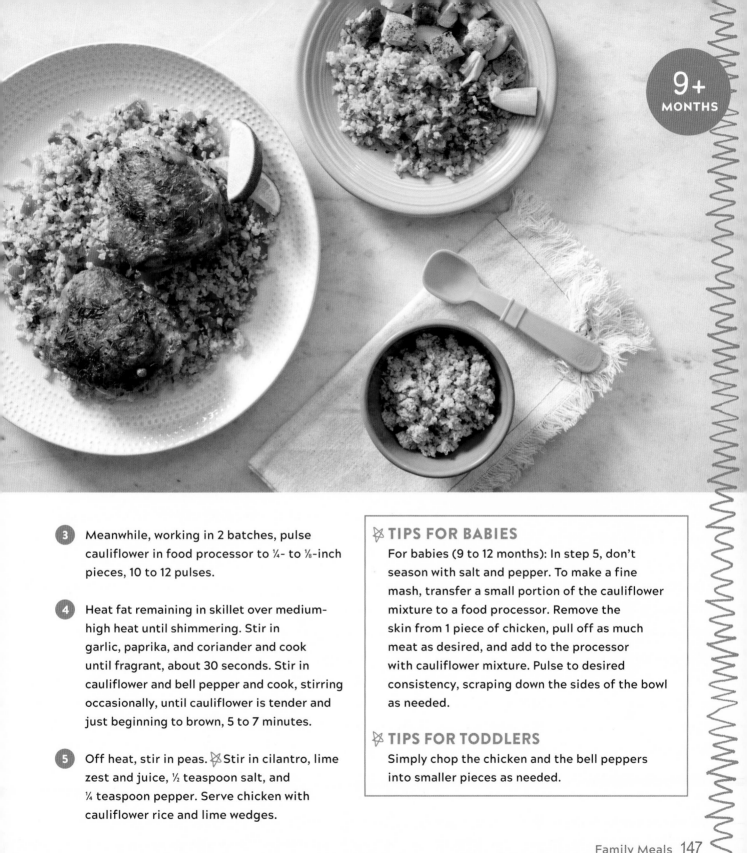

MONTHS

3 Meanwhile, working in 2 batches, pulse cauliflower in food processor to ¼- to ⅛-inch pieces, 10 to 12 pulses.

4 Heat fat remaining in skillet over medium-high heat until shimmering. Stir in garlic, paprika, and coriander and cook until fragrant, about 30 seconds. Stir in cauliflower and bell pepper and cook, stirring occasionally, until cauliflower is tender and just beginning to brown, 5 to 7 minutes.

5 Off heat, stir in peas. ⊠Stir in cilantro, lime zest and juice, ½ teaspoon salt, and ¼ teaspoon pepper. Serve chicken with cauliflower rice and lime wedges.

⊠ TIPS FOR BABIES

For babies (9 to 12 months): In step 5, don't season with salt and pepper. To make a fine mash, transfer a small portion of the cauliflower mixture to a food processor. Remove the skin from 1 piece of chicken, pull off as much meat as desired, and add to the processor with cauliflower mixture. Pulse to desired consistency, scraping down the sides of the bowl as needed.

⊠ TIPS FOR TODDLERS

Simply chop the chicken and the bell peppers into smaller pieces as needed.

Garlicky Chicken and Brown Rice Soup

Makes 8 cups
Total Time: 1 hour 30 minutes

Why This Recipe Works

We souped up (pun intended, sorry) our version of classic chicken and rice soup with brown rice, some toasty garlic, wilted spinach, and perfectly poached chicken. It's a wholesome, simple one-pot meal that packs a ton of flavor and feels healthy but not oppressively so.

✳ STORAGE INFORMATION

Soup can be refrigerated for up to 3 days or frozen for up to 1 month.

We use unsalted broth so you can make a puree appropriate for 6-month-old babies; it's important to season with salt and pepper to taste after removing the portion for babies, since otherwise it will be underseasoned for adults. If you are only feeding family members 12 months and up, you can use regular broth.

3 tablespoons extra-virgin olive oil
6 garlic cloves, minced
2 carrots, peeled and sliced ¼ inch thick
1 onion, chopped fine
1 celery rib, minced
Salt and pepper
2 teaspoons minced fresh thyme or ½ teaspoon dried
1 teaspoon tomato paste

4 cups unsalted chicken broth
2 cups water
2 bay leaves
½ cup brown rice
8 ounces boneless, skinless chicken breasts, cut into ¾-inch pieces
3 ounces (3 cups) baby spinach
¼ cup chopped fresh parsley

1 Heat oil and garlic in Dutch oven over medium-low heat, stirring occasionally, until garlic is light golden, 3 to 5 minutes. Add carrots, onion, celery, and ¼ teaspoon salt, increase heat to medium, and cook, stirring occasionally, until vegetables are just beginning to brown, 10 to 12 minutes.

2 Stir in thyme and tomato paste and cook until fragrant, about 30 seconds. Stir in broth, water, and bay leaves, scraping up any browned bits, and bring to simmer over medium-high heat. Stir in rice and return to simmer. Cover, reduce heat to medium-low, and cook until rice is tender, 40 to 45 minutes.

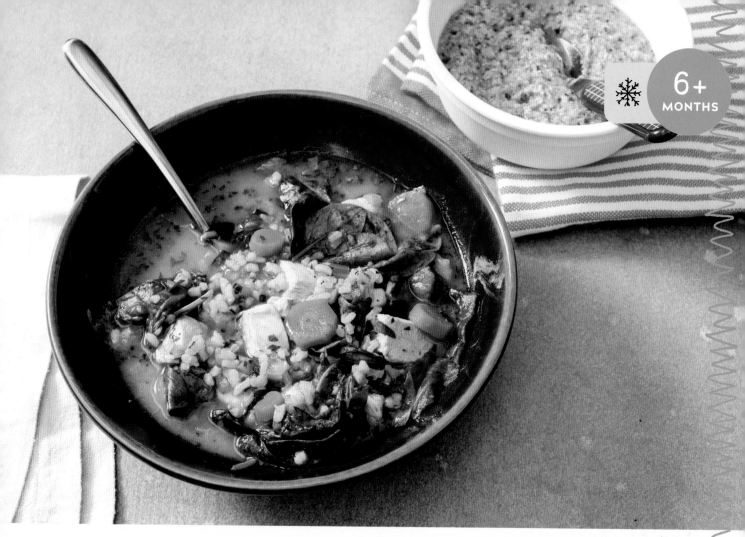

6+
MONTHS

3 Discard bay leaves. Stir in chicken and spinach and cook over low heat, stirring occasionally, until chicken is cooked through and spinach is wilted, 3 to 5 minutes.

4 ⚘ Off heat, stir in parsley and season with salt and pepper to taste. Serve.

⚘ **TIPS FOR BABIES**

For babies (6 to 12 months): In step 4, don't season with salt and pepper. Transfer a small portion of soup to a blender and process until smooth, about 1 minute.

⚘ **TIPS FOR TODDLERS**

Simply serve the soup as is, cutting chicken and spinach into smaller pieces as needed.

Turkey-Veggie Burgers with Roasted Fingerling Potatoes

Makes 4 big burgers or 8 mini burgers, plus sides
Total Time: 55 minutes

Why This Recipe Works

We wanted a great-tasting burger that we could feel good about putting into the regular family-dinner rotation. In our testing, we discovered that the secret to a juicy turkey burger was...vegetables! Adding both shredded zucchini and carrot to the patty provided moisture and a subtle sweetness. Best of all, the vegetables didn't require any precooking—adding them raw to the ground turkey gave us the juiciest results. Roasted fingerling potatoes are an easy play on french fries; a bright, tangy sauce made with lemon and herbs is great for dipping.

Be sure to use 93 percent lean ground turkey, not 99 percent fat-free ground turkey breast, or the burgers will be tough. Use the large holes of a box grater or the shredding disk of a food processor to shred the carrots and zucchini. Other fresh herbs, such as parsley, dill, cilantro, mint, or tarragon, can be used in place of the basil in the lemon-herb sauce. If you can't find fingerling potatoes, you can substitute small red or white potatoes. If you're making mini burgers, use slider buns instead of hamburger buns. You can also simply cut hamburger buns in half to fit mini burgers. Note this recipe makes 4 big burgers or 8 mini burgers, or a combination of the two!

¼ cup mayonnaise
¼ cup plain whole-milk yogurt
2 tablespoons minced fresh basil
1 tablespoon lemon juice
Salt and pepper
2 pounds fingerling potatoes, halved lengthwise

3 tablespoons extra-virgin olive oil
1 pound (93 percent) lean ground turkey
1 small zucchini, shredded (1¼ cups)
1 carrot, peeled and shredded (½ cup)
¼ cup grated Parmesan cheese
4 hamburger buns, toasted

1. Adjust oven rack to lowest position and heat oven to 450 degrees. Line rimmed baking sheet with parchment paper.

2. Mix mayonnaise, yogurt, basil, lemon juice, ⅛ teaspoon salt, and ⅛ teaspoon pepper together in small bowl. Cover and refrigerate until ready to serve.

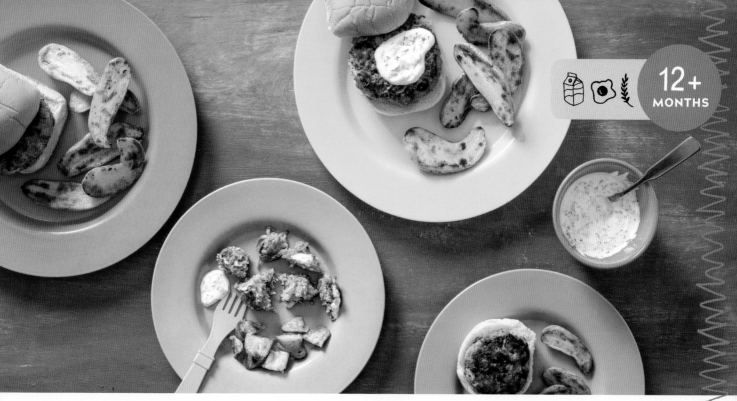

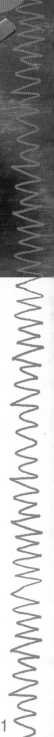

3 Toss potatoes, 2 tablespoons oil, ¼ teaspoon salt, and ¼ teaspoon pepper together in large bowl until evenly coated. Arrange potatoes on prepared baking sheet, cut side down, in even layer. Transfer to oven and cook until cut sides are crisp and skins are spotty brown, 30 to 35 minutes, rotating sheet halfway through cooking. Let potatoes cool on sheet for 5 minutes. Transfer to serving platter.

4 While potatoes roast, combine turkey, zucchini, carrot, Parmesan, and ½ teaspoon salt in large bowl and knead with your hands until thoroughly combined. ⚝ Using your hands, pat turkey mixture into four ¾-inch-thick patties, about 4 inches in diameter.

5 Heat remaining 1 tablespoon oil in 12-inch nonstick skillet over medium heat until shimmering. Add patties and cook until well browned on both sides and meat registers 165 degrees, 6 to 8 minutes per side.

6 Place burgers on buns and dollop with yogurt sauce. Serve with roasted potatoes, passing remaining sauce for dipping.

⚝ TIPS FOR TODDLERS

In step 4, divide one (or more) patty into two 3-inch patties (¾ inch thick) to make mini burgers and cook as directed. Serve on slider roll, or cut into pieces as needed. Chop potatoes into smaller pieces as needed. Serve with the dipping sauce.

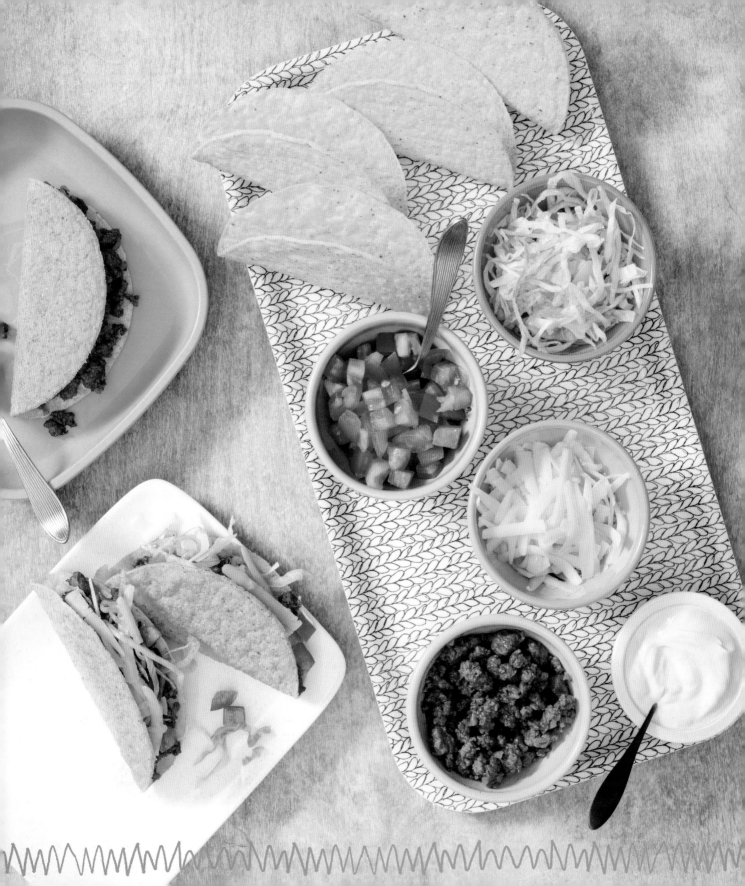

Weeknight Beef Tacos

Makes 8 to 12 tacos
Total Time: 35 minutes

Why This Recipe Works

Long live Taco Tuesday! We love ground beef tacos for family meals because they are quick and easy to make, and everyone at the table gets to pick and choose whichever toppings they like best. To ensure that the meat stayed tender and juicy, we used a long-standing test kitchen trick: raising the beef's pH by adding baking soda to the mix helps the meat proteins attract and retain more water. Our homemade taco seasoning, along with sautéed onion, salt, and umami-rich tomato paste, gave our taco filling savory depth that was far superior to any commercial taco kit.

⊠ TIPS FOR TODDLERS

If your toddler is on the pickier side, in step 2, use half of (or even omit) the spice mixture for a plainer finished taco filling. Younger toddlers may prefer soft corn tortillas to hard taco shells. Have your child pick toppings of choice.

Serve with your favorite taco toppings. Options include cilantro, chopped white onion, shredded cheese, shredded iceberg lettuce, chopped tomato, sour cream, salsa (red or green), and hot sauce.

1 tablespoon water
¼ teaspoon baking soda
12 ounces (90 percent) lean ground beef
2¼ teaspoons chili powder
2¼ teaspoons paprika
¾ teaspoon ground cumin
¾ teaspoon garlic powder
1 tablespoon canola oil
1 onion, chopped fine
¼ teaspoon salt
2 tablespoons tomato paste
8 to 12 hard taco shells or 6-inch corn tortillas

1. Stir together water and baking soda in large bowl. Add beef and mix until thoroughly combined, set aside. In small bowl, stir together chili powder, paprika, cumin, and garlic powder.

2. Heat oil in 12-inch nonstick skillet over medium heat until shimmering. Add onion and cook, stirring occasionally, until softened, about 5 minutes. ⊠Add spice mixture and salt and cook, stirring frequently, until fragrant, about 1 minute. Stir in tomato paste and cook until paste is rust-colored, 1 to 2 minutes.

3. Add beef and cook, using wooden spoon to break meat into pieces no larger than ¼ inch, until beef has just lost its raw pink color, about 5 minutes. Serve in taco shells with toppings. ⊠

✳ MAKE-AHEAD TACO NIGHT

You can make a larger batch of the taco seasoning to have on hand and make tacos quickly and easily any time. Double or triple the spices, mix until thoroughly combined, and store in an airtight container. When you're ready to cook, use 2 tablespoons of the spice mixture for every 12 ounces of ground beef.

Best Beef Stew

Makes 10 cups
Total Time: 3½ to 4 hours

Why This Recipe Works

Cooking a family dinner is often an exercise in achieving maximum flavor in the least amount of time. But there are some recipes that are worth a time investment, and beef stew is one of them. It's a one-pot dish in which low-and-slow cooking transforms simple, affordable ingredients into quintessential comfort food. During that time in the oven, the chuck-eye roast transforms from tough to tender. Onions, carrots, and potatoes soften and pick up rich, earthy sweetness from the broth and (a small amount of) red wine. Because it is a time commitment, we have scaled up the recipe to make enough to last more than one meal. This is a great make-ahead recipe that you can knock out on a Sunday or freeze for later on when life gets a little more hectic.

Try to find beef that is well marbled with white veins of fat. Meat that is too lean will come out slightly dry. Note that this recipe serves six to eight adults.

4 pounds boneless beef chuck-eye roast, pulled apart at seams, trimmed, and cut into 1- to 1½-inch pieces
Salt and pepper
3 tablespoons canola oil
2 tablespoons unsalted butter
2 onions, chopped
3 garlic cloves, minced
¼ cup all-purpose flour
1 tablespoon tomato paste
1 cup dry red wine
3½ cups beef broth
1 pound carrots, peeled and sliced 1 inch thick
2 bay leaves
1 tablespoon minced fresh thyme or 1 teaspoon dried
1½ pounds red potatoes, unpeeled, cut into 1-inch pieces
1 cup frozen peas
3 tablespoons minced fresh parsley

1. Adjust oven rack to lower-middle position and heat oven to 325 degrees. Pat beef dry with paper towels and season lightly with salt and pepper. Heat 2 tablespoons oil in Dutch oven over medium-high heat until just smoking. Add half of meat and cook, stirring occasionally, until well browned, 7 to 10 minutes, reducing heat if pot begins to scorch; transfer to bowl. Repeat with remaining 1 tablespoon oil and remaining beef.

2. Melt butter in now-empty pot over medium-low heat. Add onions and ½ teaspoon salt and cook, stirring often, until softened, 5 to 7 minutes. Stir in garlic and cook until fragrant, about 30 seconds. Stir in flour and tomato paste and cook,

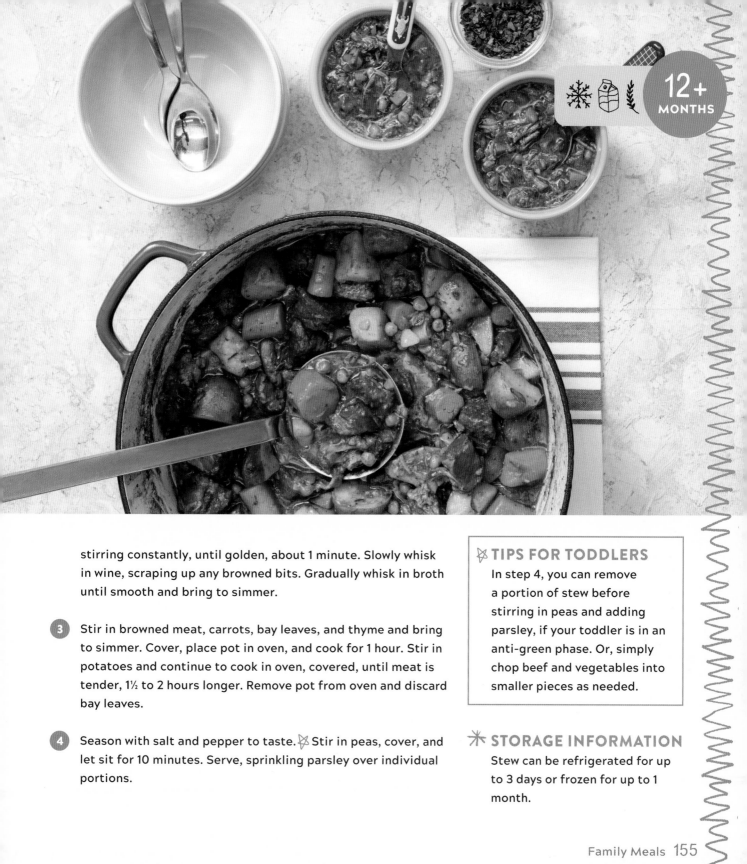

stirring constantly, until golden, about 1 minute. Slowly whisk in wine, scraping up any browned bits. Gradually whisk in broth until smooth and bring to simmer.

3 Stir in browned meat, carrots, bay leaves, and thyme and bring to simmer. Cover, place pot in oven, and cook for 1 hour. Stir in potatoes and continue to cook in oven, covered, until meat is tender, 1½ to 2 hours longer. Remove pot from oven and discard bay leaves.

4 Season with salt and pepper to taste. ⊠ Stir in peas, cover, and let sit for 10 minutes. Serve, sprinkling parsley over individual portions.

⊠ **TIPS FOR TODDLERS**

In step 4, you can remove a portion of stew before stirring in peas and adding parsley, if your toddler is in an anti-green phase. Or, simply chop beef and vegetables into smaller pieces as needed.

❋ **STORAGE INFORMATION**

Stew can be refrigerated for up to 3 days or frozen for up to 1 month.

One-Pan Pork Tenderloin with Green Beans and Potatoes

Makes 1 to 2 pork tenderloins, plus sides
Total Time: 50 minutes

Why This Recipe Works

Tender, inexpensive pork tenderloin cooks quickly and is easy to pair with a range of vegetables for a simple, satisfying one-pan meal. Small red potatoes, cut in half, cooked through in the same amount of time as the pork. Green beans generally don't take as long to cook, but when we roasted them in the center of the pan with the tenderloin on top to insulate them from the oven's intense heat, they were steamed to a perfect tender-crisp texture. Giving the beans a few extra minutes in the oven while the pork rested helped them pick up more color without drying them out. An easy garlic-chive butter added flavor to the veggies, while sweet and salty hoisin sauce helped create a caramelized exterior on the pork.

Our favorite hoisin sauce is Kikkoman's. For the best results, use potatoes that measure about 1½ inches in diameter. Note that one (12- to 16-ounce) pork tenderloin will serve two adults plus one to two kids. To serve a bigger family, use two (12- to 16-ounce) pork tenderloins of equal size, increase the hoisin to ¼ cup. In step 3, lay the tenderloins side by side, without touching, on top of the green beans.

4 tablespoons unsalted butter, softened
2 tablespoons minced fresh chives
1 garlic clove, minced
Salt and pepper
1 pound green beans, ends trimmed

2 tablespoons extra-virgin olive oil
1½ pounds small red potatoes, unpeeled, halved
1 to 2 (12- to 16-ounce) pork tenderloins, trimmed
2 tablespoons hoisin sauce

1. Adjust oven rack to lower-middle position and heat oven to 450 degrees. Combine butter, chives, garlic, ¼ teaspoon salt, and ¼ teaspoon pepper in bowl; set aside.

2. Toss green beans with 1 tablespoon oil, ¼ teaspoon salt, and ¼ teaspoon pepper in separate bowl. Arrange green bean mixture in center of rimmed baking sheet, leaving room on both sides for potatoes. Toss potatoes, remaining 1 tablespoon oil, ¼ teaspoon salt, and ¼ teaspoon pepper together in now-empty bowl. Arrange potatoes, cut side down, on either side of green beans.

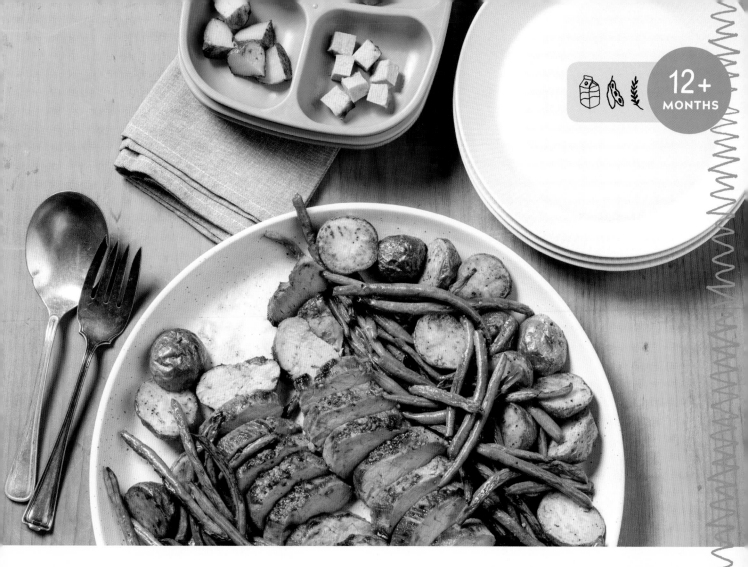

12+ MONTHS

3 Pat pork dry with paper towels and season with pepper. Brush pork all over with hoisin sauce. Lay pork lengthwise on top of green beans. Roast until pork registers 145 degrees, 20 to 25 minutes. Transfer pork to carving board and dot with 1 tablespoon reserved herb butter. Tent with aluminum foil and let rest while vegetables finish cooking.

4 Gently stir vegetables on sheet to combine. Return sheet to oven and roast until vegetables are tender and golden brown, 5 to 10 minutes longer. Remove from oven. ⚘ Add remaining herb butter to sheet and toss vegetables to coat. Transfer vegetables to platter. Cut pork into ½-inch-thick slices and serve with vegetables.

⚘ **TIPS FOR TODDLERS**

In step 4, pluck a few green beans and potatoes from the baking sheet before tossing the rest with the garlic-herb butter, if desired. Otherwise, simply chop pork, potatoes, and green beans into smaller pieces as needed.

Pork Tinga Bowls

Makes 3½ cups shredded pork, plus sides
Total Time: 2 hours and 20 minutes

Why This Recipe Works

Tinga is a classic Mexican dish in which meat, usually pork or chicken, is poached, shredded, and simmered in a spicy sauce made with tomatoes and chipotle peppers. While tinga is commonly served over tostadas, we like this weekend (but worth-it!) meal simply over rice. To keep this dish kid friendly, we hold off on adding the spicy chipotle peppers until the very end, allowing you to set aside a flavorful but mild portion for your little one(s).

✳ STORAGE INFORMATION

After step 2, pork and reserved cooking liquid can be refrigerated separately for up to 2 days. Finished pork tinga can be refrigerated for up to 2 days or frozen for up to 1 month; if frozen, thaw in refrigerator. To reheat, bring pork mixture, covered, to gentle simmer, stirring often and adjusting consistency with hot water as needed.

If you can't find Cotija cheese, substitute crumbled queso fresco or feta.

PORK

6 cups water
2 pounds boneless pork butt roast, trimmed and cut into 1-inch pieces
2 onions (1 quartered, 1 chopped fine)
5 garlic cloves (3 peeled and smashed, 2 minced)
2 bay leaves
Salt
2 tablespoons canola oil
½ teaspoon dried oregano
1 (15-ounce) can tomato sauce
1 tablespoon minced canned chipotle chile in adobo sauce

RICE AND TOPPINGS

1 tablespoon unsalted butter or canola oil
1 cup long-grain white rice, rinsed
1½ cups water
Salt
2 radishes, trimmed, halved, and sliced thin (optional)
2 ounces Cotija cheese, crumbled (½ cup) (optional)
1 avocado, halved, pitted, and cut into ½-inch pieces
¼ cup fresh cilantro leaves
Lime wedges

1 **FOR THE PORK:** Bring 6 cups water, pork, quartered onion, smashed garlic, bay leaves, and 1 teaspoon salt to simmer in large saucepan over medium-high heat, skimming off any foam that rises to surface. Reduce heat to medium-low, partially cover, and cook until pork is tender, 1¼ to 1½ hours.

2 Drain pork in fine-mesh strainer set over bowl, reserving 1 cup cooking liquid. Discard onion, garlic, and bay leaves. Return pork to now-empty saucepan and mash into rough ½-inch pieces using potato masher.

3 **FOR THE RICE:** Melt butter in medium saucepan over medium heat. Add rice and cook, stirring often, until edges begin to turn translucent, about 2 minutes. Add water and ¼ teaspoon salt and bring to boil. Cover, reduce heat to low, and simmer until liquid is absorbed and rice is tender, 16 to 18 minutes. Remove pot from heat, lay clean folded dish towel underneath lid, and let rice sit, covered, for 10 minutes.

4 **FOR THE PORK:** While rice cooks, heat oil in 12-inch nonstick skillet over medium-high heat until shimmering. Add chopped onion, oregano, and shredded pork and cook, stirring often, until pork is well browned and crisp, 7 to 10 minutes. Stir in minced garlic and cook until fragrant, about 30 seconds.

5 Stir in tomato sauce and reserved pork cooking liquid and simmer until almost all liquid has evaporated, 5 to 7 minutes. ⊠ Stir in chipotle and season with salt to taste; cover to keep warm.

6 Fluff rice with fork and divide among serving bowls. Top rice with pork. ⊠ Serve, passing radishes, Cotija, if using, avocado, cilantro, and lime wedges separately.

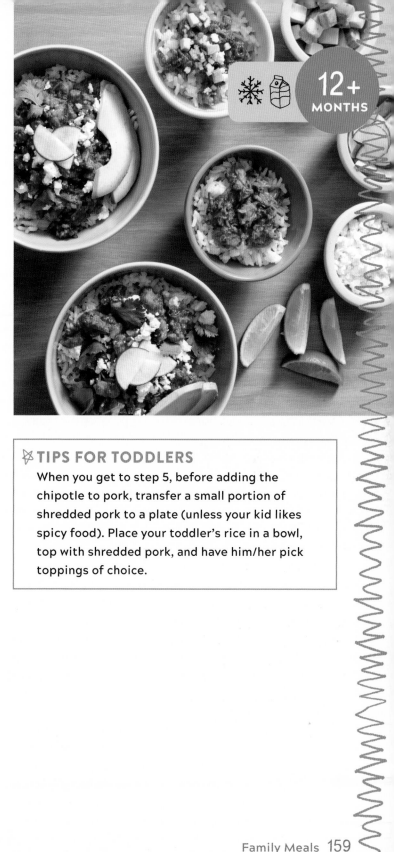

12+ MONTHS

⊠ TIPS FOR TODDLERS

When you get to step 5, before adding the chipotle to pork, transfer a small portion of shredded pork to a plate (unless your kid likes spicy food). Place your toddler's rice in a bowl, top with shredded pork, and have him/her pick toppings of choice.

Polenta with Sausage and Braised Broccolini

Makes 1 pound of sausage, plus sides
Total Time: 1 hour

Why This Recipe Works

In Italy, creamy polenta is often paired with saucy braised meat for a warming, hearty winter meal. While delicious, it's not really a weeknight meal, as traditionally prepared polenta takes over an hour to cook, and a braise takes multiple hours. To turn this dish into a midweek family dinner, we needed to cut down on cooking time. We started by adding a pinch of baking soda to the polenta cooking liquid, which helps break down the cornmeal and speeds up cooking. We then opted for Italian sausages instead of a low-and-slow protein like short ribs. After quickly browning the sausages in a skillet, we simmered them in a simple tomato sauce with onion and broccolini until the sausage was cooked and the broccolini tender.

Note that 1 pound of sausage feeds two adults plus one to two kids.

5 cups water
Pinch baking soda
Salt and pepper
1 cup coarse-ground cornmeal
2 tablespoons unsalted butter
1 tablespoon extra-virgin olive oil
1 pound sweet Italian sausage

12 ounces broccolini, trimmed and cut into 1-inch pieces
1 onion, halved and sliced thin
2 garlic cloves, minced
1 (14.5-ounce) can crushed tomatoes
¼ teaspoon red pepper flakes

1   Bring 5 cups water to boil in large saucepan over medium-high heat. Stir in baking soda and 1 teaspoon salt. Slowly pour cornmeal into water in steady stream while whisking constantly. Bring mixture to boil, whisking constantly, about 1 minute. Reduce heat to lowest possible setting, cover, and cook, whisking often, until tender, about 30 minutes. Off heat, stir in butter and adjust consistency with extra hot water as needed. Season polenta with salt and pepper to taste.

2   Meanwhile, heat oil in 12-inch skillet over medium heat until shimmering. Add sausages and cook until browned on all sides, about 6 minutes. Transfer sausages to plate. Increase heat to medium-high, add broccolini, onion, and ¼ teaspoon salt, and cook, stirring occasionally, until vegetables begin to soften

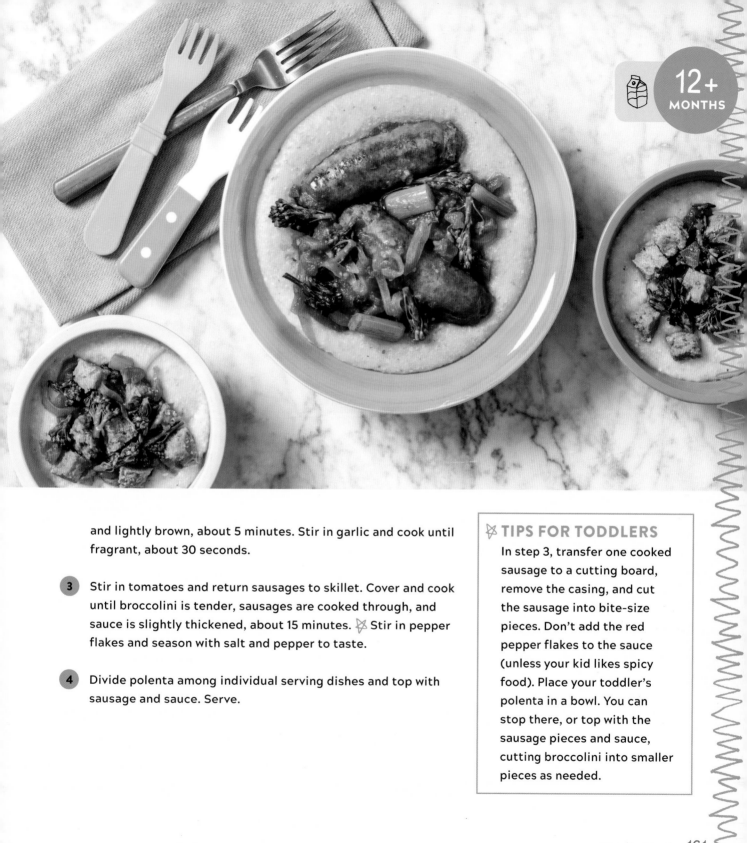

and lightly brown, about 5 minutes. Stir in garlic and cook until fragrant, about 30 seconds.

3 Stir in tomatoes and return sausages to skillet. Cover and cook until broccolini is tender, sausages are cooked through, and sauce is slightly thickened, about 15 minutes. ✗ Stir in pepper flakes and season with salt and pepper to taste.

4 Divide polenta among individual serving dishes and top with sausage and sauce. Serve.

✗ TIPS FOR TODDLERS

In step 3, transfer one cooked sausage to a cutting board, remove the casing, and cut the sausage into bite-size pieces. Don't add the red pepper flakes to the sauce (unless your kid likes spicy food). Place your toddler's polenta in a bowl. You can stop there, or top with the sausage pieces and sauce, cutting broccolini into smaller pieces as needed.

Lamb Meatballs with Lemony Couscous and Harissa Yogurt

Makes 20 meatballs, plus sides
Total Time: about 50 minutes

Why This Recipe Works

We wanted to create a recipe for meatballs with modern flavors that will still only take about an hour to get on the table. We started with lamb and aromatic spices. Making a quick mixture of bread crumbs and Greek yogurt (officially called a panade!), plus adding an egg yolk, helped bind the meatballs together and kept them from drying out. We sautéed some chopped spinach in the flavorful fat left behind in the skillet after searing the meatballs and stirred it into the light, lemony couscous. A touch of harissa (a potent chili paste commonly used in North African cooking) brought just a little bit of heat to our yogurt dipping sauce.

Harissa can vary in spiciness from brand to brand, so add it to taste in step 1.

1 cup plain Greek yogurt
1¾ cups water
¼ cup minced fresh mint
¼ cup extra-virgin olive oil
2 to 4 teaspoons harissa
2 garlic cloves, minced
Salt and pepper
1½ cups couscous
3 tablespoons panko bread crumbs
1 pound ground lamb
1 large egg yolk
1 teaspoon ground cumin
¾ teaspoon ground cinnamon
5 ounces (5 cups) baby spinach, roughly chopped
3 tablespoons lemon juice, plus lemon wedges for serving

1. Combine ⅔ cup yogurt, 2 tablespoons water, 1 tablespoon mint, 1 tablespoon oil, harissa, if using, half of garlic, and ¼ teaspoon salt in small bowl. Cover and refrigerate until ready to use.

2. Heat 1 tablespoon oil in medium saucepan over medium-high heat until shimmering. Add couscous and cook, stirring frequently, until grains are just beginning to brown, 3 to 5 minutes. Stir in 1½ cups water and ¼ teaspoon salt. Cover, remove saucepan from heat, and let sit until couscous is tender, about 7 minutes.

3. Meanwhile, mash panko, remaining ⅓ cup yogurt, and remaining 2 tablespoons water together with fork in large bowl to form paste. Add ground lamb, 2 tablespoons mint, egg yolk, cumin, cinnamon, ¼ teaspoon salt, ⅛ teaspoon pepper, and

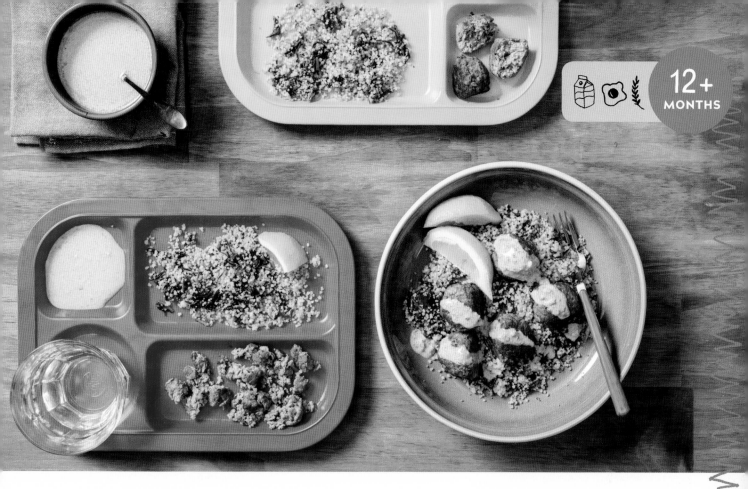

remaining garlic and knead with your hands until thoroughly combined. Using wet hands, roll heaping tablespoons of lamb mixture into 20 tightly packed meatballs.

4. Heat 1 tablespoon oil in 12-inch nonstick skillet over medium-high heat until just smoking. Add meatballs and cook until well browned on all sides and cooked through, 8 to 10 minutes; transfer to serving platter and tent with aluminum foil.

5. Pour off all but 1 tablespoon fat from skillet. Add spinach and cook over medium heat, stirring occasionally, until wilted and uniformly dark green, about 1 minute. Transfer to serving bowl.

6. Fluff couscous with fork and transfer to bowl with spinach. Stir in lemon juice, remaining 1 tablespoon mint, and remaining 1 tablespoon oil. Season with salt and pepper to taste. ⭐ Serve meatballs with yogurt sauce, couscous, and lemon wedges.

⭐ TIPS FOR TODDLERS

The harissa in the yogurt sauce in step 1 does make it spicy. Reserve some plain yogurt (or yogurt sauce with everything but the harissa) for your kid, if desired. In step 6, simply chop up the meatballs and serve them with the couscous and yogurt sauce.

California-Style Fish Tacos with Cabbage Slaw

Makes 8 to 12 tacos, plus toppings
Total Time: 50 minutes

Why This Recipe Works

Baja- or California-style fish tacos have become a popular menu offering at taquerias across the United States and for good reason: mild white fish, crunchy cabbage, and creamy white sauce, all piled onto a corn tortilla (or two), come together to deliver an irresistible combination of flavors and textures. For kids who might be a bit skeptical of fish, these tacos are a great way to introduce it—layered with their favorite toppings, of course. The fish featured in California-style fish tacos is usually beer-battered and deep fried, but for less mess and a quicker weeknight cooking option, we opted to simply pan-sear and flake apart the fillets. We made a quick pickle of red onions and jalapeños to add crunch and tang (the jalapeños can be omitted for the spicy averse!). Store-bought coleslaw mix was a convenient shortcut for the cabbage topping.

Serve with your favorite taco toppings; we like chopped cilantro, radishes, and hot sauce. Use 6-ounce fillets to make 8 tacos or 8-ounce fillets to make 12 tacos. Note that most adults will eat 2 to 3 tacos.

1 small red onion, halved and sliced thin
1 jalapeño chile, stemmed and sliced into thin rings (optional)
1 cup white wine vinegar
¼ cup lime juice
1 tablespoon sugar
Salt and pepper
3 cups (8¼ ounces) coleslaw mix
¼ cup mayonnaise
¼ cup sour cream
1 tablespoon milk
2 (6- to 8-ounce) skinless white fish fillets, such as cod, haddock, or halibut, 1 inch thick
1 tablespoon canola oil
8 to 12 (6-inch) corn tortillas, warmed
1 avocado, pitted and chopped

1. Combine onion and jalapeño, if using, in small bowl. Bring vinegar, 2 tablespoons lime juice, sugar, and 1 teaspoon salt to boil in small saucepan. Pour vinegar mixture over onion mixture and let sit for at least 30 minutes. (Pickled onions can be refrigerated for up to 2 days.)

2. Meanwhile, toss coleslaw mix, 1 tablespoon lime juice, ¼ teaspoon salt, and ⅛ teaspoon pepper together in separate bowl; set aside.

3. Whisk together mayonnaise, sour cream, milk, and remaining

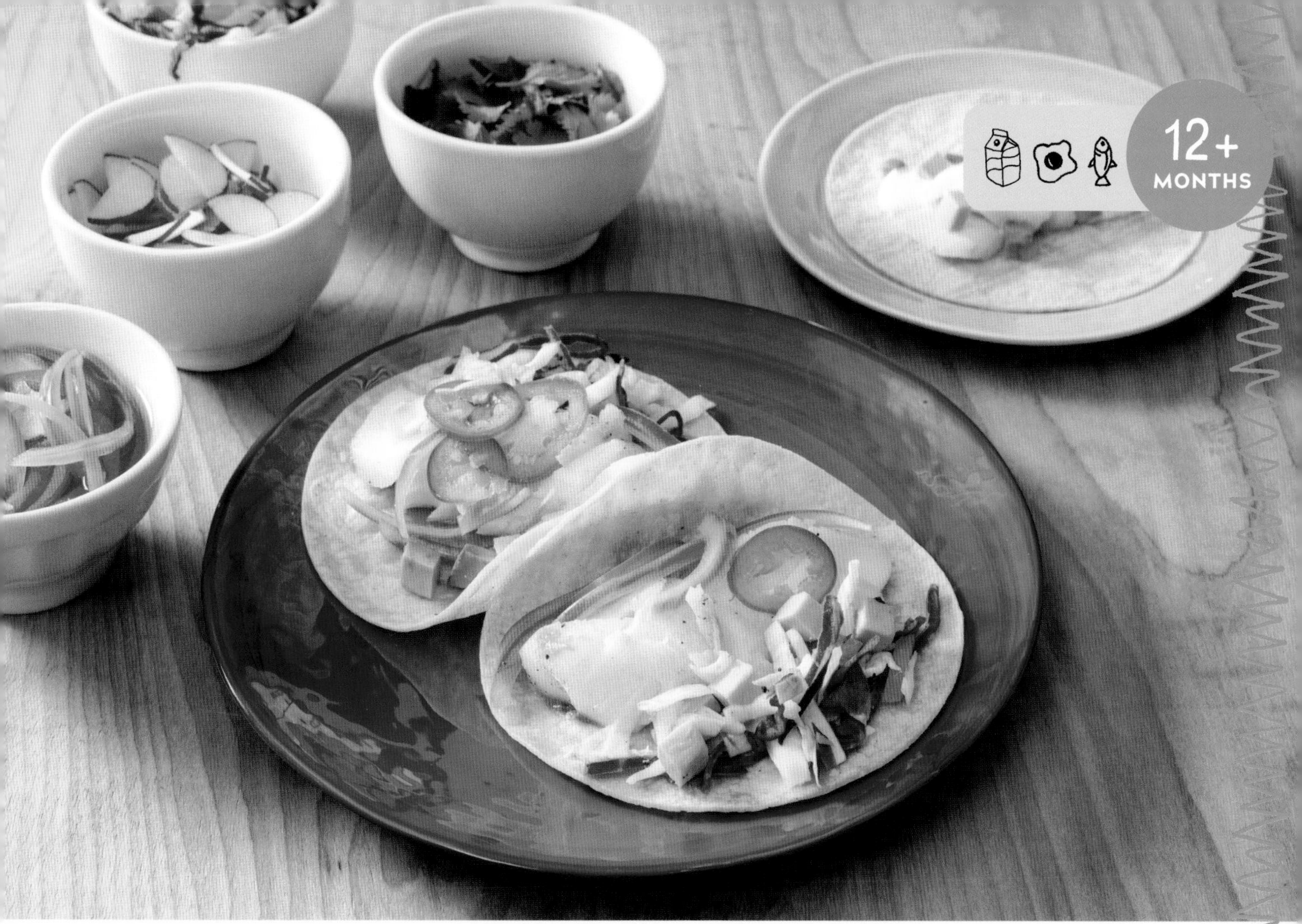

1 tablespoon lime juice in small bowl; set aside. (Sauce can be refrigerated for up to 2 days.)

4 Pat fish dry with paper towels and season with salt and pepper. Heat oil in 10-inch nonstick skillet over medium heat until shimmering. Add fish and cook until both sides are lightly browned and fish registers 140 degrees, 4 to 6 minutes per side. Transfer fish to plate and let cool slightly, about 2 minutes.

5 Using 2 forks, flake fish into 1-inch pieces. Divide fish evenly among tortillas. Top with pickled onions, coleslaw mixture, sauce, and avocado. Serve.

TIPS FOR TODDLERS

In step 1, omit the jalapeños from the pickled onions (unless your toddler really likes spicy food). When you get to step 5, place your toddler's fish in a warm tortilla and have him/her pick toppings of choice.

Oven-Roasted Salmon with Mango-Mint Salsa and Quinoa

Makes 2 to 4 salmon fillets, plus sides
Total Time: 1 hour

Why This Recipe Works

Salmon is rich and mild tasting and can have a silky, almost buttery texture. Roasting salmon brings out some of its best qualities and is also a quick, hands-off way to prepare it. We start with a preheated baking sheet, which allows us to render some of the salmon's fat and firm up its exterior, and then we immediately lowered the temperature to gently cook the fillets through. A sweet mango-mint salsa was the perfect bright balance to the rich fish, and a nutty quinoa pilaf with fresh snap peas and lime rounded out the meal.

If using wild salmon, cook it until it registers 120 degrees (see "Wild versus Farmed Salmon," right). If you buy unwashed quinoa, rinse the grains in a fine-mesh strainer and drain well. There are 3 types of quinoa on the market: white, black, and red. Be sure to buy white quinoa for this recipe, as it has the softest texture of the three quinoas. Note that 2 salmon fillets will serve one adult plus one to two kids. Cook the number of salmon fillets that feed your family.

1 mango, peeled, pitted, and cut into ¼-inch pieces
2 shallots, minced
1 teaspoon grated lime zest plus ¼ cup juice, plus lime wedges for serving
¼ cup chopped fresh mint
¼ cup extra-virgin olive oil
1 garlic clove, minced
Salt and pepper
1½ cups white quinoa
1¾ cups water
2 to 4 (6- to 8-ounce) skin-on salmon fillets, 1½ inches thick
8 ounces sugar snap peas, strings removed and sliced thin on the bias

1 Adjust oven rack to lowest position, place foil-lined rimmed baking sheet on rack, and heat oven to 500 degrees. Combine mango, 1 tablespoon shallot, 3 tablespoons lime juice, 2 tablespoons mint, 1 tablespoon oil, garlic, and ¼ teaspoon salt in small bowl; set aside.

2 Heat 2 tablespoons oil in medium saucepan over medium heat until shimmering. Add remaining shallot and ¾ teaspoon salt and cook, stirring often, until softened, 2 to 3 minutes.

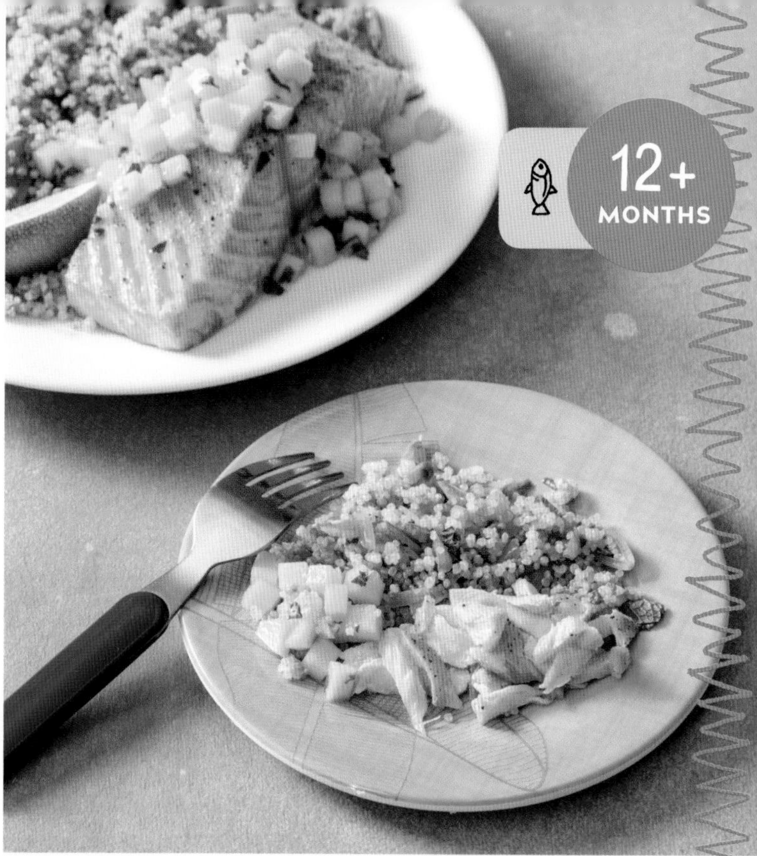

12+ MONTHS

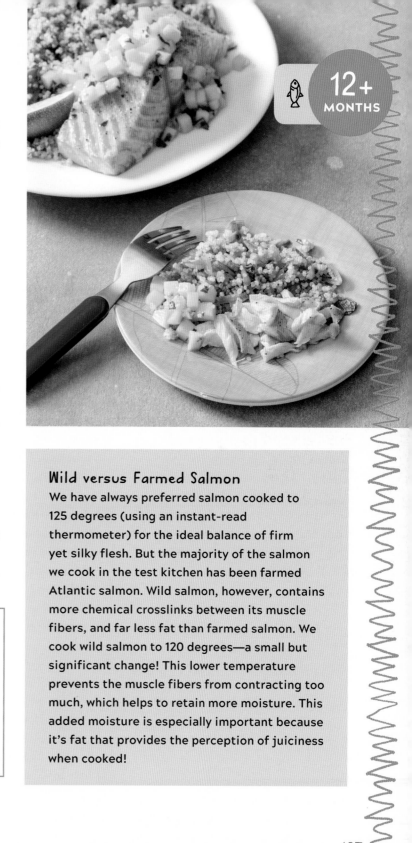

3. Stir in quinoa and water, increase heat to medium-high, and bring to simmer. Cover, reduce heat to low, and simmer until grains are just tender and liquid is absorbed, 18 to 20 minutes, stirring once halfway through cooking. Remove saucepan from heat, uncover, and let cool for 15 minutes.

4. While quinoa is cooling, pat salmon dry with paper towels and season with salt and pepper. Reduce oven temperature to 275 degrees and remove baking sheet. Carefully place salmon, skin side down, on hot sheet, return to oven, and roast until center is still translucent when checked with tip of paring knife and registers 125 degrees (for medium-rare), 9 to 13 minutes. Slide fish spatula along underside of fillets and transfer to serving platter, leaving skin behind; discard skin.

5. Fluff quinoa with fork and stir in snap peas, lime zest, remaining 1 tablespoon lime juice, remaining 2 tablespoons mint, and remaining 1 tablespoon oil. Season with salt and pepper to taste. Serve salmon with mango salsa, quinoa pilaf, and lime wedges.

TIPS FOR TODDLERS

In step 5, reserve some quinoa and snap peas before adding in all the other green stuff, if desired. Place your toddler's fish on a small plate and flake it into small pieces. Top with mango salsa, and serve with quinoa, cutting the snap peas into smaller pieces as needed.

Wild versus Farmed Salmon

We have always preferred salmon cooked to 125 degrees (using an instant-read thermometer) for the ideal balance of firm yet silky flesh. But the majority of the salmon we cook in the test kitchen has been farmed Atlantic salmon. Wild salmon, however, contains more chemical crosslinks between its muscle fibers, and far less fat than farmed salmon. We cook wild salmon to 120 degrees—a small but significant change! This lower temperature prevents the muscle fibers from contracting too much, which helps to retain more moisture. This added moisture is especially important because it's fat that provides the perception of juiciness when cooked!

Bucatini All'Amatriciana

Makes up to 1 pound of sauced pasta
Total Time: 40 minutes

Why This Recipe Works

Amatriciana sauce takes everything we love about classic tomato sauce and turns things up to an 11 without adding a laundry list of ingredients or a bunch of complicated steps. Our recipe features pancetta, which we crisp in the skillet and then use the rendered fat to give the dish savory meatiness. All these ingredients can be kept on hand in your fridge and pantry for weeks if not months, making Amatriciana a great option for evenings when you don't have the time or desire to make a run to the grocery store. *Buon appetito!*

We have provided a range for the amount of red pepper flakes in this recipe so you can adjust heat levels to your preference. There is also a range for the amount of bucatini so you can adjust according to how many people you are feeding. You can substitute spaghetti, penne, or rigatoni for the bucatini. If you make a smaller amount of pasta, you may have extra sauce, which you can save for later.

1 teaspoon extra-virgin olive oil
6 ounces pancetta, cut into ¼-inch pieces
2 ounces Pecorino Romano cheese, finely grated (1 cup)
2 tablespoons tomato paste
⅛ to ¼ teaspoon red pepper flakes
½ cup red wine (optional)
1 (28-ounce) can crushed tomatoes
12 to 16 ounces bucatini

1. Heat oil in 12-inch skillet over medium-low heat until shimmering. Add pancetta and cook, stirring frequently, until fat renders and pancetta is crispy, 10 to 12 minutes. Using slotted spoon, transfer pancetta to bowl. Off heat, transfer 2 tablespoons fat from skillet and half of Pecorino to separate small bowl and smear together to form paste, leaving remaining fat in skillet.

2. Return skillet to medium heat, stir in tomato paste and red pepper flakes, and cook, stirring constantly, for 20 seconds. Stir in wine, if using, and cook for 30 seconds. Stir in tomatoes and rendered pancetta and bring to simmer. Cook, stirring often, until sauce is thickened, 10 to 12 minutes.

3. Meanwhile, bring 4 quarts water to boil in large Dutch oven. Add bucatini and cook, stirring often, until al dente. Reserve 1 cup cooking water, then drain pasta and return to pot.

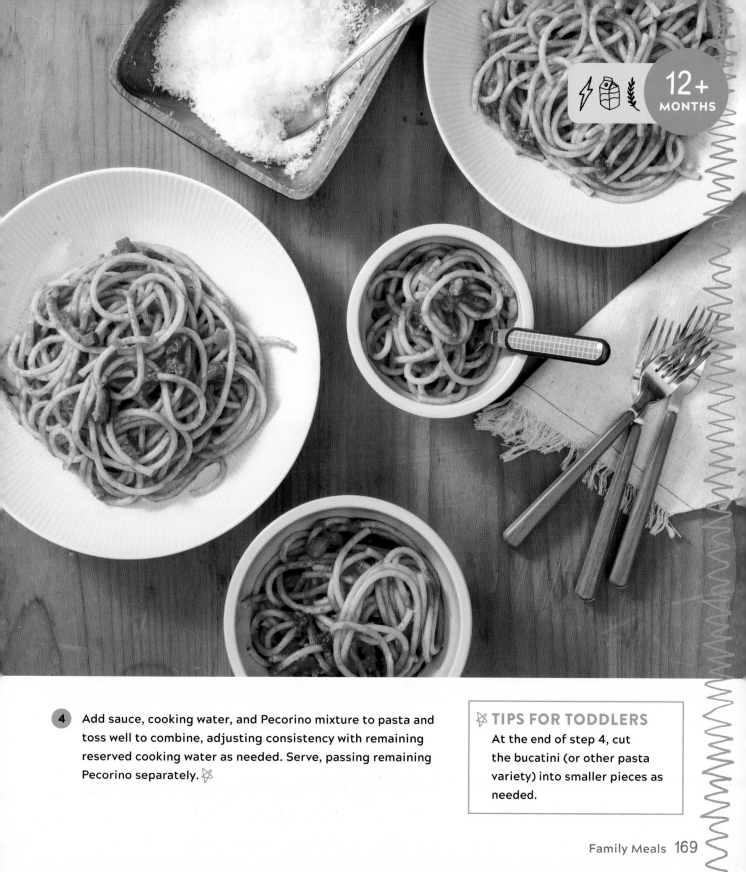

4　Add sauce, cooking water, and Pecorino mixture to pasta and toss well to combine, adjusting consistency with remaining reserved cooking water as needed. Serve, passing remaining Pecorino separately. �

✻ TIPS FOR TODDLERS

At the end of step 4, cut the bucatini (or other pasta variety) into smaller pieces as needed.

Skillet Lasagna

Makes 1 small lasagna
Total Time: 1 hour

Why This Recipe Works

To get our lasagna fix without spending hours in the kitchen, we wanted to see if we could make the entire dish, from start to finish, in a 12-inch skillet. (Spoiler: we did!) We liked meatloaf mix—a blend of ground beef, pork, and veal—for its deep, meaty flavor. Canned tomatoes made a quick and easy sauce, and thinning the diced tomatoes with some water gave us just enough liquid to cook the dried pasta right in the sauce (no precooking and draining of noodles required). For the cheese, we stirred grated Parmesan into the sauce and dropped dollops of ricotta over the noodles and covered the pan briefly so they'd melt. A final sprinkle of Parmesan and basil brought the lasagna flavors home.

Meatloaf mix is sold prepackaged in many supermarkets. If it's unavailable, you can use ground beef instead. Do not substitute no-boil lasagna noodles for the traditional, curly-edged lasagna noodles here. You will need a 12-inch nonstick skillet with a tight-fitting lid for this recipe. Note that 1 lasagna serves four to six adults.

1 (28-ounce) can diced tomatoes
Water
1 tablespoon extra-virgin olive oil
1 onion, chopped fine
Salt and pepper
3 garlic cloves, minced
1 pound meatloaf mix

10 curly-edged lasagna noodles, broken into 2-inch lengths
1 (8-ounce) can tomato sauce
1 ounce Parmesan cheese, grated (½ cup), plus extra for serving
8 ounces (1 cup) whole-milk ricotta cheese
3 tablespoons chopped fresh basil

1. Place tomatoes in 4-cup liquid measuring cup. Add water until mixture measures 4 cups.

2. Heat oil in 12-inch nonstick skillet over medium heat until shimmering. Add onion and ½ teaspoon salt and cook until softened, about 5 minutes. Stir in garlic and cook until fragrant, about 30 seconds. Add meat and cook, breaking up meat into small pieces with wooden spoon, until it is no longer pink, about 5 minutes.

3. Scatter pasta over meat; do not stir. Pour tomato mixture and tomato sauce over pasta and bring to simmer. Reduce heat to medium-low, cover, and simmer, stirring occasionally, until pasta is tender, 20 to 25 minutes.

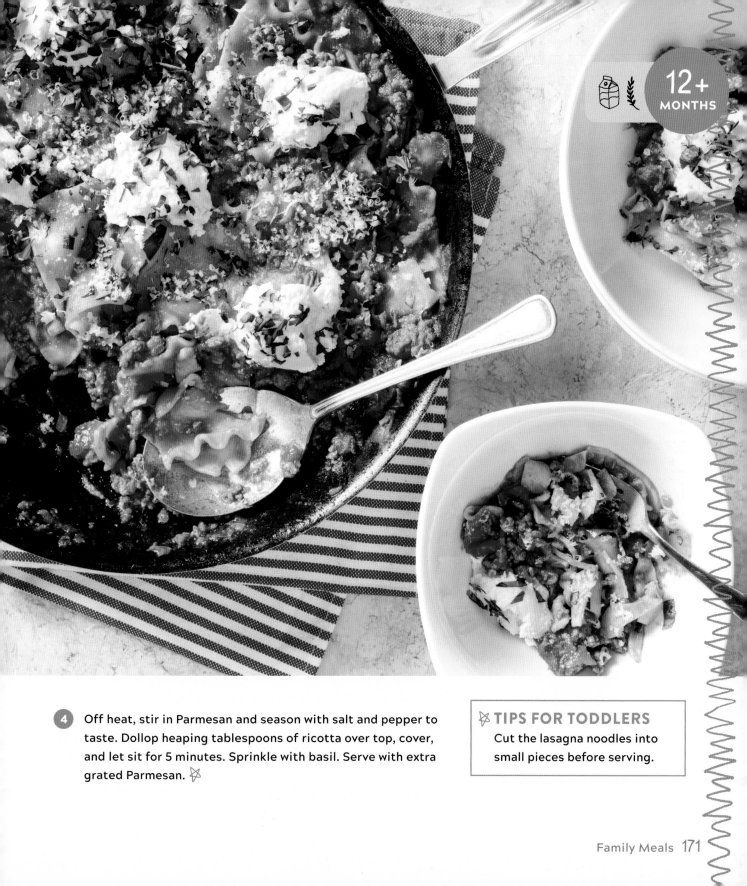

4 Off heat, stir in Parmesan and season with salt and pepper to taste. Dollop heaping tablespoons of ricotta over top, cover, and let sit for 5 minutes. Sprinkle with basil. Serve with extra grated Parmesan.

⊠ TIPS FOR TODDLERS
Cut the lasagna noodles into small pieces before serving.

Macaroni and Cheese with Swiss Chard

Makes 8 ounces pasta
Total Time: 45 minutes

Why This Recipe Works

For a version of mac and cheese that's miles beyond a powdered cheese packet but still uses a simple stovetop preparation, we turned to a powerful secret ingredient: American cheese. American cheese contains special emulsifying salts that keep the cheese extra smooth when melted. This meant we could skip the fussy step of making a béchamel sauce, which is what is traditionally used to keep aged cheeses from breaking and curdling. Because American cheese is mild in flavor, we combined it with some extra-sharp cheddar plus a bit of Dijon mustard. We help make it more of a well-rounded meal by stirring in some sautéed Swiss chard at the end of cooking. On top of it all goes crunchy, cheesy, toasted panko bread crumbs.

Use a 5-ounce block of American cheese from the deli counter, not presliced cheese. Because the macaroni is cooked in a measured amount of liquid, we don't recommend using different shapes or sizes of pasta in this recipe; stick to elbow macaroni. Note that this recipe feeds two adults plus one to two kids.

⅓ cup panko bread crumbs
2 tablespoons extra-virgin olive oil
Salt and pepper
2 tablespoons grated Parmesan cheese
1¾ cups water
1¾ cups whole milk
8 ounces elbow macaroni
5 ounces American cheese, shredded (1¼ cups)
½ teaspoon Dijon mustard
5 ounces extra-sharp cheddar cheese, shredded (1¼ cups)
1 pound Swiss chard, stemmed and cut into 1-inch pieces

1 Combine panko, 1 tablespoon oil, ⅛ teaspoon salt, and ⅛ teaspoon pepper in 12-inch nonstick skillet until panko is evenly moistened. Cook over medium heat, stirring frequently, until evenly browned, 3 to 4 minutes. Off heat, sprinkle Parmesan over panko mixture and stir to combine. Transfer panko mixture to small bowl and set aside.

2 Bring water and milk to boil in medium saucepan over high heat. Stir in macaroni and reduce heat to medium-low. Cook, stirring frequently, until macaroni is tender, 6 to 8 minutes. Add American cheese and mustard and cook, stirring constantly, until cheese is completely melted, about 1 minute. Off heat, stir in cheddar until evenly distributed but not melted. Cover saucepan and let sit for 5 minutes.

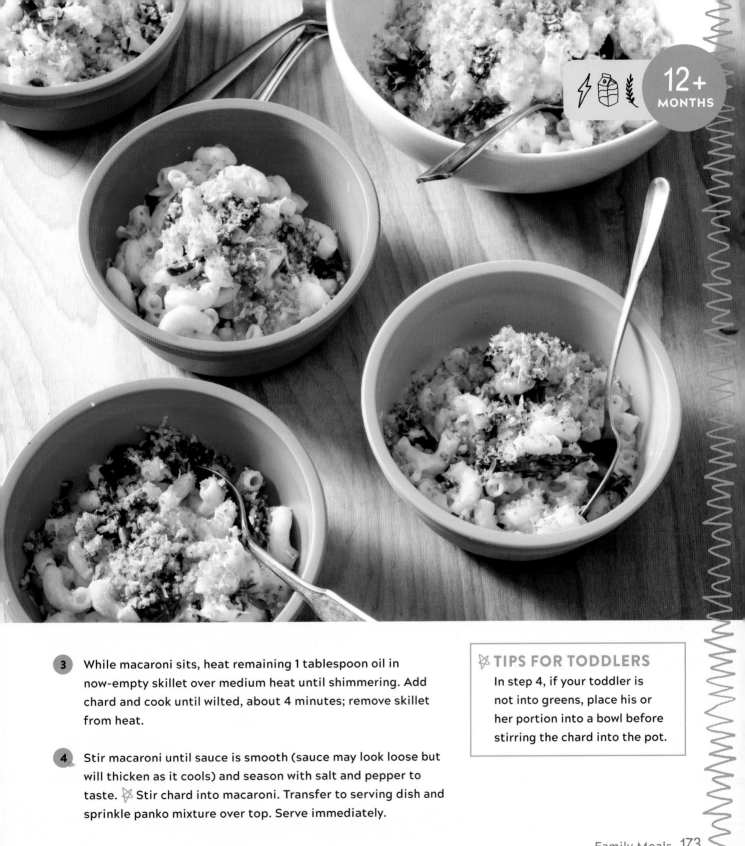

3   While macaroni sits, heat remaining 1 tablespoon oil in now-empty skillet over medium heat until shimmering. Add chard and cook until wilted, about 4 minutes; remove skillet from heat.

4   Stir macaroni until sauce is smooth (sauce may look loose but will thicken as it cools) and season with salt and pepper to taste. ✫ Stir chard into macaroni. Transfer to serving dish and sprinkle panko mixture over top. Serve immediately.

✫ TIPS FOR TODDLERS

In step 4, if your toddler is not into greens, place his or her portion into a bowl before stirring the chard into the pot.

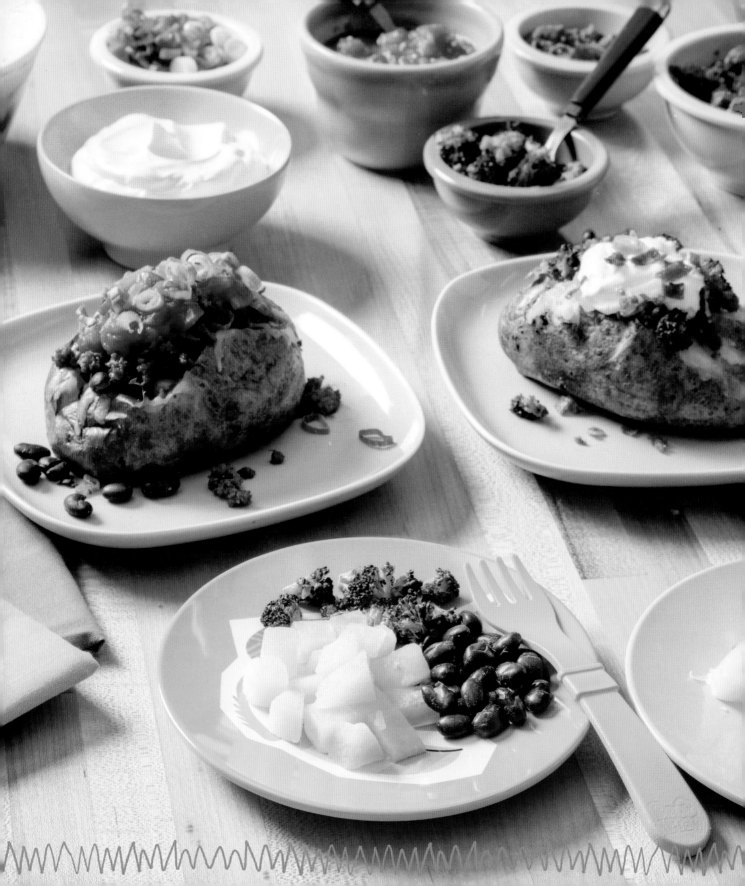

Baked Potato Bar

Makes 2 to 4 potatoes, plus toppings
Total Time: 1 hour to 1 hour 15 minutes

Why This Recipe Works

While tasty on its own, sure, the real purpose of a baked potato is to be a vehicle for toppings. On top of our fluffy spuds go veggies and proteins of all kinds, offering endless mix-and-match opportunities. Best of all, baked potatoes are relatively hands-off, leaving plenty of time to build your DIY topping bar while they cook. For the best baked potatoes, we found that dipping them in salty water before baking ensured an evenly-seasoned exterior, and brushing them with oil toward the end of cooking rendered them browned and crisp. Baking the potatoes until they reached 205 degrees (yes, we took our potatoes' temperatures) ensured they were light and fluffy from edge to center.

Open up the potatoes immediately after removal from the oven in step 3 so steam can escape. You can make one or both of the following toppings while the potatoes bake, or serve with your favorite toppings, such as sour cream, minced chives, sliced scallions, shredded cheese, salsa, crumbled bacon, or black beans.

Salt and pepper
2 to 4 (7- to 9-ounce) russet potatoes, unpeeled, each lightly pricked with fork in 6 places
1 tablespoon canola oil
1 or 2 topping recipes (recipes follow, pages 176 and 177)

1. Adjust oven rack to middle position and heat oven to 450 degrees. Dissolve 2 tablespoons salt in ½ cup water in large bowl. Place potatoes in bowl and toss so exteriors of potatoes are evenly moistened. Transfer potatoes to wire rack set in rimmed baking sheet and bake until center of largest potato registers 205 degrees, 45 minutes to 1 hour. (This is a good time to prepare your toppings.)

2. Remove potatoes from oven and brush tops and sides with oil. Return potatoes to oven and continue to bake for 10 minutes.

3. Remove potatoes from oven and, using paring knife, carefully make 2 slits, forming an X, in each potato. Hold ends with clean dish towel and squeeze slightly to push flesh up and out. Season with salt and pepper to taste. Serve immediately with toppings. ⊗

> ⊗ **TIPS FOR TODDLERS**
> Have your toddler pick his/her toppings of choice. Feel free to scoop out the potato flesh and discard the skin if your toddler would prefer, or just cut everything into smaller pieces.

CHORIZO TOPPING

Makes enough for 4 potatoes
Total Time: 30 minutes

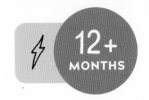

Juicy, highly seasoned Mexican chorizo makes for a great baked potato topping, but it can be hard to find, so we devised a quick method for making our own. If you don't have ancho chile powder, or would like a less-spicy version, substitute milder chili powder for the ancho chile powder.

2 tablespoons canola oil
1½ teaspoons smoked paprika
1 teaspoon ground coriander
1 teaspoon dried oregano
¾ teaspoon ancho chile powder
Pinch ground allspice

Salt and pepper
2 tablespoons cider vinegar
1 teaspoon sugar
1 garlic clove, minced
8 ounces ground pork

1. Combine oil, paprika, coriander, oregano, chile powder, allspice, ½ teaspoon salt, and ¼ teaspoon pepper in 12-inch nonstick skillet. Cook over medium heat, stirring constantly, until mixture is bubbling and fragrant, about 3 minutes.

2. Off heat, carefully stir in vinegar, sugar, and garlic (mixture will sputter). Let stand until steam subsides and skillet cools slightly, about 5 minutes. Add pork to skillet. Mash and mix with rubber spatula until spice mixture is evenly incorporated into pork.

3. Return skillet to medium heat and cook, mashing and stirring until pork has broken into fine crumbles and juices are bubbling, about 3 minutes. Simmer until pork is cooked through, about 2 minutes. Season with salt and pepper to taste. Serve.

PAN-ROASTED BROCCOLI TOPPING

Makes enough for 4 potatoes
Total Time: 25 minutes

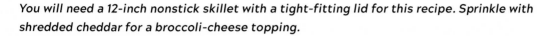

You will need a 12-inch nonstick skillet with a tight-fitting lid for this recipe. Sprinkle with shredded cheddar for a broccoli-cheese topping.

1 tablespoon canola oil	**Salt and pepper**
3 cups broccoli florets, cut into ½-inch pieces	**2 tablespoons unsalted butter**
	1 small shallot, minced
2 tablespoons water	**1 garlic clove, minced**

1 Heat oil in 12-inch nonstick skillet over medium-high heat until just smoking. Add broccoli and cook, without stirring, until florets just begin to brown, about 2 minutes.

2 Add water, ⅛ teaspoon salt, and ⅛ teaspoon pepper and cover skillet. Cook until broccoli is bright green but still crisp, about 2 minutes.

3 Uncover, reduce heat to medium, and stir in butter and shallot. Cook, stirring frequently, until shallot is golden and softened, 2 to 3 minutes. Stir in garlic and cook until fragrant, about 30 seconds. Off heat, season with salt and pepper to taste. Serve.

Vegetable Fried Rice

Makes 6 cups
Total Time: 1 hour and 15 minutes

Why This Recipe Works

While it is a takeout food staple, fried rice can easily be made at home, and it's a great vegetable delivery system for young eaters. This dish is all about the texture of the rice. Unlike the sticky and tender plain white rice, the grains in fried rice are separate and slightly crispy. Restaurants achieve this texture by using leftover cooked white rice, because rice dries out over time. Drier rice means the grains are able to sear rather than steam in the hot pan. We don't expect you to have a ready stash of leftover rice, so instead we've engineered a hack that uses less water than normal, as well as a little vegetable oil to keep grains from sticking to each other. Scrambled eggs provide protein, while bok choy, peas, and bean sprouts lend crunch. Fresh shiitake mushrooms stand in for meat here, while a simple sauce made with soy sauce and oyster sauce boosts the savory flavor even more. If you do happen to have 4 cups leftover cooked rice available, skip step 1 and proceed with the recipe starting at step 2.

3 tablespoons canola oil
1 cup jasmine or long-grain white rice, rinsed
1⅓ cups water
3 tablespoons oyster sauce
1 tablespoon soy sauce
3 large eggs, beaten lightly
2 heads baby bok choy (4 ounces each), cut into ¾-inch pieces
1 cup frozen peas, thawed
2 garlic cloves, minced
1 teaspoon grated fresh ginger
4 ounces shiitake mushrooms, stemmed and sliced ¼ inch thick
1 cup bean sprouts (about 2½ ounces)
5 scallions, sliced thin

1 Heat 1 tablespoon oil in large saucepan over medium heat until shimmering. Add rice and stir to coat grains with oil, about 30 seconds. Add water, increase heat to high, and bring to boil. Reduce heat to low, cover, and simmer until all liquid is absorbed, 15 to 18 minutes. Off heat, remove lid and place clean folded dish towel underneath lid. Let sit until rice is just tender, about 10 minutes. Spread cooked rice onto rimmed baking sheet and let cool for 10 minutes. Transfer to refrigerator and chill until ready to use. (You should have about 4 cups cooked rice; cooked rice can be refrigerated in airtight container for up to 24 hours.)

2 Combine oyster sauce and soy sauce in small bowl; set aside.

3 Heat 2 teaspoons oil in 12-inch nonstick skillet over medium heat until shimmering. Add eggs and cook without stirring until they just begin to set, about 30 seconds, then scramble and break into small pieces with wooden spoon; continue to cook, stirring constantly, until eggs are cooked through but not browned, 30 seconds to 1 minute longer. Transfer eggs to separate small bowl and set aside. Wipe out skillet.

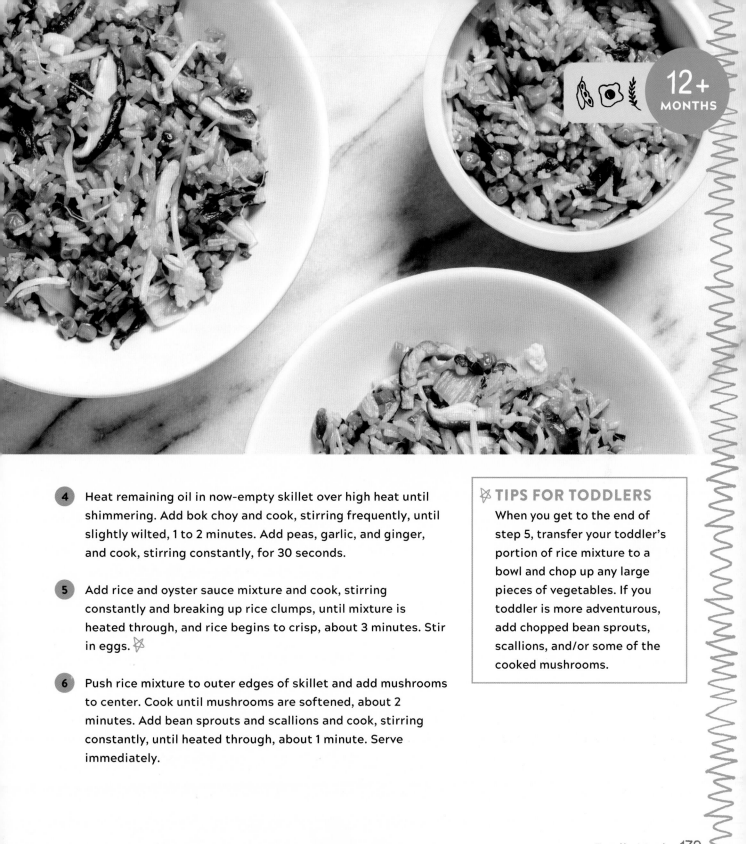

4 Heat remaining oil in now-empty skillet over high heat until shimmering. Add bok choy and cook, stirring frequently, until slightly wilted, 1 to 2 minutes. Add peas, garlic, and ginger, and cook, stirring constantly, for 30 seconds.

5 Add rice and oyster sauce mixture and cook, stirring constantly and breaking up rice clumps, until mixture is heated through, and rice begins to crisp, about 3 minutes. Stir in eggs.

6 Push rice mixture to outer edges of skillet and add mushrooms to center. Cook until mushrooms are softened, about 2 minutes. Add bean sprouts and scallions and cook, stirring constantly, until heated through, about 1 minute. Serve immediately.

⚘ TIPS FOR TODDLERS

When you get to the end of step 5, transfer your toddler's portion of rice mixture to a bowl and chop up any large pieces of vegetables. If you toddler is more adventurous, add chopped bean sprouts, scallions, and/or some of the cooked mushrooms.

Korean Rice Bowl (Bibimbap)

Makes up to 4½ cups rice, plus toppings
Total Time: 1 hour

Why This Recipe Works

Bibimbap is one of the quintessential dishes of Korean cuisine and the grandmother to the now-trendy grain bowls. *Bibimbap* translates from Korean to "mixed rice," and rice is really the only nonnegotiable ingredient in the dish, although most versions include a runny egg with a spicy-sweet sauce made with the fermented pepper paste *gochujang*. The other components are really a matter of taste. Bibimbap makes for a great clear-out-the-fridge meal that can be adapted to work with ingredients you already have on hand—it's an especially great dish when you want your kids to make their own choices. Balancing different flavors, textures, and temperatures is part of the fun of making this dish.

❋ **STORAGE INFORMATION**
Chile sauce can be refrigerated for up to 3 days. Marinated spinach can be refrigerated for up to 24 hours.

Here are some ideas for alternative vegetable toppings to the ones provided in the recipe: bean sprouts, pickled cucumbers, sautéed mushrooms, sliced radishes, chopped kale, steamed green peas, roasted broccoli. If you would like to add more protein to your bibimbap, shredded rotisserie chicken, seared tofu, or beef bulgogi are all great options. Note that 2 eggs will serve one adult plus one to two kids. Cook the number of eggs that feed your family.

CHILE SAUCE
- ¼ cup gochujang
- 3 tablespoons water
- 2 tablespoons toasted sesame oil
- 1 teaspoon sugar

RICE
- 1¾ cups water
- 1½ cups short-grain white rice, rinsed
- ¼ teaspoon salt

MARINATED SPINACH, EGGS, AND TOPPINGS
- 1 tablespoon soy sauce
- 1 tablespoon toasted sesame oil
- 1 tablespoon sesame seeds
- 1 garlic clove, minced
- 1 teaspoon sugar
- 10 ounces (10 cups) baby spinach
- 2 teaspoons canola oil
- 2 to 4 large eggs
- 3 scallions, sliced thin
- 2 carrots, peeled and shredded
- ¾ cup kimchi
- 1 sheet toasted nori, cut into ½-inch pieces (optional)

1 **FOR THE CHILE SAUCE:** Whisk gochujang, water, sesame oil, and sugar together in small bowl. Cover and set aside.

2 **FOR THE RICE:** Bring water, rice, and salt to boil in medium saucepan over high heat. Cover, reduce heat to low, and cook for 15 minutes. Remove rice from heat and let sit, covered, until tender, about 10 minutes.

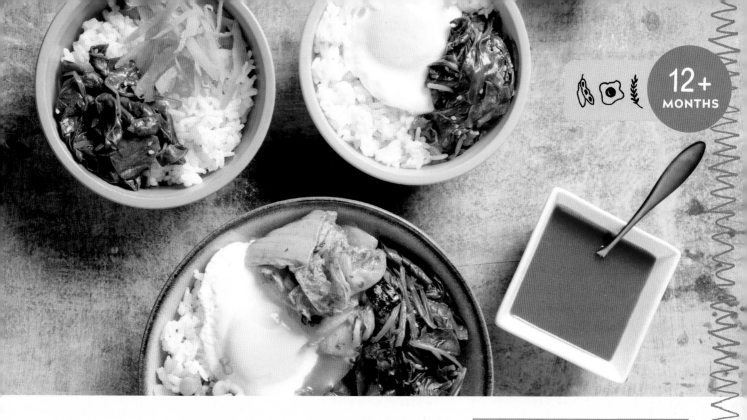

3 **FOR THE MARINATED SPINACH, EGGS, AND TOPPINGS:**
Meanwhile, whisk soy sauce, sesame oil, sesame seeds, garlic, and sugar together in medium bowl; set aside. Bring 10 cups water to boil in large saucepan over high heat. Add spinach and cook, stirring frequently, for 1 minute. Drain spinach in colander set in sink and run under cold water for 30 seconds. Gently press spinach with rubber spatula against colander to release all excess liquid. Add spinach to bowl with soy sauce mixture and toss to combine. Cover and set aside.

4 Heat canola oil in 12-inch nonstick skillet over low heat for 5 minutes. Crack eggs into small bowl. Pour eggs into skillet; cover and cook (about 2 minutes for runny yolks, 2½ minutes for soft but set yolks, and 3 minutes for firmly set yolks).

5 Meanwhile, divide rice between individual serving bowls. ⚜ Divide toppings between each bowl, arranging marinated spinach, scallions, carrots, kimchi, and nori, if using, in small piles around edge of bowl. Drizzle 1 to 2 tablespoons chile sauce in center of each bowl, and top with fried egg. Serve, mixing ingredients together thoroughly before eating.

> ⚜ **TIPS FOR TODDLERS**
>
> In step 5, place your toddler's rice in a bowl and have him/her pick toppings of choice. Omit the chile sauce (unless they really like spicy food!) and replace it with 1 teaspoon sesame oil.

Black Bean Burgers with Roasted Carrot Fries

Makes 4 big burgers or 8 mini burgers, plus sides
Total Time: 50 minutes

Why This Recipe Works

Veggie burgers are a great vegetarian meal, but making them at home is often more work than they're worth. These simple black bean burgers are easy to make: just combine canned beans with a few complementary ingredients and shape the mixture into patties. The food processor makes quick work of the beans, while some scallions and chili powder lend a boost of flavor and an egg to keep the mixture cohesive. We turned to ground tortilla chips to hold our patties together without drying them out, while adding the subtle flavor of toasted corn. Sticking with the Southwestern flavor profile, we made a quick sauce for our burgers from salsa and sour cream. We served them alongside sweet roasted carrot "fries."

A standard 15-ounce can of black beans will yield 1½ cups of beans, drained; you will need 2 cans. Drain the beans thoroughly after rinsing. If you're making mini burgers, use slider buns instead of hamburger buns. You can also simply cut hamburger buns in half to fit mini burgers. Note this recipe makes 4 big burgers or 8 mini burgers, or a combination of the two!

¼ **cup sour cream**
2 **tablespoons salsa**
2 **ounces tortilla chips, crushed (1 cup)**
4 **scallions, chopped coarse**
2 **cups drained black beans, rinsed**
1 **large egg**
1 **tablespoon chili powder**
Salt and pepper

1½ **pounds carrots, peeled and cut into 3-by-½-inch pieces**
3 **tablespoons extra-virgin olive oil**
1 **tablespoon honey**
1 **small head Bibb lettuce (6 ounces), leaves separated**
4 **hamburger buns, toasted**

1 Adjust oven rack to middle position and heat oven to 450 degrees. Line rimmed baking sheet with aluminum foil. Combine sour cream and salsa in bowl. Cover and refrigerate until ready to serve.

2 Process tortilla chips in food processor until very finely ground, about 1 minute. Add scallions and pulse until finely chopped, about 10 pulses. Add beans, egg, chili powder, ¼ teaspoon salt, and ¼ teaspoon pepper and pulse until beans are finely chopped, 10 to 15 pulses.

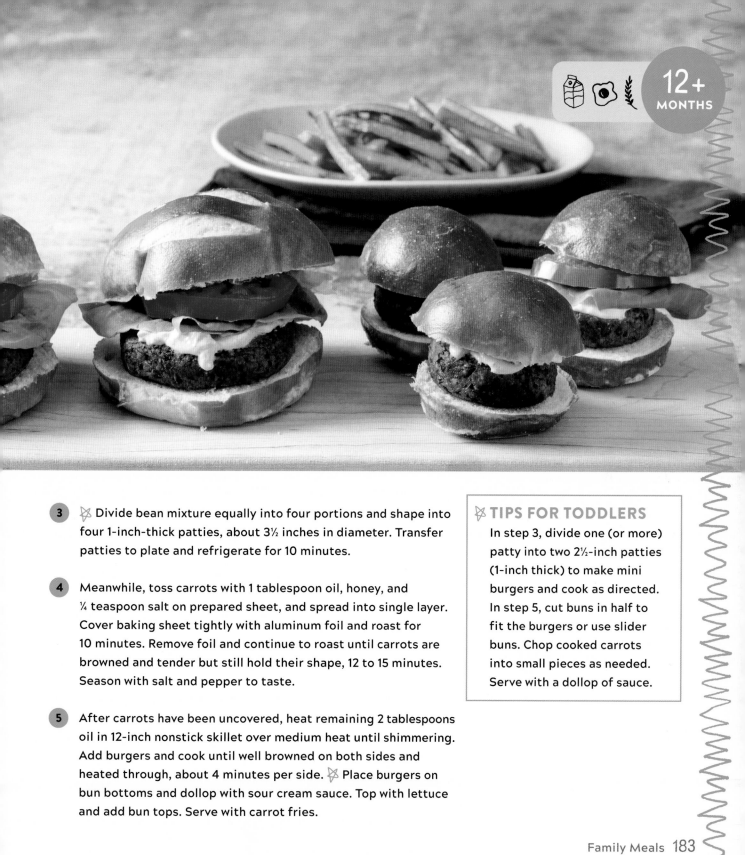

3 ⊠ Divide bean mixture equally into four portions and shape into four 1-inch-thick patties, about 3½ inches in diameter. Transfer patties to plate and refrigerate for 10 minutes.

4 Meanwhile, toss carrots with 1 tablespoon oil, honey, and ¼ teaspoon salt on prepared sheet, and spread into single layer. Cover baking sheet tightly with aluminum foil and roast for 10 minutes. Remove foil and continue to roast until carrots are browned and tender but still hold their shape, 12 to 15 minutes. Season with salt and pepper to taste.

5 After carrots have been uncovered, heat remaining 2 tablespoons oil in 12-inch nonstick skillet over medium heat until shimmering. Add burgers and cook until well browned on both sides and heated through, about 4 minutes per side. ⊠ Place burgers on bun bottoms and dollop with sour cream sauce. Top with lettuce and add bun tops. Serve with carrot fries.

> ⊠ **TIPS FOR TODDLERS**
>
> In step 3, divide one (or more) patty into two 2½-inch patties (1-inch thick) to make mini burgers and cook as directed. In step 5, cut buns in half to fit the burgers or use slider buns. Chop cooked carrots into small pieces as needed. Serve with a dollop of sauce.

Red Lentil Soup with Arugula and Fennel Salad

Makes 8 cups soup, plus side
Total Time: 1 hour

Why This Recipe Works

Consider the red lentil. This bright legume is a great building block for vegetarian soups—and cooks in less than 20 minutes. Because lentils break down so readily during cooking, you get a pureed soup without having to bust out your blender. We added North African spices to complement the earthiness of the lentils in this soup. A simple arugula, fennel, and pita chip salad tossed with a bright yogurt-based dressing rounds out this vegetable-driven dinner.

✳ STORAGE INFORMATION

Soup can be refrigerated for up to 3 days. Thin soup with water, if desired, when reheating.

This recipe calls for chicken broth; if you prefer to keep this meal vegetarian, you can substitute vegetable broth. We use unsalted broth so you can make a puree appropriate for 6- to 12-month-old babies; it's important to season with salt and pepper to taste after removing the portion for babies, since otherwise it will be underseasoned for adults. If you are only feeding folks ages 12 months and up, you can use regular broth.

¼ cup extra-virgin olive oil
1 large onion, chopped fine
Salt and pepper
¾ teaspoon ground coriander
½ teaspoon ground cumin
¼ teaspoon ground ginger
⅛ teaspoon ground cinnamon
1 tablespoon tomato paste
2 garlic cloves, minced
4 cups unsalted chicken broth
2 cups water
10½ ounces (1½ cups) red lentils, picked over and rinsed
3 tablespoons lemon juice
1½ teaspoons dried mint, crumbled
1 teaspoon paprika
2 tablespoons plain yogurt
3 ounces (3 cups) baby arugula
1 small fennel bulb, stalks discarded, bulb halved, cored, and sliced thin
2 ounces pita chips, broken into 1-inch pieces (1 cup)
¼ cup chopped fresh cilantro

1 Heat 2 tablespoons oil in large saucepan over medium heat until shimmering. Add onion and ¼ teaspoon salt and cook, stirring occasionally, until softened, about 5 minutes. Stir in coriander, cumin, ginger, cinnamon, and ⅛ teaspoon pepper and cook until fragrant, about 2 minutes. Stir in tomato paste and half of garlic and cook for 1 minute.

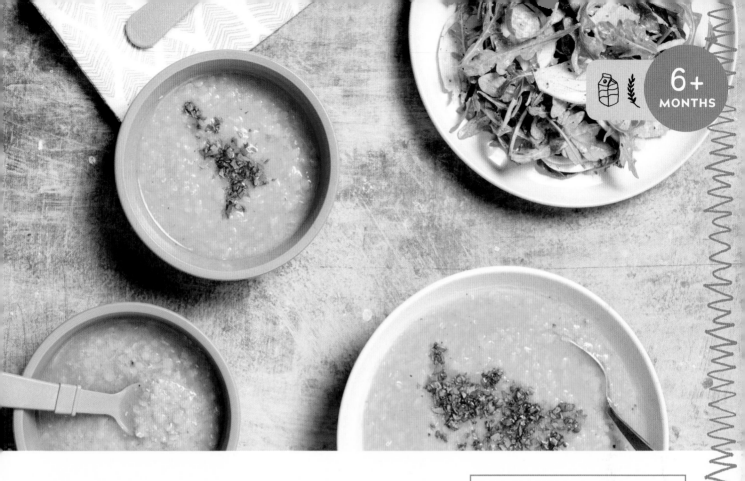

2. Stir in broth, water, and lentils and bring to vigorous simmer. Cook, stirring occasionally, until lentils are soft and about half are broken down, about 15 minutes.

3. Whisk soup vigorously until broken down to coarse puree, about 30 seconds. ✻ Off heat, stir in 2 tablespoons lemon juice and season with salt to taste. Cover to keep warm.

4. Heat remaining 2 tablespoons oil in 8-inch skillet over medium heat until shimmering. Off heat, stir in remaining garlic, mint, and paprika and transfer to large bowl. Whisk in yogurt, remaining 1 tablespoon lemon juice, and ¼ teaspoon salt until combined. Add arugula, fennel, and pita chips to bowl and toss to combine. Ladle soup into individual bowls and sprinkle with cilantro. Serve with salad.

✻ TIPS FOR BABIES
For babies (6 to 12 months): In step 3, don't season with lemon juice and salt. Transfer a small portion of soup to a bowl and serve.

✻ TIPS FOR TODDLERS
Simply serve the soup as is, sprinkling with cilantro, if desired. We know salads can be tricky for this age; this component might just be for the adult(s) in the room.

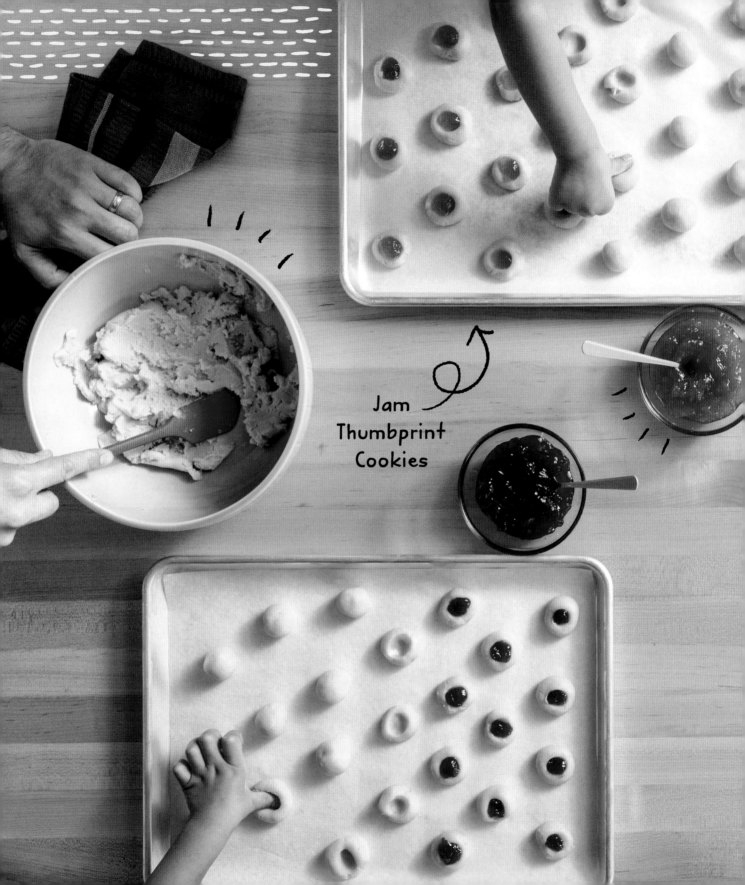

Jam
Thumbprint
Cookies

COOKING with YOUR KIDS

2+ YEARS

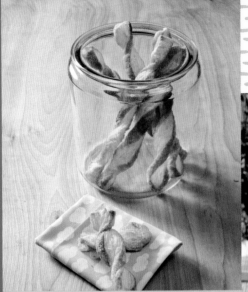

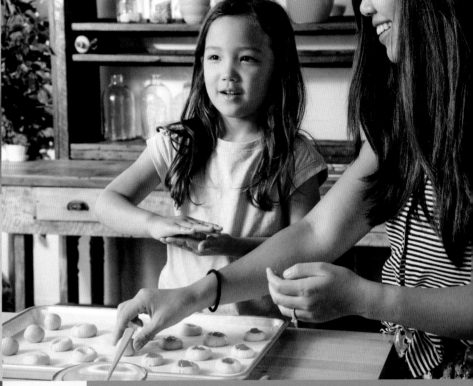

"My 3-year-old loved getting into the kitchen to help prep this dish, and he was so proud that he made dinner! He really earned a sense of accomplishment with this meal."

—Parent of 3-year-old, on Cheese Calzones

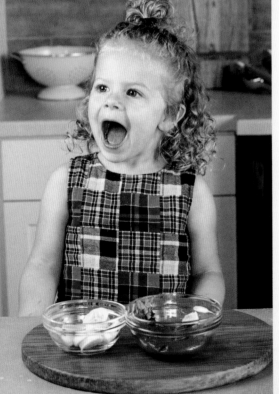

"My daughter was eating the filling straight from the bowl! She enjoyed helping. She helped me pour the sauce in and sprinkle cheese, though she can't quite mix yet and wasn't great at rolling."

—Parent of 18-month-old, on Bean, Cheese, and Spinach Enchiladas

ALL ABOUT COOKING WITH YOUR KIDS

You're home with your kids. You need something to do. We suggest heading to the kitchen.

You may have a toddler, a preschooler, an older kid—or all of the above! Cooking is an achievable and engaging hands-on activity for you all to do together—with delicious results. Plus, it's a wonderful way to involve children (and get them interested) in the process of getting food from the store to the pantry to the table. Cooking is a gateway to learning about numbers, from counting (1, 2, 3, 4 dumplings!) to measuring (the difference between 1 cup and ⅓ cup). Working with food is also an opportunity to introduce descriptive words, ones that will help your kids to talk about food for their entire lives. You can start by describing how things taste (salty, sweet, bitter, or sour), how things smell (cheesy, bright, sweet, or buttery), how things feel (crunchy, cold, or spicy), and how they look (fluffy, dense, or green).

An added bonus? Research has shown that getting kids involved in cooking (or gardening or grocery shopping) makes them more willing to try new foods.

Note that the age range for each of these recipes pertains to cooking—not eating—ability.

We've developed each of these recipes with tiny humans (and shorter attention spans) in mind, giving suggestions for what your kids can do to help. What they actually do will depend on their ages, their interests, and their attention spans.

Fluffy Whole-Wheat Pancakes

Makes 15 pancakes
Total Time: 25 minutes

Why This Recipe Works

Yes, whole-wheat pancakes sound healthy. And they are! But they are also light, fluffy, flavorful—and a wonderful recipe for small arms to stir and stir and stir. Recipes for pancakes made with white flour advise undermixing the batter—overmix and your pancakes will be like barely edible hockey pucks. Why? During mixing, the proteins in white flour come together to form gluten, a protein network that gets denser with every stir—and a thick network will make for tough pancakes. Whole-wheat flour, however, contains fewer gluten-forming proteins and also contains the wheat bran, which is sharp and cuts through any gluten that does form. The result? You can stir this batter all day and will still end up with tender pancakes. Whisk away!

For the best flavor, store whole-wheat flour in the freezer. If you have an electric griddle, set the temperature to 350 degrees and cook up to 8 pancakes at a time.

2 cups (11 ounces) whole-wheat flour
2 tablespoons sugar
1½ teaspoons baking powder
½ teaspoon baking soda
¾ teaspoon salt
2¼ cups buttermilk
5 tablespoons plus 2 teaspoons vegetable oil
2 large eggs

1. Whisk flour, sugar, baking powder, baking soda, and salt together in large bowl. Whisk buttermilk, 5 tablespoons oil, and eggs together in separate bowl. Make well in center of flour mixture and pour in buttermilk mixture; whisk until smooth. (Mixture will be thick; do not add more buttermilk.)

2. Heat 1 teaspoon oil in 12-inch nonstick skillet over medium heat until shimmering. Using paper towels, carefully wipe out oil, leaving thin film on bottom and sides of pan. Using ¼-cup dry measuring cup or 2-ounce ladle, portion batter into pan in 3 places. Gently spread each portion into 4½-inch circles. Sprinkle pancakes with any add-ins, if desired (see "What to Add to Your Pancakes," right).

3. Cook until edges are set, first side is golden brown, and bubbles on surface are just beginning to break, 2 to 3 minutes. Using thin, wide spatula, flip pancakes and continue to cook until second side is golden brown, 1 to 2 minutes longer. Serve pancakes immediately (or transfer to wire rack in oven—see "Keeping Pancakes Warm," right). Repeat with remaining batter, using remaining 1 teaspoon oil as necessary.

WHAT TO ADD TO YOUR PANCAKES

You can customize pancakes with any number of fun add-ins. Try chocolate chips, chopped nuts, shredded coconut, sliced bananas, blueberries, or raspberries. Simply sprinkle each pancake with 1 tablespoon of add-ins after spreading pancakes into the skillet in step 2.

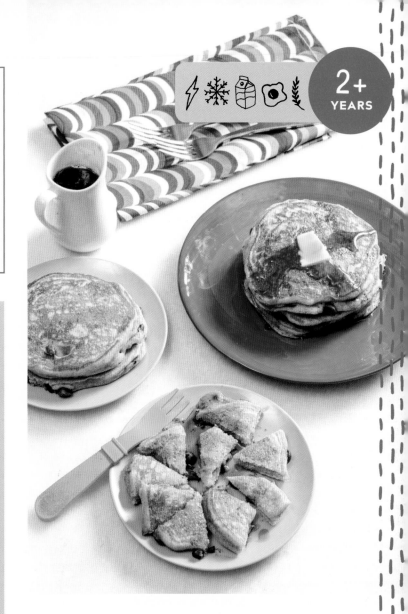

Keeping Pancakes Warm

You can't make all the pancakes at once (you would need a very large skillet). There are two ways to guarantee everyone eats warm pancakes. One option is to simply serve them as soon as they're cooked. The downside is that the cook doesn't get to sit down and eat with everyone else (since he or she is still cooking). The second option is easy: Adjust the oven rack to the middle position and heat the oven to 200 degrees before you start cooking. Spray a wire rack set in a rimmed baking sheet with vegetable oil spray and place it in the oven. As soon as your pancakes are cooked, place them on the baking sheet in the oven. They'll stay warm until all are cooked and it's time to eat.

✳ STORAGE INFORMATION

You can freeze any leftover pancakes for up to one month for a quick breakfast or snack. Stack cooled pancakes with parchment paper between them, put stack of pancakes in a zipper-lock bag, and freeze. To serve, heat pancakes one at a time in microwave until warmed through, about 30 seconds.

HOW YOUR CHILD CAN HELP

✓ Make batter in step 1
✓ Pick out and sprinkle add-ins onto pancakes in step 2 ("What to Add to Your Pancakes," above)

Crêpes with Nutella and Banana

Makes 8 crêpes
Total Time: 40 minutes

Why This Recipe Works

In some circles, *crêpe* is French for "delicious." We agree with that notion, but we might also contend that it's French for "a great way to bring adults and littles together in the kitchen." Crêpes are fun to make and delicious to eat. The first step in these delicate, pancake-like treats is to make sure the pan is properly heated. A tiny test crêpe (see step 3) will show you that the pan is the correct temperature if it's golden brown after 20 seconds. It's also important to use just enough batter to coat the bottom of the pan, using a tilt-and-shake motion to distribute it evenly. To avoid singed fingertips, loosen the crêpe with a rubber spatula before grasping its edge, and then carefully flip it. Voilà!

To allow for practice, this recipe yields a little extra batter. If you want to make crêpes ahead of time or all at once before filling, stack cooked crêpes on wire rack. When ready to fill, transfer stack of crêpes to large microwave-safe plate and invert second plate over crepes. Microwave on high power until crêpes are warm, 30 to 60 seconds. Remove top plate and fill crêpes.

½ **teaspoon vegetable oil**
⅔ **cup (3⅓ ounces) all-purpose flour**
1 **teaspoon sugar**
⅛ **teaspoon salt**
1 **cup whole milk**
2 **large eggs**

1½ **tablespoons unsalted butter, melted and cooled**
8 **teaspoons Nutella spread**
3 **bananas, cut into ¼-inch-thick slices**

1. Place oil in 10-inch nonstick skillet and heat over low heat for at least 10 minutes.

2. While skillet is heating, whisk together flour, sugar, and salt in large bowl. In separate bowl, whisk together milk and eggs. Add half of milk mixture to dry ingredients and whisk until smooth. Add melted butter and whisk until incorporated. Whisk in remaining milk mixture until smooth.

3. Using paper towel, wipe out skillet, leaving thin film of oil on bottom and sides. Increase heat to medium and let skillet heat for 1 minute. After 1 minute, test heat of skillet by placing 1 teaspoon batter in center and cook for 20 seconds. If mini crêpe is golden brown on bottom, skillet is properly heated; if it is too light or too dark, adjust heat accordingly and retest.

4. Pour scant ¼ cup batter into far side of pan and tilt and shake gently until batter evenly covers bottom of pan.

Cook crêpe without moving it until top surface is dry and crêpe starts to brown at edges, about 25 seconds. Loosen crêpe from side of pan with rubber spatula, and then gently slide spatula underneath edge of crêpe, grasp edge with fingertips, and flip. Cook until second side is lightly spotted, about 20 seconds.

5 Transfer cooked crêpe to plate. Spread 1 teaspoon Nutella over top half, followed by 8 to 10 banana slices (see "Filling Crêpes," below). Fold crêpe into quarters. Serve.

6 Return pan to medium heat and heat for 10 seconds before repeating with remaining batter and filling to make 7 more crêpes.

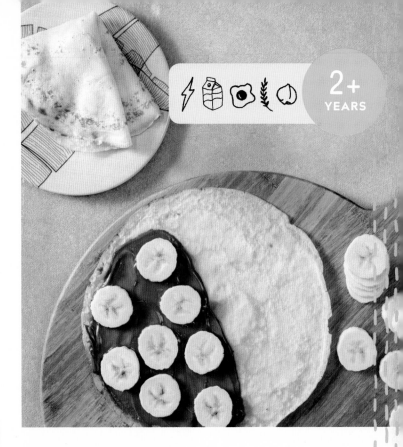

CRÊPES WITH LEMON AND SUGAR

Omit Nutella and bananas. In step 5, sprinkle ½ teaspoon sugar over top half of each crêpe. Fold into quarters. Serve with lemon wedges.

CRÊPES WITH JAM AND POWDERED SUGAR

Omit Nutella and bananas. In step 5, spread 1 teaspoon of your favorite jam over top half of each crêpe. Fold into quarters and dust with powdered sugar.

FILLING CRÊPES

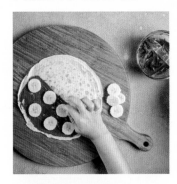

1 Spread 1 teaspoon Nutella over top half of crêpe followed by 8 to 10 banana slices.

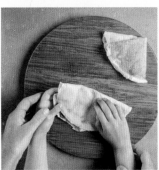

2 Fold crêpe into quarters.

French Toast Sticks

Makes 12 sticks
Total Time: 25 minutes

Why This Recipe Works

To make a breakfast favorite even more toddler-friendly, we cut the slices of bread into small, easy-to-hold sticks. For a thicker and more custardy French toast, we started with challah rather than sandwich bread. It allowed the rich egg mixture to really soak in without becoming soggy (it's also important to toast the bread—see "Why Toast the Bread First?," right). We think these French toast sticks are sweet enough on their own, but feel free to serve them with maple syrup, powdered sugar, or fruit.

HOW YOUR CHILD CAN HELP
✓ Whisk together custard mixture in step 2
✓ Dip bread sticks in custard in step 3

To prevent the butter from clumping during mixing, heat the milk in a microwave or small saucepan until it is warm to the touch (about 80 degrees). This recipe is easy to double if serving a crowd.

6 slices challah,
  ½ inch thick
1 cup whole milk, warmed
2 tablespoons packed light
  brown sugar
2 large egg yolks

2 tablespoons unsalted
  butter, melted, plus
  1 tablespoon for cooking
2 teaspoons vanilla extract
½ teaspoon ground
  cinnamon
¼ teaspoon salt

1. Toast challah slices in toaster until light golden brown, about 1 minute. Cut each slice of challah in half lengthwise to form 2 roughly 1½-inch-wide sticks to make 12 sticks total.

2. Whisk milk, sugar, yolks, 2 tablespoons melted butter, vanilla, cinnamon, and salt in shallow bowl until well blended.

3. Working with 1 stick at a time, soak bread in milk mixture until saturated but not falling apart, about 3 seconds per side. Remove stick, allowing excess milk mixture to drip off, and transfer to rimmed baking sheet. Repeat with remaining sticks.

4. Melt ½ tablespoon butter in 12-inch nonstick skillet over medium-low heat. Place 6 soaked sticks in skillet and cook until golden brown, 2 to 3 minutes per side. Transfer French toast sticks to plate. Wipe out skillet with paper towels. Repeat with remaining ½ tablespoon butter and remaining 6 soaked sticks. Serve.

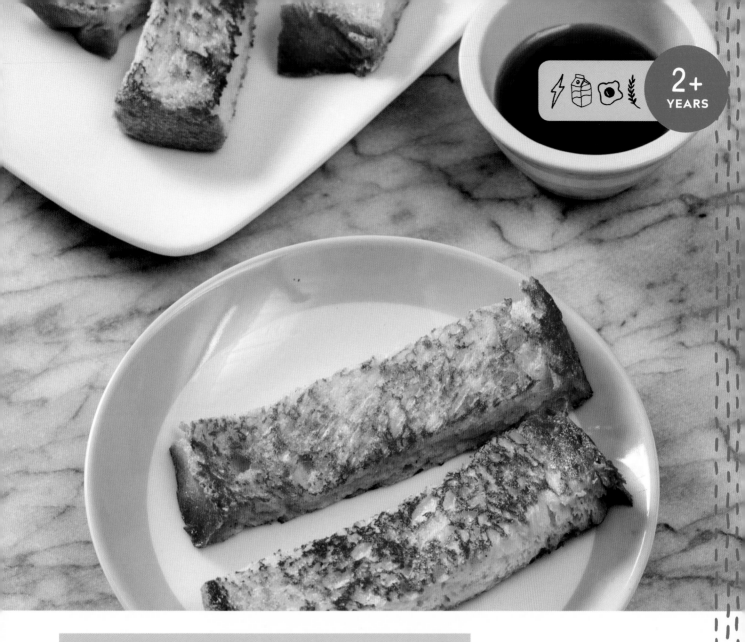

Why Toast the Bread First?

It may seem counterintuitive to toast bread before dipping it into a liquid mixture. Oddly enough, we found that drying out the bread first enabled it to absorb *more* of the custard mixture than fresh bread that we hadn't toasted first. This step also made the bread easier to handle during the dipping process; without toasting, the bread became limp and fragile once soaked in custard.

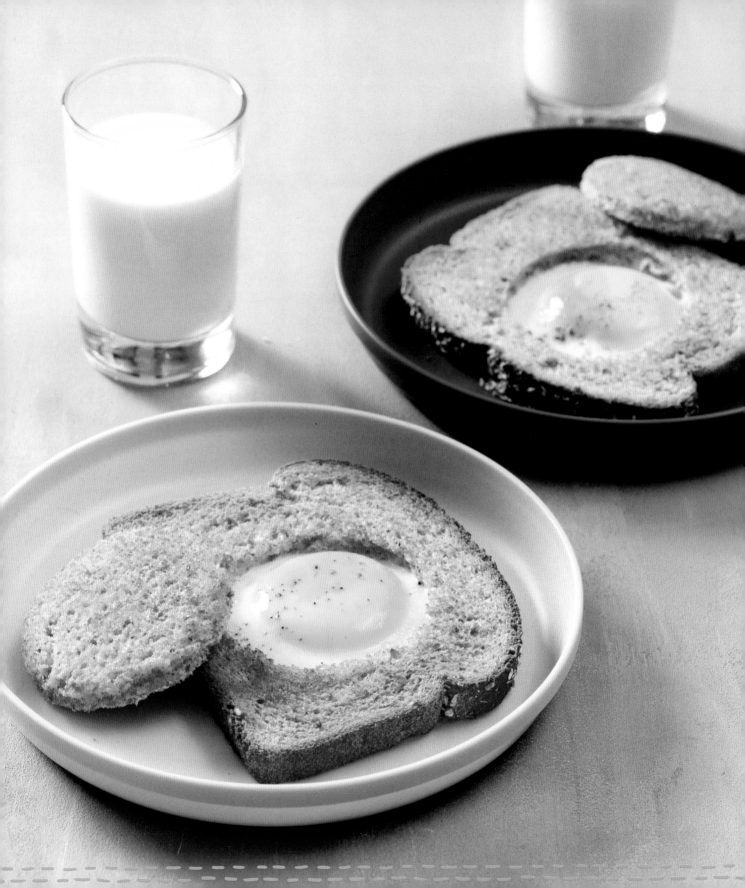

Eggs in a Hole

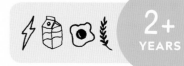

Makes 3 toasts
Total Time: 20 minutes

Why This Recipe Works

There aren't many classic breakfast dishes that can be described as whimsical. Even fewer that are also easy to make. Behold: Eggs in a Hole! Toddlers can make the holes in the toast and practice their egg-cracking skills (maybe have a couple extra eggs on hand, just in case). Unlike most recipes for Eggs in a Hole that call for cracking eggs into a preheated skillet, we assemble the toast and eggs in a cold skillet before cooking, making it safe for kids to help with this task, too.

HOW YOUR CHILD CAN HELP

✓ Butter toast in step 1
✓ Cut out toast circles in step 2
✓ Crack eggs into toast holes in step 3
✓ Sprinkle with salt and pepper in step 3

This recipe is easy to double; just let the skillet cool in between batches. If you don't have a biscuit cutter, cut the toast holes with a sturdy drinking glass. To make handling eggs easier for your toddler, crack each egg into a small bowl before pouring it into the hole.

3 slices hearty white or wheat sandwich bread
2 tablespoons unsalted butter, softened
3 large eggs
Salt and pepper

1. Toast bread in toaster until lightly browned, 1 to 2 minutes. Spread ½ tablespoon butter evenly over 1 side of each piece of toast.

2. Using 2½-inch biscuit cutter, cut and remove circle from each piece of bread; reserve toast circles.

3. Place pieces of toast, buttered side down, in 12-inch nonstick skillet. Divide remaining ½ tablespoon butter among 3 holes in toast. Crack 1 egg into each hole. Season eggs with salt and pepper.

4. Cover skillet and cook over medium-low heat until whites are set and yolks still jiggle, about 8 minutes, or 9 minutes for set yolks. Serve with buttered toast circles.

Cinnamon Twists

Makes 10 twists
Total Time: 30 minutes, plus thawing time

Why This Recipe Works

This cinnamon-kissed, flaky breakfast treat has a high payoff for a minimal amount of work. Store-bought puff pastry dough—an MVP from the frozen food aisle—provides a premade base for melted butter, cinnamon, and sugar. Your child will love winding the strips of dough into twists. Everyone will love eating them.

HOW YOUR CHILD CAN HELP
✓ Make sugar mixture in step 1
✓ Brush pastry with butter and sprinkle pastry with sugar mixture in step 2
✓ Twist pastry strips in step 3

Be sure to let puff pastry thaw completely before using; otherwise it can crack and fall apart. To thaw frozen puff pastry, allow it to sit either in the refrigerator for 24 hours or on the counter for 30 minutes to 1 hour.

3 tablespoons sugar
1 teaspoon ground cinnamon
1 (9½-by-9-inch) sheet puff pastry, thawed
2 tablespoons unsalted butter, melted and cooled

1 Adjust oven rack to upper-middle position and heat oven to 425 degrees. Line rimmed baking sheet with parchment paper. Combine sugar and cinnamon in bowl.

2 Roll pastry into 10-inch square on lightly floured counter. Brush pastry with 1 tablespoon melted butter, then sprinkle evenly with 1½ tablespoons sugar mixture. Flip pastry over and repeat with remaining 1 tablespoon melted butter and remaining 1½ tablespoons sugar mixture.

3 Cut pastry into ten 1-inch-wide strips. Working with one strip at a time, twist strip several times (see "Making Twists," right); transfer twists to prepared baking sheet.

4 Bake twists until fully puffed and golden, 10 to 14 minutes, rotating sheet halfway through baking. Transfer twists to wire rack and let cool slightly. Serve warm or at room temperature.

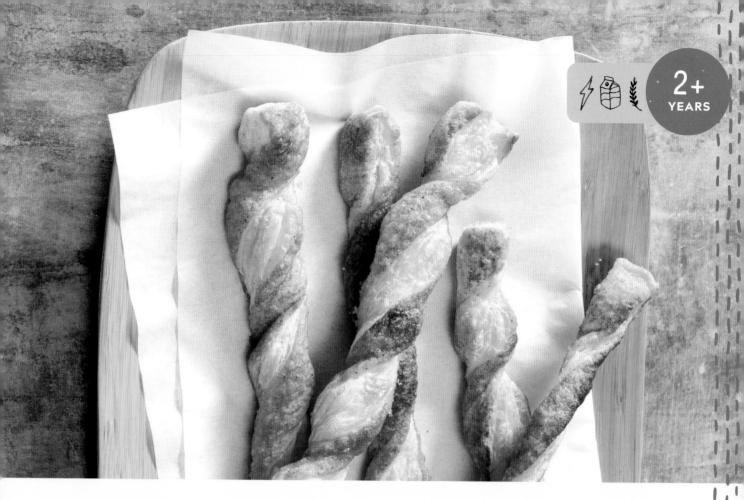

MAKING TWISTS

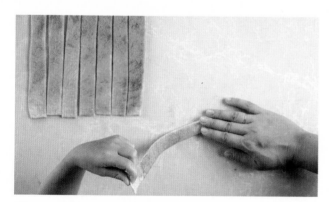

(1) Working with one strip of dough at a time, hold one end of dough on counter and lift the other up.

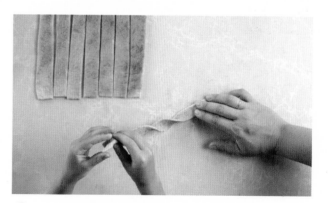

(2) Twist dough several times and transfer twist to prepared baking sheet.

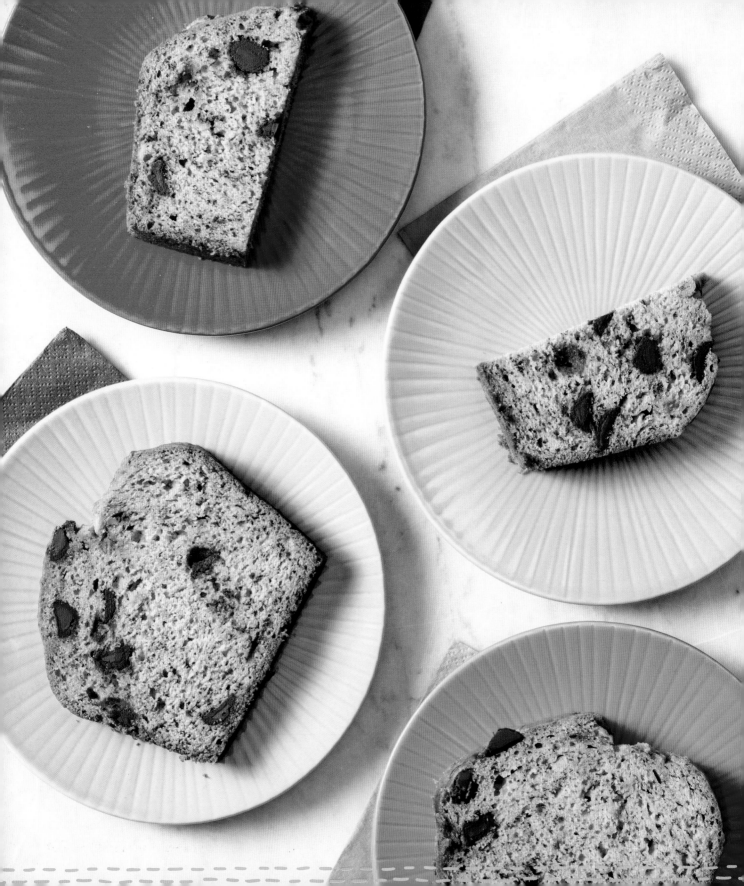

Chocolate-Chip Banana Bread

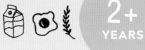

Makes 1 loaf
Total Time: 1 hour and 20 minutes, plus cooling time

Why This Recipe Works

This sweet quick bread is packed with banana flavor and studded with chocolate. The key to great banana bread is ripe bananas. During ripening, some of the starch in bananas converts to sugar, making the baked banana bread sweeter, moister (sugar acts like a liquid in baked goods), and more banana flavored. It's worth keeping frozen ripe bananas on hand so you can make this tasty snack bread whenever you want. The two biggest challenges in this recipe? Keeping the chocolate chips from "disappearing" before they make it into the batter and waiting for the bread to bake and cool.

HOW YOUR CHILD CAN HELP
✓ Make batter in steps 1 and 2 (mashing bananas is a favorite)

Our preferred loaf pan measures 8½ by 4½ inches; if you use a 9-by-5-inch loaf pan, start checking for doneness 5 minutes earlier than advised in the recipe.

2 cups (10 ounces) all-purpose flour
⅔ cup (4⅔ ounces) sugar
¾ teaspoon baking soda
½ teaspoon salt
3 large very ripe bananas
6 tablespoons unsalted butter, melted and cooled
2 large eggs
¼ cup plain whole-milk yogurt
1 teaspoon vanilla extract
⅔ cup chocolate chips

1. Adjust oven rack to lower-middle position and heat oven to 350 degrees. Grease 8½-by-4½-inch loaf pan. Whisk flour, sugar, baking soda, and salt together in large bowl.

2. In separate bowl, use potato masher to mash bananas until smooth. Whisk in melted butter, eggs, yogurt, and vanilla until well combined. Gently fold banana mixture into flour mixture with rubber spatula until just combined (do not overmix). Fold in chocolate chips.

3. Scrape batter into prepared pan and smooth top. Bake until golden brown and toothpick inserted into center comes out with few crumbs attached, about 55 minutes, rotating pan halfway through baking.

4. Let bread cool in pan on wire rack for 10 minutes. Remove bread from pan and let cool completely on rack, about 1 hour. Serve.

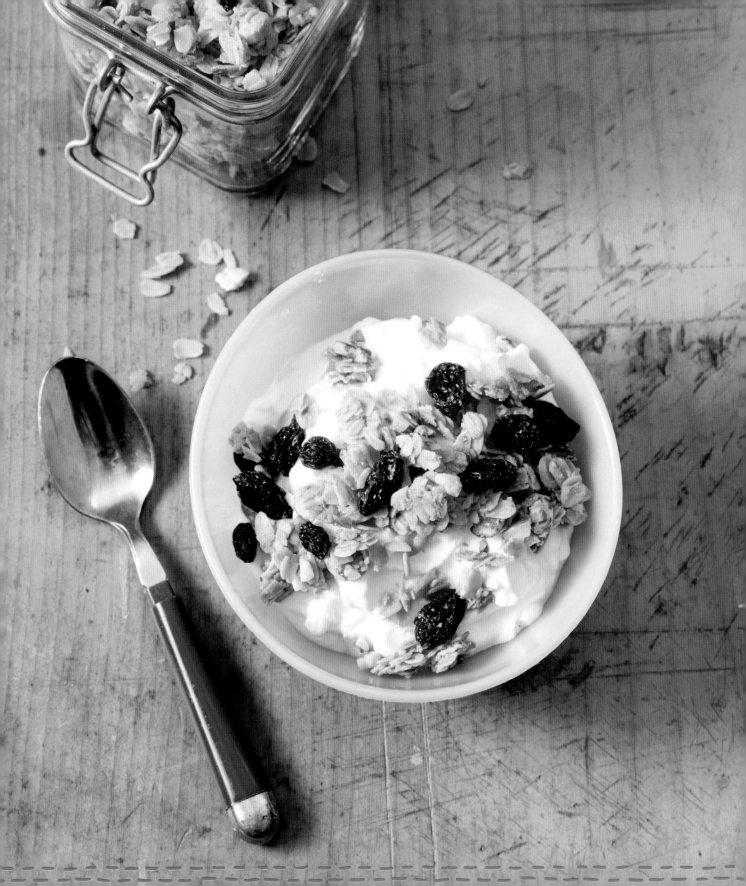

Almond-Raisin Granola

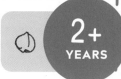

2+ YEARS

Makes 9 cups
Total Time: 1 hour, plus cooling time

Why This Recipe Works

One of the most important steps in one of our favorite granola recipes is to firmly pack the granola mixture inside a rimmed baking sheet before baking. Our preferred tools? The palms of our hands. Or, more specifically, the palms of our kids' hands! Packing the granola firmly helps create large, satisfying clusters (fan favorite for all ages) in the finished granola. Once baked, we had a sheet of granola "bark" that our kid helpers could break into crunchy pieces.

HOW YOUR CHILD CAN HELP
✓ Make oat mixture in step 2
✓ Press oat mixture with hands in step 3
✓ Break cooled granola into pieces in step 4

✳ STORAGE INFORMATION
Granola can be stored in airtight container for up to 2 weeks.

Do not use quick oats here. We prefer to chop the almonds by hand for superior crunch. (A food processor will chop whole nuts unevenly.) You can substitute an equal amount of slivered or sliced almonds, if desired. You can also substitute an equal amount of your favorite dried fruit for the raisins in step 4; coarsely chop larger dried fruits such as apricots.

½ **cup canola oil**
⅓ **cup maple syrup**
⅓ **cup packed (2⅓ ounces) light brown sugar**
4 **teaspoons vanilla extract**
½ **teaspoon salt**

5 **cups (15 ounces) old-fashioned rolled oats**
2 **cups (10 ounces) raw almonds, chopped coarse**
2 **cups (10 ounces) raisins**

1 Adjust oven rack to upper-middle position and heat oven to 325 degrees. Line rimmed baking sheet with parchment paper and spray with vegetable oil spray.

2 Whisk oil, maple syrup, sugar, vanilla, and salt together in large bowl. Fold in oats and almonds until thoroughly combined.

3 Transfer oat mixture to prepared sheet and spread across entire surface of sheet in even layer. Place second sheet of parchment paper over oat mixture. Use your palms to press down firmly on oat mixture until very compact.

4 Bake until lightly browned, 35 to 40 minutes, rotating sheet halfway through baking. Transfer sheet to wire rack and let granola cool completely, about 1 hour. Break cooled granola into pieces of desired size. Stir in raisins and serve.

Strawberry Fruit Leather

Makes 12 strips
Total Time: 1 hour, plus 4½ to 5½ hours baking and cooling time

Why This Recipe Works

We were after a fruit leather that was pleasantly chewy (not tough), delicately sweet (not cloying), and full of fruit flavor (not bland). After dehydrating dozens of different kinds of fruit, our tasting team unanimously chose strawberry as the favorite. We tested our way through batch after batch of pureed strawberries, sugar, and a variety of thickening agents, and we found that simply adding Granny Smith apples, which are high in natural pectin, to the pureed strawberry-sugar mixture gave our finished fruit leather a firm yet tender texture and bright, fruity flavor. Paper backings on the strips not only help with storage but also invoke childhood memories for the adult cooks in the room. Have fun rolling them up, or just eat them straight!

✳ STORAGE INFORMATION

Cut and rolled fruit leather can be stored in airtight container for up to 2 weeks.

You will need a rimless baking sheet for this recipe to ensure even cooking. You can substitute an equal amount of defrosted frozen strawberries for the fresh strawberries.

Vegetable oil spray
1¼ pounds strawberries, hulled and chopped
2 large Granny Smith apples (8 ounces each), peeled, cored, and chopped
¼ cup sugar

1 Adjust oven rack to middle position and heat oven to 200 degrees. Line rimless baking sheet with parchment paper and spray with vegetable oil spray.

2 Place strawberries in blender followed by apples. Pulse until fruit is finely chopped, about 10 pulses, scraping down blender jar as needed. Add sugar and process until very smooth, about 3 minutes, scraping down blender jar as needed.

3 Transfer strawberry mixture to large saucepan and bring to boil over medium-high heat. Reduce heat to medium-low and simmer, adjusting heat as needed and whisking often, until mixture has thickened and reduced to 2 cups, about 30 minutes.

4 Pour strawberry mixture onto center of prepared baking sheet and use offset spatula to spread into 11-by-14-inch rectangle. Gently jiggle and tap baking sheet on counter to create smooth, even layer.

5 Bake until mixture has set, center feels dry but slightly tacky to touch, and fruit leather peels away from parchment cleanly, 4 to 5 hours.

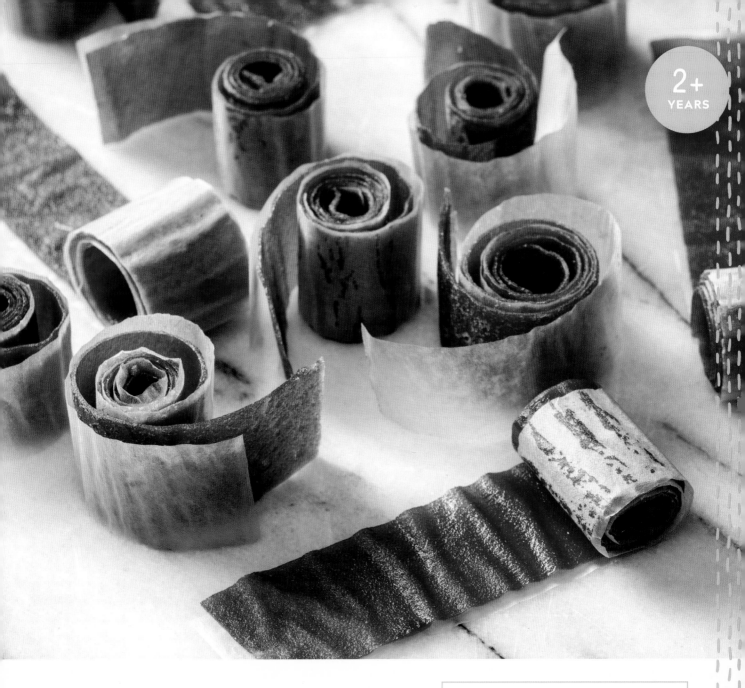

6 Transfer baking sheet to wire rack and let cool completely, about 30 minutes. Use scissors to cut fruit leather (along with parchment paper backing) crosswise into twelve 1-inch strips, trimming away any dry edges as needed. Roll strips into rolls, if desired.

HOW YOUR CHILD CAN HELP
- ✓ Add chopped fruit to blender jar in step 2
- ✓ Cut fruit leather into strips (or whatever shapes they like!) with scissors and roll up strips in step 6

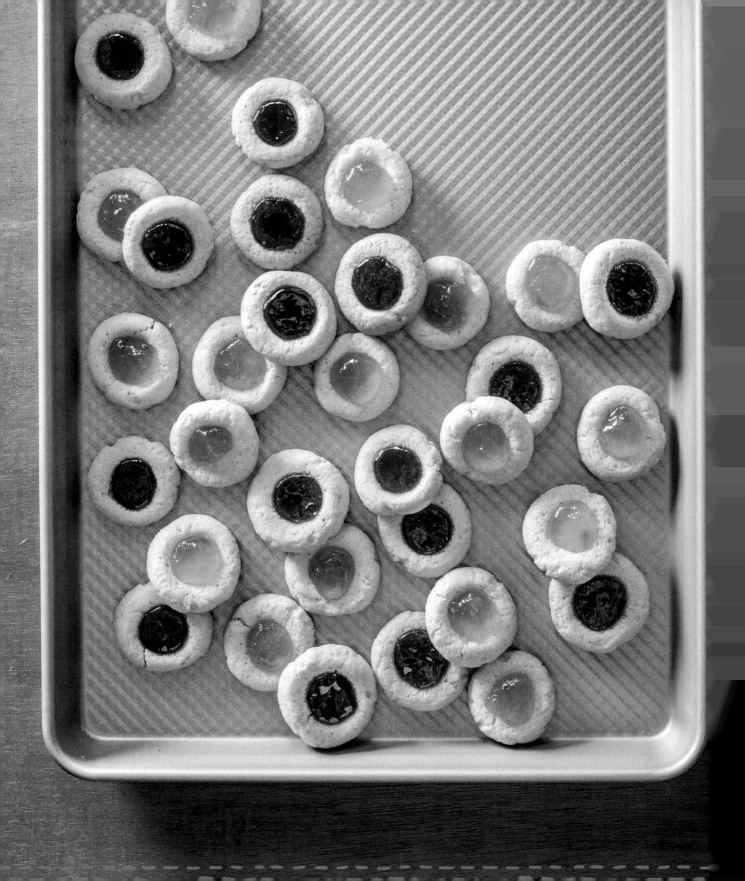

Jam Thumbprint Cookies

2+ YEARS

Makes 24 cookies
Total Time: 45 minutes, plus cooling time

Why This Recipe Works

The joy of making thumbprint cookies with your kids is twofold: toddlers can fill the center indent with any kind of jam they want, and they get to stick their fingers into cookie dough...on purpose. We love the tender crumb of the cookie, which we achieved by adding a little cream cheese to the buttery dough.

HOW YOUR CHILD CAN HELP
✓ Make dough in step 2
✓ Roll dough into balls in step 3
✓ Make thumbprints in dough balls and fill with jam in step 3

You can use any flavor jam you like in this recipe.

1⅛ cups (5⅔ ounces) all-purpose flour
¼ teaspoon salt
¼ teaspoon baking soda
⅛ teaspoon baking powder
6 tablespoons unsalted butter, softened
⅓ cup (2⅓ ounces) sugar
1½ ounces cream cheese, softened
1 large egg yolk
¾ teaspoon vanilla extract
⅓ cup seedless jam

1. Adjust oven rack to middle position and heat oven to 350 degrees. Line rimmed baking sheet with parchment paper.

2. Whisk flour, salt, baking soda, and baking powder together in medium bowl. Combine butter and sugar in large bowl and stir together with wooden spoon until well blended, about 1 minute. Add cream cheese, egg yolk, and vanilla and stir until combined. Add flour mixture to butter mixture and stir until just incorporated.

3. Working with 2 teaspoons dough at a time, roll dough into balls and space them 1 inch apart on prepared sheet (you should have 24 balls). Using thumb, make indentation in center of each dough ball. Fill each indentation with heaping ½ teaspoon jam.

4. Bake until light golden brown, 15 to 18 minutes, rotating sheet halfway through baking. Let cookies cool on sheet for 10 minutes, then transfer to wire rack. Let cookies cool completely before serving.

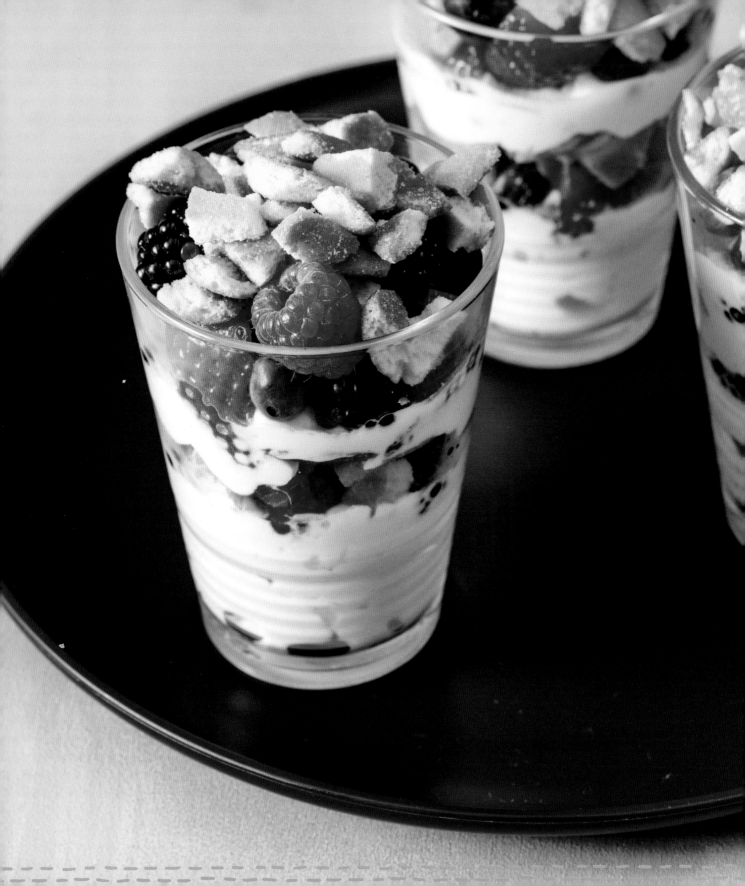

Cookie and Berry Trifle

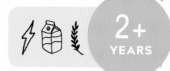

2+ YEARS

Makes four 8-ounce trifles
Total Time: 15 minutes

Why This Recipe Works

Trifles have the potential to be showstopping holiday desserts. They can also be so simple to make that a toddler can participate in almost every step. (And often, they're both!) One of the most satisfying parts of this layered cookie, berry, and cream dessert is crushing up the cookies—a perfect job for your little helper. Plus, assembling the layers in a clear glass or cup is a great way to get creative. Make them all identical or have fun and mix it up.

HOW YOUR CHILD CAN HELP
✓ Crush cookies in step 2
✓ Toss berries together in step 2
✓ Assemble trifles in step 3

Mascarpone is a soft, creamy cow's-milk cheese from Italy that's both slightly sweet and slightly tangy. Mascarpone is usually sold in small containers in the refrigerated section of your market due to its short shelf life. You can crumble 7 graham crackers instead of using Nilla Wafers, if desired. You will need four 8-ounce parfait glasses or glass tumblers for this recipe. If using a handheld electric mixer, increase mixing times by about 1 minute.

3 ounces (⅓ cup) mascarpone cheese
¼ cup (1¾ ounces) sugar
½ teaspoon vanilla extract
⅛ teaspoon salt
¾ cup heavy cream
1½ cups (3 ounces) Nilla Wafer cookies
10 ounces (2 cups) blackberries, blueberries, raspberries, and/or hulled and quartered strawberries

1. Using stand mixer fitted with whisk attachment, whip mascarpone, sugar, vanilla, and salt on medium-high speed until smooth, about 1 minute, scraping down bowl as needed. Reduce speed to low and gradually add cream until combined. Increase speed to medium-high and whip until stiff peaks form, 1 to 2 minutes.

2. Place cookies in large zipper-lock bag and crush into roughly ½-inch pieces with hands or rolling pin. Gently toss berries together in bowl.

3. Spoon ¼ cup cream mixture into each of four 8-ounce parfait glasses or glass tumblers. Top with ¼ cup berries, followed by 2 tablespoons cookies. Repeat layering process with remaining cream mixture, berries, and cookies. Serve.

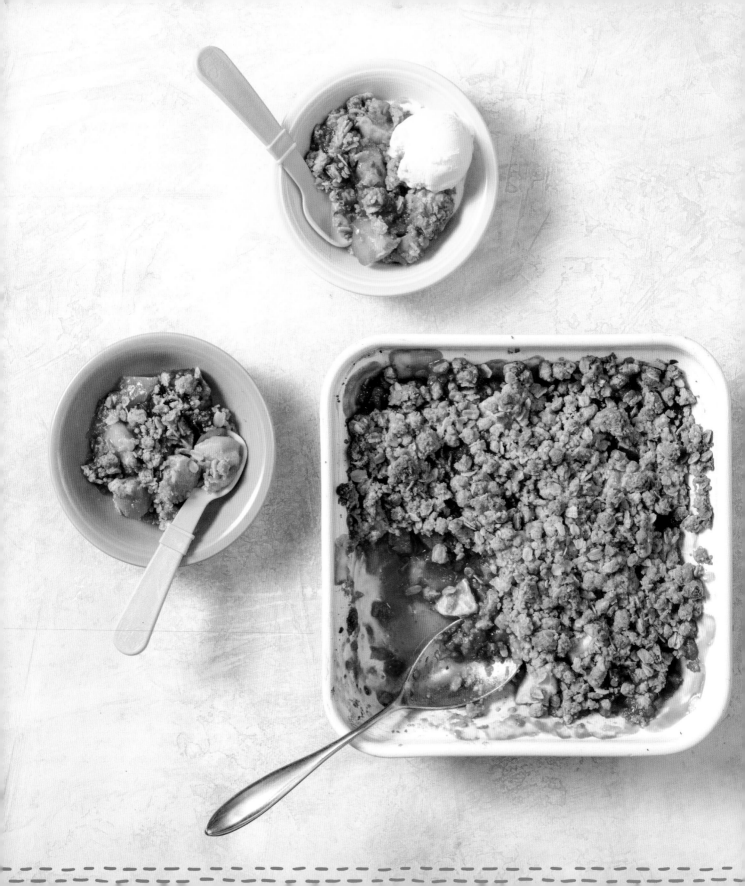

Apple-Raspberry Crisp

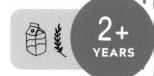

Makes one 8-inch square crisp
Total Time: 1 hour, plus cooling time

Why This Recipe Works

Most fruit crisp recipes call for making the oat-butter topping in a food processor. But where's the fun in that? Instead, we use an old-school kitchen tool: our fingers. Using melted butter and a combination of your and your toddler's digits, you can squish and crumble this topping together in just a few minutes. We used a mixture of apples and raspberries, thickened with a touch of cornstarch, for a brightly colored, tasty fruit filling.

HOW YOUR CHILD CAN HELP
✓ Make crisp topping in step 2
✓ Toss fruit filling together in step 3
✓ Sprinkle topping over fruit in step 3

We like Golden Delicious apples in this recipe, but any sweet, crisp apple such as Honeycrisp or Braeburn can be substituted.

⅔ cup (3⅓ ounces) all-purpose flour
½ cup (1½ ounces) old-fashioned rolled oats
¼ cup packed (1¾ ounces) light brown sugar
½ teaspoon ground cinnamon
¼ teaspoon salt
5 tablespoons unsalted butter, melted and cooled
¼ cup (1¾ ounces) granulated sugar
1 tablespoon cornstarch
2½ pounds Golden Delicious apples, peeled, cored, and cut into 1-inch pieces
6 ounces (1¼ cups) raspberries

1 Adjust oven rack to lower-middle position and heat oven to 375 degrees.

2 Stir flour, oats, brown sugar, cinnamon, and ⅛ teaspoon salt together in medium bowl. Drizzle with melted butter and toss with fork or fingers until evenly moistened and mixture forms small pea-size clumps.

3 Combine granulated sugar, cornstarch, and remaining ⅛ teaspoon salt in large bowl. Add apples and raspberries to bowl and toss to coat. Transfer apple mixture to 8-inch square baking dish. Sprinkle oat topping evenly over apple mixture.

4 Bake until filling is bubbling around edges and topping is golden brown, about 45 minutes. Cool on wire rack for at least 30 minutes before serving.

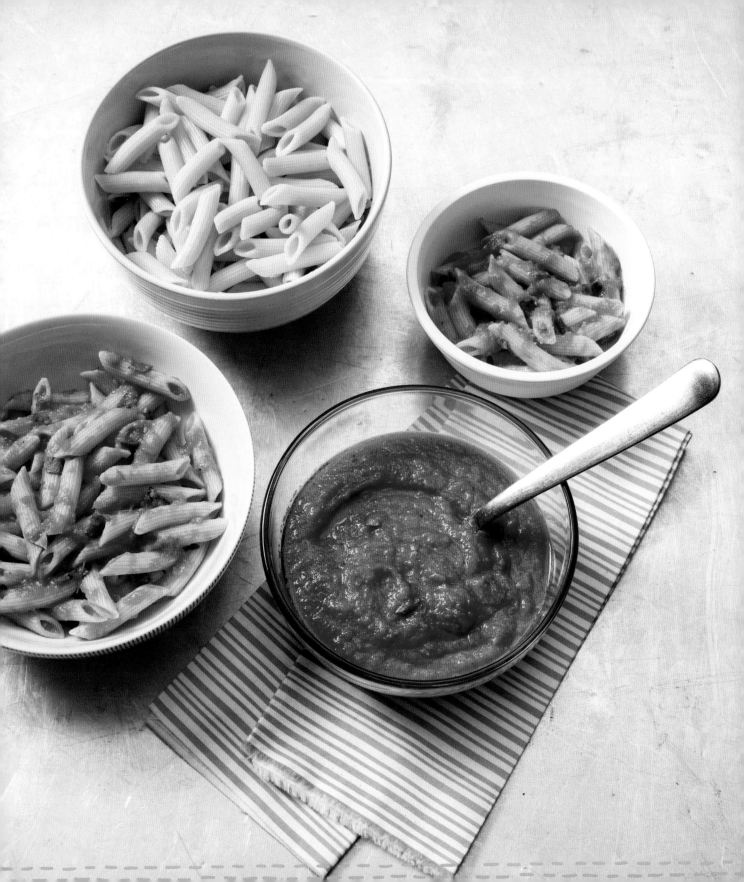

Hand-Squished Roasted Tomato Sauce

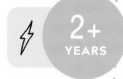

2+ YEARS

Makes 2 cups; enough for 12 ounces pasta
Total Time: 45 minutes

Why This Recipe Works

Tomatoes are filled with flavor—and a lot of water. To make a thick, savory tomato sauce without simmering this fruit (yes, a fruit!) on the stovetop for a long time, we start with our hands. Squeezing out all the extra water and seeds from the fresh tomatoes before roasting them with garlic guarantees a fun time for your toddler. (Just make sure your child is wearing something that washes easily!) Once blended, the sauce has just the right amount of smooth and velvety body without ever hitting the stovetop.

HOW YOUR CHILD CAN HELP

✓ Squeeze tomatoes in step 2
✓ Combine tomatoes with oil and garlic and arrange on baking sheet in step 2
✓ Tear basil leaves into pieces for step 4

2½ pounds vine-ripe tomatoes, cored and halved
4 garlic cloves, peeled and smashed
2 tablespoons extra-virgin olive oil
2 teaspoons sugar
Salt
¼ cup fresh basil leaves, torn

1. Adjust oven rack to upper-middle position and heat oven to 425 degrees. Line rimmed baking sheet with parchment paper.

2. Working over bowl, squeeze each tomato half to remove seeds and excess juice; discard seeds and juice. Transfer tomatoes to large bowl. Stir in garlic, 1 tablespoon oil, sugar, and 1 teaspoon salt; transfer to prepared sheet, arranging tomatoes cut side up in even layer.

3. Bake until tomatoes are very soft and starting to brown around edges, 20 to 25 minutes. Transfer sheet to wire rack and let tomatoes cool slightly, about 5 minutes.

4. Carefully transfer tomatoes, garlic, and any accumulated juices from sheet to food processor. Process until smooth, about 1 minute, scraping down bowl as needed. Transfer sauce to clean bowl and stir in remaining 1 tablespoon oil and basil. Season with salt to taste. Serve.

Baked Arancini

Makes 12 arancini
Total Time: 1 hour and 45 minutes

Why This Recipe Works

Arancini are heavenly balls of risotto stuffed with meat, cheese, or peas, coated in bread crumbs, and then deep fried. In other words, too much work when your cooking partner is a kid. For our streamlined version, we started with a hands-free risotto technique—just cook the rice and broth together, stir a few times along the way, and you're done. Really! Then we chilled the rice to firm it up and get it ready for filling. Here's where your child comes in: forming the rice balls, poking holes in the balls and filling them with cheese, and coating the balls in bread crumbs before baking.

HOW YOUR CHILD CAN HELP
✓ Rub panko mixture with fingers in step 5
✓ Roll risotto into balls and fill with mozzarella in step 6
✓ Coat balls in panko mixture in step 7

We chose a simple filling of cubed mozzarella, but for more adventurous eaters, you can substitute ¼ cup diced ham, chopped baby spinach, or frozen peas for half of mozzarella; use 1 teaspoon ham, spinach, or peas in place of one piece of cheese in step 6.

2¼ cups chicken broth
3 tablespoons extra-virgin olive oil
1 shallot, minced
Salt and pepper
¾ cup Arborio rice
¼ cup dry white wine

1 ounce Parmesan cheese, grated (½ cup)
⅓ cup panko bread crumbs
2 ounces mozzarella cheese, cut into 24 pieces (about ½-inch cubes)

1. Bring broth to boil in medium saucepan over high heat. Cover and reduce heat to low. Heat 1 tablespoon oil in large saucepan over medium heat until shimmering. Add shallot and ¼ teaspoon salt and cook until softened, about 3 minutes. Add rice and cook, stirring frequently, until grains are translucent around edges, about 3 minutes.

2. Add wine and cook, stirring constantly, until fully absorbed, 2 to 3 minutes. Stir in 2 cups hot broth and bring to boil; reduce heat to low, cover, and simmer until almost all liquid has been absorbed and rice is tender, 16 to 18 minutes, stirring twice during cooking.

3. Uncover and stir gently and constantly until risotto becomes creamy, about 1 minute. Remove saucepan from heat and stir in ¼ cup Parmesan. Transfer risotto to large bowl, spread in thin layer, and let cool to room temperature, about 10 minutes. Transfer bowl to refrigerator and chill risotto until firm, at least 1 hour and up to 24 hours.

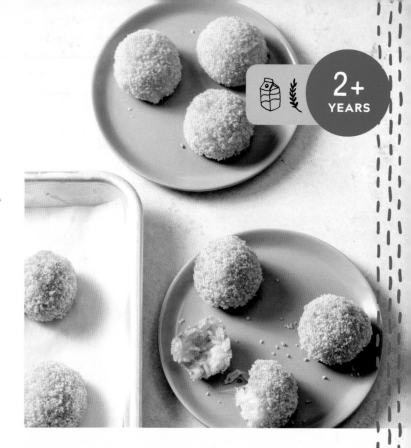

4 Adjust oven rack to middle position and heat oven to 425 degrees. Line rimmed baking sheet with parchment paper.

5 Combine panko and remaining ¼ cup Parmesan in shallow dish. Drizzle with remaining 2 tablespoons oil and rub mixture between your fingers until well combined and no clumps remain; set aside.

6 Divide risotto into 12 equal portions (about 2 tablespoons each). Using lightly moistened hands, roll each portion into ball. Use your finger to make a hole in each ball, then fill each hole with 2 pieces of mozzarella (see "Filling and Coating Arancini," below). Carefully press risotto together to seal hole and reshape into ball.

7 Roll each ball in panko mixture to coat thoroughly, pressing lightly to help crumbs adhere. Arrange balls evenly on prepared sheet.

8 Bake arancini until crisp and lightly browned, about 25 minutes, rotating sheet halfway through baking. Let arancini cool slightly, about 5 minutes. Serve warm.

TOMATO-BASIL BAKED ARANCINI

Substitute 1 tablespoon tomato paste for wine in step 2 and cook until fragrant, about 30 seconds. Add pinch of shredded fresh basil to mozzarella in each ball in step 6.

FILLING AND COATING ARANCINI

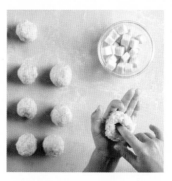

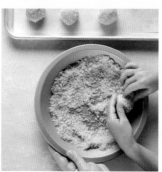

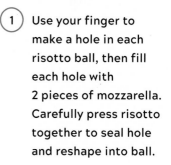

1 Use your finger to make a hole in each risotto ball, then fill each hole with 2 pieces of mozzarella. Carefully press risotto together to seal hole and reshape into ball.

2 Roll each ball in panko mixture to coat thoroughly, pressing lightly to help crumbs adhere. Arrange balls evenly on prepared sheet.

Veggie Dumplings

Makes 24 dumplings
Total Time: 1 hour and 15 minutes

Why This Recipe Works

Making these Chinese-style dumplings (a.k.a. pot stickers) is a great rainy-day activity (or, let's be real, an any-day activity). To be sure our vegetarian dumplings were free of excess moisture (which would make them soggy), we first salted and drained the cabbage and carrots. Brushing the edges of the dumpling wrapper with water helped them seal properly. A sequence of browning, steaming, and then cranking up the heat produced pot stickers with a pleasing balance between soft and crispy textures.

We prefer to use round gyoza wrappers in this recipe, but (slightly thinner) round or square wonton wrappers can be used in their place. If using square wrappers, fold diagonally into a triangle before pinching to seal; for round or square wonton wrappers, adjust steaming time in step 5 to 6 minutes. Serve with soy sauce for dipping, if desired.

½ **head napa cabbage, minced (3 cups)**
2 **carrots, peeled and shredded (1⅓ cups)**
½ **teaspoon salt**
4 **scallions, sliced thin**
1 **tablespoon soy sauce, plus more for serving**
2 **teaspoons toasted sesame oil**
1 **teaspoon grated fresh ginger**
1 **garlic clove, minced**
24 **(3½-inch) round gyoza wrappers**
2 **tablespoons canola oil**
1 **cup water, plus extra for brushing**

1. Toss cabbage and carrots with salt in colander and let drain in sink for 20 minutes; press gently to squeeze out excess moisture.

2. Transfer drained cabbage and carrots to medium bowl. Stir in scallions, soy sauce, sesame oil, ginger, and garlic.

3. Working with 4 wrappers at a time (cover others with moist paper towel), place scant tablespoon vegetable filling in center of each wrapper. Brush edges of wrappers with water. Fold wrappers in half and pinch dumplings closed, pressing out any air pockets (see "Shaping Dumplings," right). Transfer to baking sheet and cover with damp dish towel. Repeat with remaining wrappers and filling to make a total of 24 dumplings.

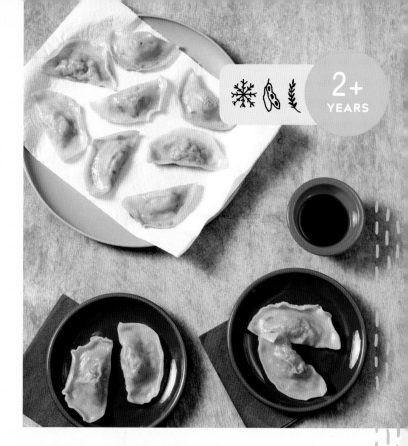

4   Brush 1 tablespoon oil over bottom of 12-inch nonstick skillet and arrange half of dumplings in skillet, flat side facing down (they may overlap). Cook over medium heat, without moving them, until golden brown on bottom, 3 to 4 minutes.

5   Reduce heat to low, add ½ cup water, and cover. Cook until most of water is absorbed and wrappers are slightly translucent, 8 to 10 minutes. Uncover, increase heat to medium, and cook, without stirring dumplings, until bottoms are well browned and crisp, 1 to 2 minutes; transfer to paper-towel-lined plate.

6   Wipe out skillet with paper towels and repeat with remaining oil, dumplings, and water.

HOW YOUR CHILD CAN HELP

✓ Make filling in steps 1 and 2
✓ Brush wrappers with water in step 3
✓ Fold, pinch, and seal dumplings in step 3

✳ STORAGE INFORMATION

Uncooked dumplings can be refrigerated for up to 24 hours or frozen for up to 1 month. To freeze, prepare dumplings through step 3 and place filled, uncooked dumplings in freezer in single layer on plate until frozen, then transfer to storage bag. There's no need to thaw frozen dumplings; just add about 5 minutes to steaming time.

SHAPING DUMPLINGS

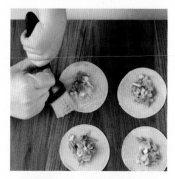

1   Working with 4 wrappers at a time (cover others with moist paper towel), place scant tablespoon of filling in center of each wrapper. Brush edges of wrappers with water.

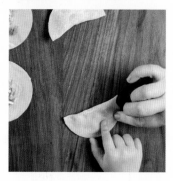

2   Fold wrapper in half and pinch dumpling closed, pressing out any air pockets.

Cheese Calzones

Makes 2 calzones
Total Time: 45 minutes, plus cooling time

Why This Recipe Works

Pizza gets way more attention than calzones, especially in the world of kids. But dough that's easy to shape, simple to cook, and filled with delicious melted cheese? Yes, please. To simplify the calzone-making process, we used store-bought pizza dough and jarred marinara sauce for dipping. We rolled out, assembled, and sealed up the calzones on a baking sheet before putting them in the oven. And voilà! Handheld pizza pockets for everyone.

HOW YOUR CHILD CAN HELP
- ✓ Make cheese filling in step 2
- ✓ Shape dough in step 3
- ✓ Fill calzone and seal dough in step 4
- ✓ Brush tops of calzones with egg wash in step 5

Our favorite jarred marinara sauce is Rao's Homemade Marinara Sauce.

6 ounces (¾ cup) whole-milk ricotta cheese
4 ounces mozzarella cheese, shredded (1 cup)
1 ounce Parmesan cheese, grated (½ cup)
1 garlic clove, minced
½ teaspoon dried oregano
⅛ teaspoon pepper
1 pound pizza dough, room temperature
1 large egg, lightly beaten
1 cup jarred marinara sauce, warmed

1 Adjust oven rack to lower-middle position and heat oven to 500 degrees. Line baking sheet with parchment paper.

2 Combine ricotta, mozzarella, Parmesan, garlic, oregano, and pepper in bowl.

3 Place dough on lightly floured counter and divide in half. Press and roll one piece of dough into 9-inch round of even thickness. Transfer to one side of prepared sheet and reshape as needed. Repeat shaping with remaining piece of dough and transfer to other side of prepared sheet.

4 Divide cheese filling between dough rounds, spreading over half of each round and leaving 1-inch border. Brush edges with beaten egg. Fold dough over filling (see "Shaping Calzones," right). Using fingers, pinch edges of dough together to seal. Then fold ½ inch of dough up and press again firmly to crimp dough.

5 Using sharp paring knife, cut 5 steam vents, each about 1½ inches long, in top of each calzone. Brush tops with beaten egg.

6 Bake calzones until golden brown, 13 to 15 minutes, rotating sheet halfway through baking. Transfer calzones to wire rack and discard parchment. Let cool for 10 minutes. Serve with marinara for dipping.

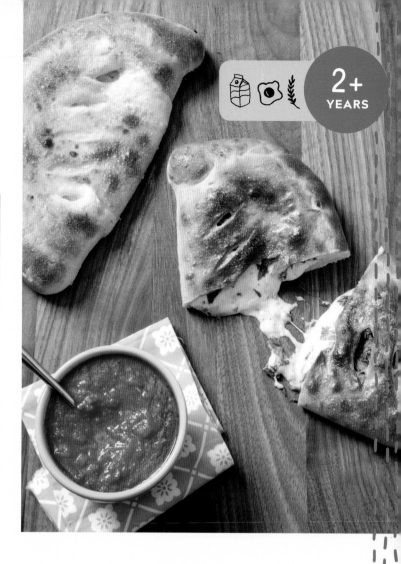

BELL PEPPER CALZONES
Microwave 1 chopped bell pepper in covered bowl until softened, 2 to 3 minutes. Let cool slightly, about 5 minutes. Divide microwaved pepper in half and sprinkle over each cheese filling mound in step 4.

PEPPERONI CALZONES
Arrange 12 thin slices pepperoni (¾ ounce) over each cheese filling mound in step 4.

SPINACH CALZONES
Chop 2 cups baby spinach. Arrange 1 cup chopped baby spinach over each cheese filling mound in step 4.

SHAPING CALZONES

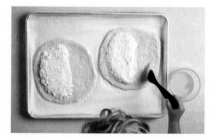

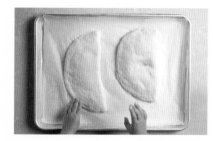

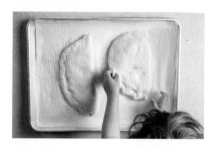

1 Divide cheese filling between dough rounds, spreading over half of each round and leaving 1-inch border. Brush edges with beaten egg.

2 Fold dough over filling. Using fingers, pinch edges of dough together to seal.

3 Fold ½ inch of dough up and press again firmly to crimp dough.

Bean, Cheese, and Spinach Enchiladas

Makes 12 enchiladas
Total Time: 1 hour and 20 minutes

Why This Recipe Works

Enchiladas don't need to be complicated. Our vegetarian version is simple but flavorful— with lots of mashing, mixing, brushing, and rolling for your little helpers to do. A great enchilada isn't possible without a great sauce; we start with canned tomato sauce and then flavor it with sautéed onion plus garlic, chili powder, and cumin. For the filling, we smashed some canned black beans to create a quick "refried" bean base, and then we added some whole beans, creamy Monterey Jack cheese, spinach, and just enough sauce to bind it all together.

HOW YOUR CHILD CAN HELP

✓ Make filling in step 3
✓ Brush tortillas with oil in step 4
✓ Roll up tortillas in step 5
✓ Sprinkle enchiladas with cheese in step 5

Serve with your favorite enchilada garnishes, such as sour cream, diced avocado, sliced radishes, shredded romaine lettuce, or lime wedges.

3 tablespoons canola oil
1 onion, chopped fine
Salt and pepper
3 garlic cloves, minced
2 teaspoons ground chili powder
1½ teaspoons ground cumin
3 (8-ounce) cans tomato sauce
½ cup water
2 (15-ounce) cans black beans, rinsed
8 ounces Monterey Jack cheese, shredded (2 cups)
3 ounces baby spinach, chopped (3 cups)
12 (6-inch) corn tortillas
2 tablespoons chopped fresh cilantro

1 Adjust oven rack to middle position and heat oven to 400 degrees. Heat 1 tablespoon oil in medium saucepan over medium heat until shimmering. Add onion and ½ teaspoon salt and cook until softened, 5 to 7 minutes. Stir in garlic, chili powder, and cumin and cook until fragrant, about 30 seconds. Stir in tomato sauce and water. Bring to a simmer and cook until slightly thickened, about 5 minutes. Remove saucepan from heat.

2 Spread ½ cup sauce over bottom of 13-by-9-inch baking dish. Let remaining sauce cool to room temperature, about 10 minutes.

3 Place half of beans in large bowl and use potato masher to mash beans until smooth but some pieces remain. Stir in remaining whole beans, 1 cup cheese, spinach, and ½ cup cooled sauce. Season with salt and pepper to taste.

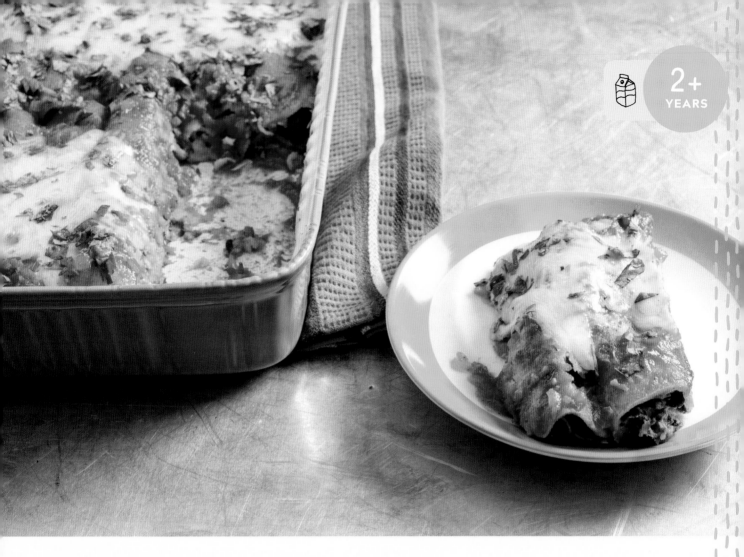

4 Brush both sides of tortillas with remaining 2 tablespoons oil.
   Stack tortillas, wrap in damp dish towel, and place on plate;
   microwave until warm and pliable, about 1 minute.

5 Spread ¼ cup bean filling across center of each tortilla. Roll
   each tortilla tightly around filling and place seam side down
   in baking dish. Pour remaining sauce over top of enchiladas to
   cover completely. Sprinkle remaining 1 cup cheese over top of
   enchiladas.

6 Cover dish tightly with greased aluminum foil. Bake until
   enchiladas are heated through and cheese is melted, about
   25 minutes. Let cool for 5 minutes, sprinkle with cilantro,
   and serve.

Parmesan Bread Shapes

Makes 12 bread sticks
Total Time: 30 minutes, plus rising time

Why This Recipe Works

Start with store-bought pizza dough, butter, garlic, and Parmesan cheese. End with the best bread sticks—or twists or coils or any other shape. We cut the dough into 12 strips, which gave us pieces just the right size for young hands to create fanciful shapes. After brushing the dough with melted butter flavored with a hint of garlic and sprinkling them with Parmesan cheese, they only needed to bake for 10 minutes. A final brushing with garlic butter added a burst of savory flavor and helped keep the twists tender as they cooled.

✳ STORAGE INFORMATION

Bread sticks can be stored at room temperature for up to 2 days. To serve, reheat in 350-degree oven for 5 minutes.

Serve with Hand-Squished Roasted Tomato Sauce (page 213) or your favorite dip. Make sure to let the pizza dough come to room temperature before shaping the dough.

Vegetable oil spray
1 pound pizza dough, room temperature
4 tablespoons unsalted butter, melted and cooled
⅛ teaspoon garlic powder
1 ounce Parmesan cheese, grated (½ cup)

1 Line rimmed baking sheet with parchment paper and spray parchment with vegetable oil spray. Spray countertop lightly with vegetable oil spray. Transfer dough to greased counter and press and stretch dough into 12-by-6-inch rectangle, with long side parallel to counter edge. Using pizza cutter or chef's knife, cut dough crosswise at 1-inch intervals into 12 strips; cover loosely with greased plastic.

2 Working with one piece of dough at a time (keep remaining pieces covered), stretch and roll into 14-inch rope. Shape each rope into desired shapes (see "Two Options for Bread Shapes," right).

3 Arrange shaped pieces of dough on prepared sheet about 1 inch apart. Cover loosely with greased plastic and let rise until nearly doubled in size, 1 to 1½ hours.

4 Adjust oven rack to middle position and heat oven to 450 degrees. In small bowl, stir together melted butter and garlic powder. Brush shaped dough with 2 tablespoons garlic butter and sprinkle each with 2 teaspoons grated Parmesan.

5 Bake until bread sticks are golden brown, about 10 minutes, rotating sheet halfway through baking. Transfer bread sticks to wire rack. Brush with remaining 2 tablespoons garlic butter and let cool for 10 minutes. Serve warm.

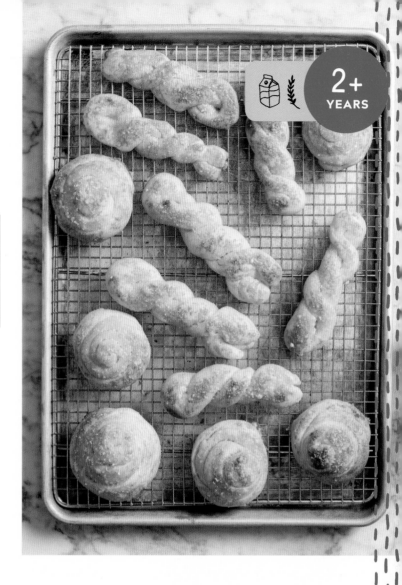

HOW YOUR CHILD CAN HELP
✓ Stretch, roll, and shape dough in step 2
✓ Make garlic butter in step 4
✓ Brush dough shapes with garlic butter and sprinkle with cheese in step 4

TWO OPTIONS FOR BREAD SHAPES

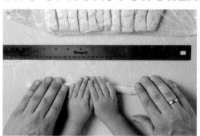

1 Stretch and roll each piece of dough into 14-inch rope.

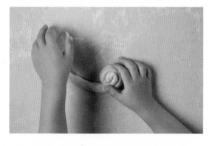

2A Coil rope of dough into spiral, tucking end underneath.

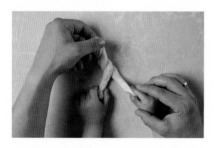

2B Shape rope into U shape. Wrap ends over each other three times to create twist, then pinch ends together.

Whole-Wheat Sesame Crackers

Makes 30 crackers
Total Time: 1 hour, plus cooling time

Why This Recipe Works

Toddlers and snack crackers are like peanut butter and jelly—practically inseparable. Traditionally, homemade crackers are made by rolling dough out into a flat, thin, even layer and then cutting it into uniform shapes. That can be tricky even for an adult, so instead we smushed little mounds of dough—with the help of plastic wrap (to avoid sticking) and a drinking glass—until they became flat disks. Kids can participate in every step, from mixing to smushing, for these frustration- and rolling pin–free snacks.

HOW YOUR CHILD CAN HELP
✓ Make dough in steps 2 and 3
✓ Roll dough into balls in step 4
✓ Press dough balls flat in step 5

1 cup (5½ ounces) whole-wheat flour
2 tablespoons sesame seeds
1 tablespoon sugar
½ teaspoon salt
4 tablespoons unsalted butter, cut into ¼-inch pieces and chilled
5 tablespoons cold water

1. Adjust oven racks to lower-middle and upper-middle positions and heat oven to 350 degrees. Line 2 rimless baking sheets with parchment paper.

2. Whisk flour, sesame seeds, sugar, and salt together in large bowl. Add butter to flour mixture. Using your fingertips, work butter into flour mixture until it resembles coarse meal with a few slightly larger butter lumps.

3. Add water and stir with rubber spatula until dough forms. Knead in bowl using your hands just until dough comes together, about 30 seconds. Shape dough into disk and wrap dough in plastic wrap; refrigerate until dough is slightly chilled and no longer sticky, about 20 minutes.

4. Working with 1 heaping teaspoon dough at a time, roll dough into balls and space them evenly on prepared sheets (about 15 dough balls per sheet). Cover sheets loosely with plastic wrap.

5. With plastic still in place, use bottom of drinking glass to press each dough ball very flat and thin and about 2½ inches in diameter (see "Shaping Crackers," right). Peel away and discard plastic wrap.

6. Bake until crackers are browned around edges, 20 to 24 minutes, switching and rotating sheets halfway through baking. Let crackers cool completely on sheets. Serve.

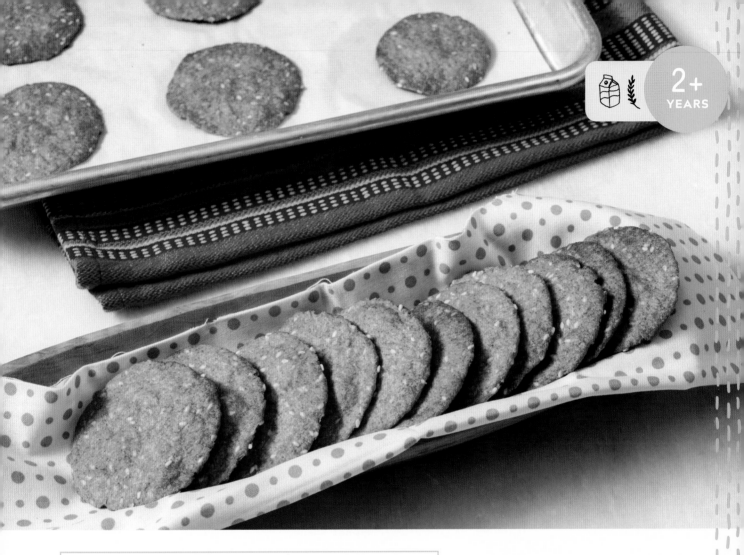

WHOLE-WHEAT EVERYTHING CRACKERS

Reduce sesame seeds to 1½ teaspoons. Add 1½ teaspoons poppy seeds, 1½ teaspoons dried minced garlic, and 1½ teaspoons dried minced onion to flour mixture in step 2.

WHOLE-WHEAT SEA SALT CRACKERS

Reduce salt in dough to ¼ teaspoon. Sprinkle 1 teaspoon sea salt flakes evenly over crackers before baking in step 6.

SHAPING CRACKERS

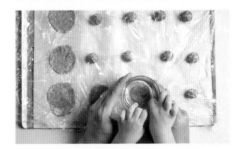

With plastic still in place, use bottom of drinking glass to press each dough ball very flat and thin and about 2½ inches in diameter.

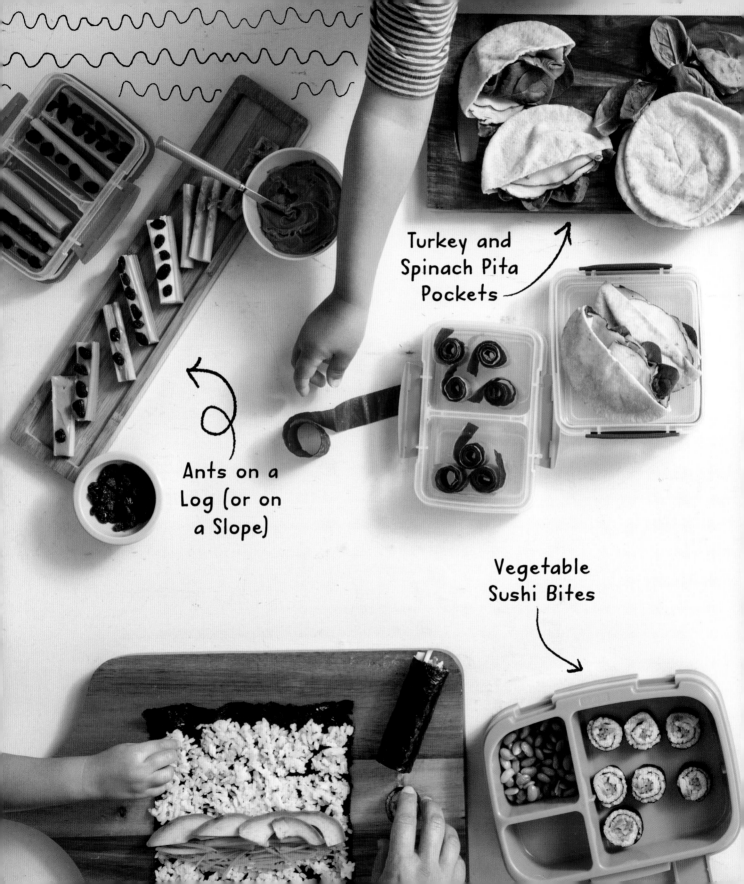

Turkey and Spinach Pita Pockets

Ants on a Log (or on a Slope)

Vegetable Sushi Bites

LUNCHES for PRESCHOOL (and Beyond)

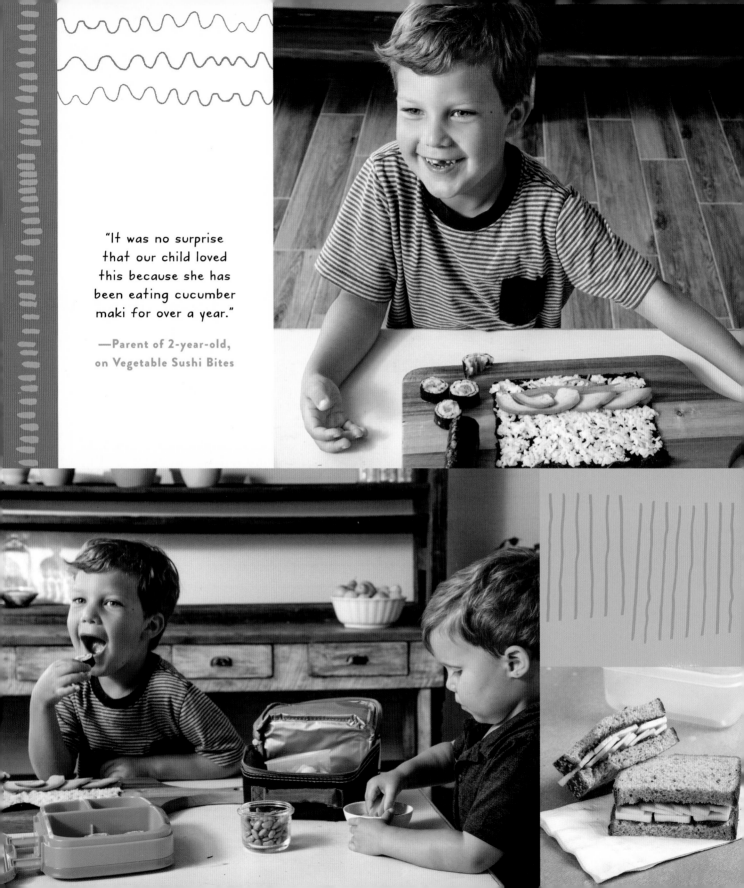

"It was no surprise that our child loved this because she has been eating cucumber maki for over a year."

—Parent of 2-year-old, on Vegetable Sushi Bites

ALL ABOUT LUNCHES FOR PRESCHOOL (and Beyond)

The pack-a-lunch struggle is real. To pack a lunch perfectly means packing a lunch your kid will enjoy (or at least consume) and that is healthy enough that *you're* not packing on any guilt. To do this, you need to balance a seemingly implausible number of conflicting desires. Not to mention all the other little questions: raw versus cooked, bento box versus paper bag, thermos versus ice pack, hot versus room temperature. Who has the energy for creativity? Or even the time to Google "what to pack for preschool lunch"?

We've got you. We created a chapter of recipes ready to go into your kiddo's lunch box (or to eat at home). Some are simple and fast (but still fun), like our Cream Cheese Sandwich with Carrots and Bell Pepper (page 231). Others take a bit more work up front but provide special lunches all week, like our Indian-Style Potato Hand Pies (page 252). All are easily portable, created with a healthy mix of ingredients in mind, and are meant to be eaten at room temperature (minus a hot soup for your favorite kid-friendly thermos).

Like most recipes in this book, these are not recipes just for kids. If you're not packing some Mini Falafels with Yogurt Sauce (page 243) and Vegetable Sushi Bites (page 248) in your own lunch box in the near future, we'd be surprised.

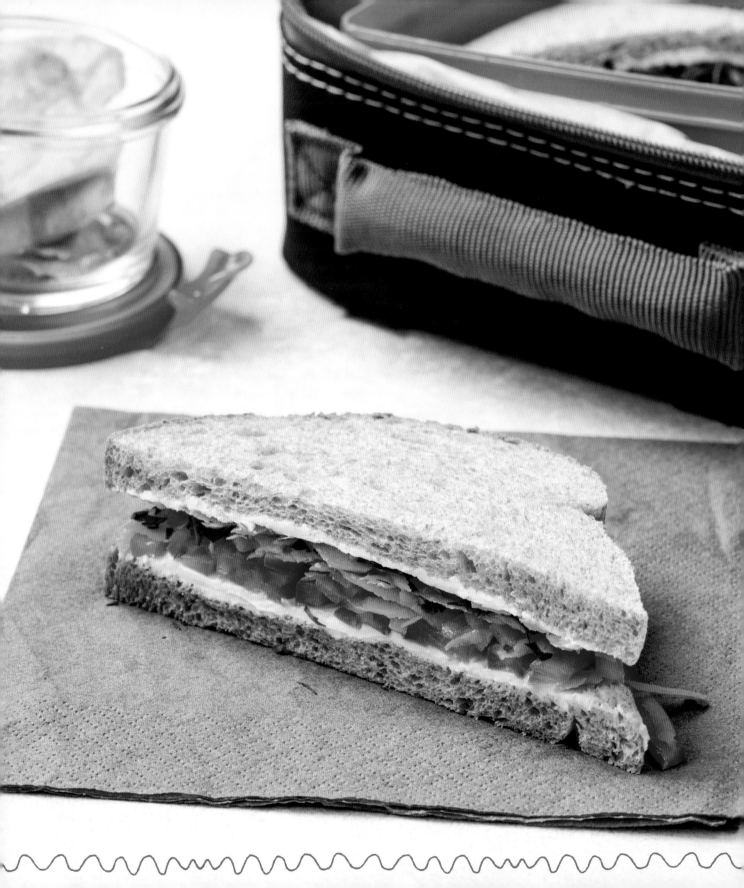

Cream Cheese Sandwich with Carrots and Bell Pepper

Makes 1 sandwich
Total Time: 10 minutes

Why This Recipe Works

Cream cheese is not just for bagels. It makes a wonderful base for a veggie-packed (but still very kid-friendly) sandwich. Carrot and bell peppers are naturally sweet and a nice, crunchy contrast to the thick, creamy cream cheese. Shredding the vegetables makes them easy to eat, especially for tiny humans. Chopped fresh parsley adds a pop of green. What's better than kids having their vegetables and eating them, too?

Other types of bread can be substituted for whole-wheat bread.

2 tablespoons cream cheese
2 slices hearty whole-wheat sandwich bread
½ small red bell pepper, sliced thin
1 tablespoon chopped fresh parsley
1 small carrot, peeled and shredded (½ cup)
Salt and pepper

1. Spread 1 tablespoon cream cheese over each slice of bread. Arrange bell pepper in even layer on one slice of bread, followed by parsley, and then carrots. Season with salt and pepper to taste.

2. Top with remaining slice of bread, with cream cheese on inside. Cut sandwich in half. Serve or pack in lunch box.

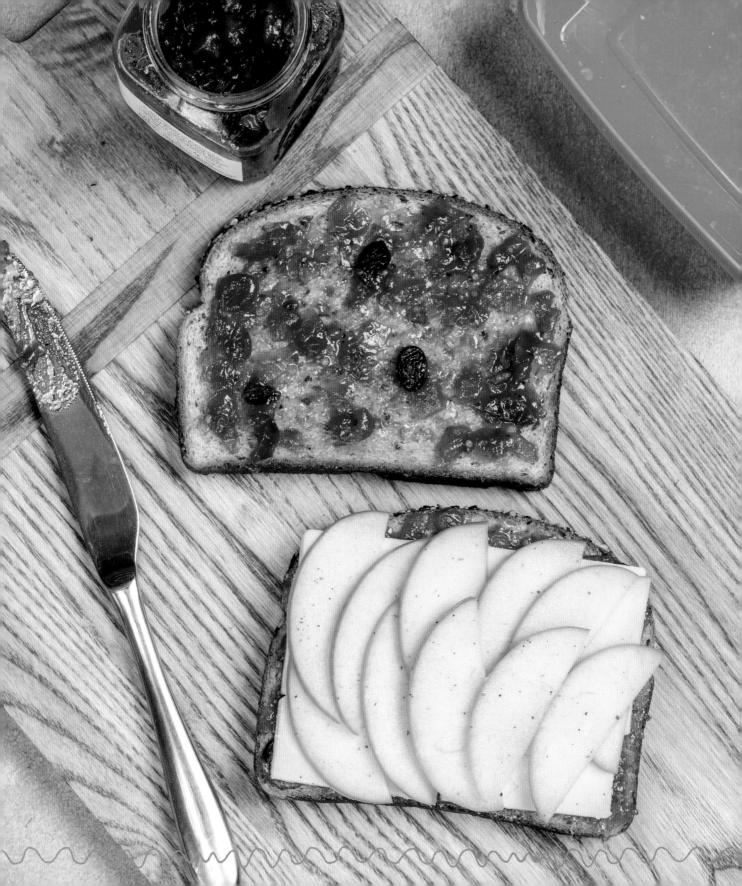

Cheddar Cheese, Chutney, and Apple Sandwich

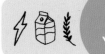

2+ YEARS

Makes 1 sandwich
Total Time: 10 minutes

Why This Recipe Works

This simple sandwich is all about balancing flavors and textures. Sweet and gooey apple chutney plays off tart and crisp Granny Smith apples, while sharp and creamy cheddar cheese keeps this lunch from veering into dessert territory. Think of this as a special kids' cheese plate between two pieces of bread.

Different brands of store-bought apple chutneys vary widely. For this sandwich, we recommend using a chutney with a complementary fruit ingredient like cranberry, rather than a spice-forward one such as ginger. Other types of bread can be substituted for the multigrain bread.

2 tablespoons apple chutney
2 slices hearty multigrain
    sandwich bread
2 ounces sharp (or
    extra-sharp) cheddar
    cheese, cut into ¼-inch-
    thick pieces

¼ Granny Smith apple,
    sliced thin
Salt and pepper

1. Spread 1 tablespoon chutney evenly over each slice of bread. Arrange cheese slices in even layer on one slice of bread, followed by apple. Season with salt and pepper to taste.

2. Top with remaining bread slice, with chutney on inside. Cut in half. Serve or pack in lunch box.

Hummus and Cucumber Lavash Roll-Up

Makes 1 sandwich
Total Time: 10 minutes

Why This Recipe Works

Hummus is a hit with all ages, and we use a healthy amount as the base in this wrap made with lavash, a Middle Eastern flatbread. We toss sweet cherry tomatoes and crunchy cucumbers with a little extra-virgin olive oil, and then we put them all on a bed of crisp romaine lettuce. This is a salad that kids *should* pick up with their hands.

Lavash can often be found near the tortillas in the supermarket. These flatbreads are often sold in a 12-by-9-inch size; to make this roll-up manageable for kids, we recommend cutting flatbreads of this size in half (save the other half for another day). A tortilla can be used in place of lavash.

¼ cucumber, cut into ¼-inch pieces (¼ cup)
2 cherry tomatoes, cut into eighths
1 teaspoon extra-virgin olive oil
Salt and pepper
1 (12-by-9-inch) lavash, cut in half
¼ cup plain hummus
¼ cup shredded romaine lettuce

1. Toss cucumber, cherry tomatoes, and oil together in small bowl. Season with salt and pepper to taste.

2. Lay one lavash half on clean counter with short edge of lavash parallel to counter edge (save other half for later use). Spread hummus evenly over lavash, leaving ½-inch border around edge. Arrange lettuce in even layer over bottom third of lavash, then top with cucumber-tomato mixture.

3. Fold up bottom of lavash over filling (see "Rolling a Wrap," right), followed by sides, then roll tightly into cylinder. Cut sandwich in half. Serve or pack in lunch box.

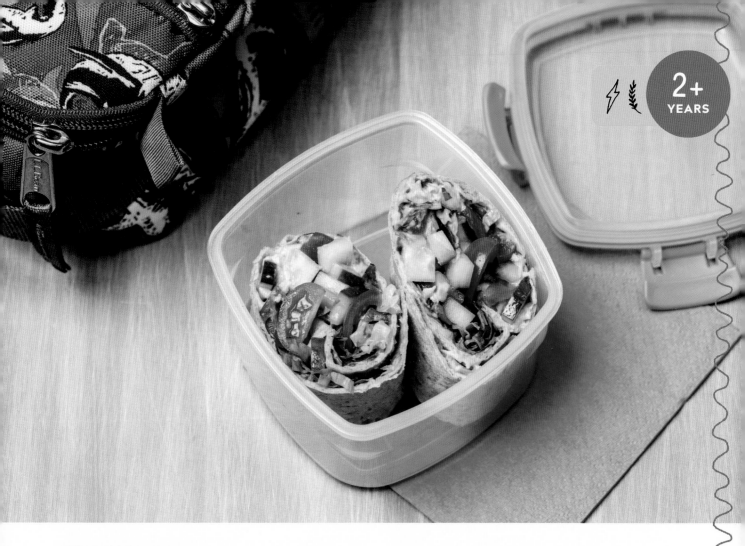

2+ YEARS

ROLLING A WRAP

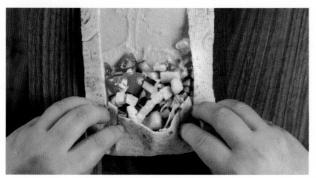

(1) Fold up bottom of lavash over filling, followed by sides. Hold ends of lavash and begin to roll forward.

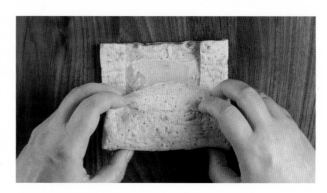

(2) Continue to roll tightly into cylinder.

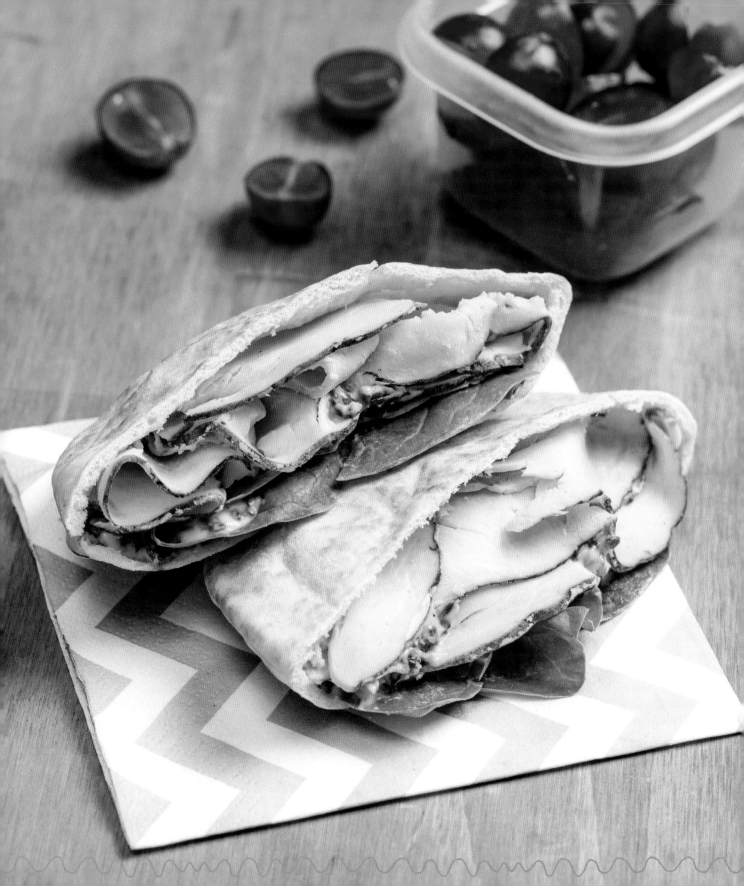

Turkey and Spinach Pita Pockets

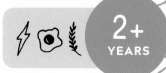

2+ YEARS

Makes 1 sandwich
Total Time: 5 minutes

Why This Recipe Works

Turkey sandwiches are always a good option to have in your packed-lunch repertoire, and this jazzed-up version couldn't be simpler to make. The magic comes with a simple flavor addition: we punch up regular mayonnaise with just a little finely chopped sun-dried tomatoes and spread that inside pita bread. Sliced turkey and baby spinach round out the sandwich. We understand that lunch often needs to be easy and quick, but it should always be tasty.

If you don't have sun-dried tomatoes, you can substitute a few drops of sriracha or even a little ketchup to add some pep to your regular mayonnaise.

1 tablespoon mayonnaise
1 teaspoon finely chopped oil-packed sun-dried tomatoes

1 (5-inch) pita bread
2 slices turkey breast
½ cup baby spinach

1 Stir mayonnaise and sun-dried tomatoes together in small bowl. Cut pita in half. Spread mayonnaise mixture evenly on inside of each pita bread half.

2 Stuff each half of pita bread with turkey and spinach. Serve or pack in lunch box.

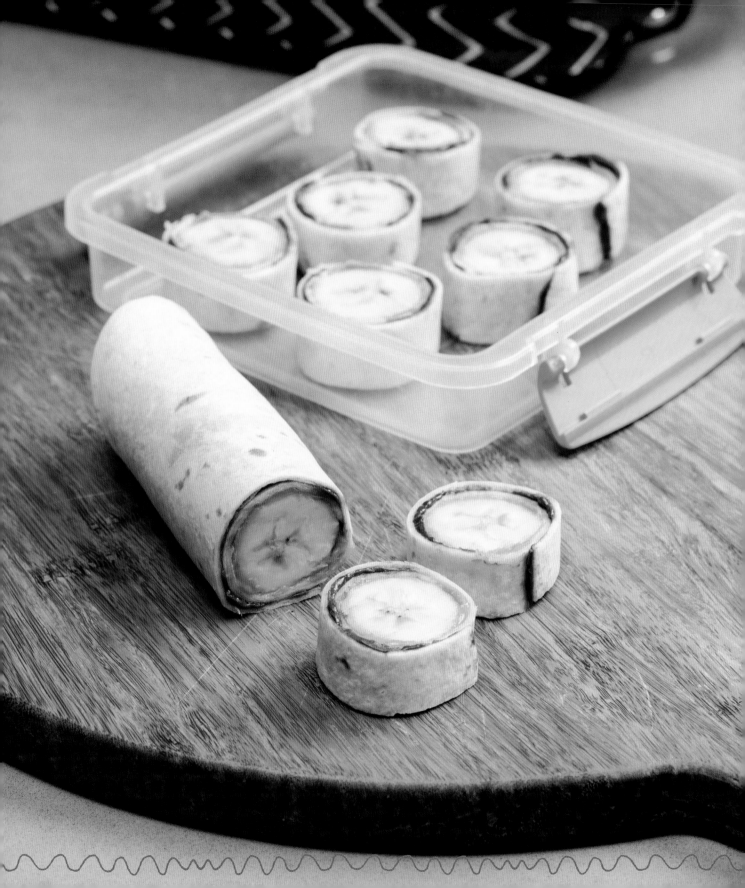

Almond Butter, Nutella, and Banana "Sushi Rolls"

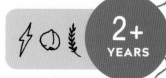

2+ YEARS

Makes 1 roll
Total Time: 5 minutes

Why This Recipe Works

For a sweet treat, it's hard to beat the combination of creamy almond butter, rich Nutella, and banana. We often use these ingredients as a filling for crêpes (see page 192), but for lunch we wrap them in a flour tortilla before slicing them into *maki*-size bites. Who can say no to dessert sushi?

Other nut butters can be substituted for almond butter.

1 tablespoon almond butter
1 (8-inch) flour tortilla

1 tablespoon Nutella spread
1 small ripe banana, peeled and ends trimmed

1. Spread almond butter evenly over half of tortilla, then spread Nutella evenly over other half of tortilla. Place banana on top of almond butter, along edge closest to you.

2. Fold bottom edge of tortilla up and over banana, then continue to roll tortilla tightly around banana into cylinder (see "Rolling 'Sushi,'" below). Cut into 6 even pieces. Serve or pack in lunch box.

ROLLING "SUSHI"

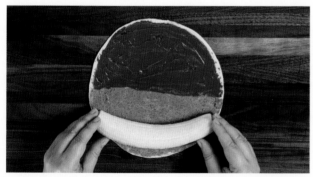

1. Place banana on top of almond butter across width of tortilla, along edge closest to you.

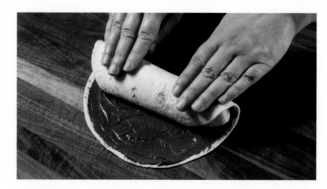

2. Roll tortilla tightly around banana to form cylinder.

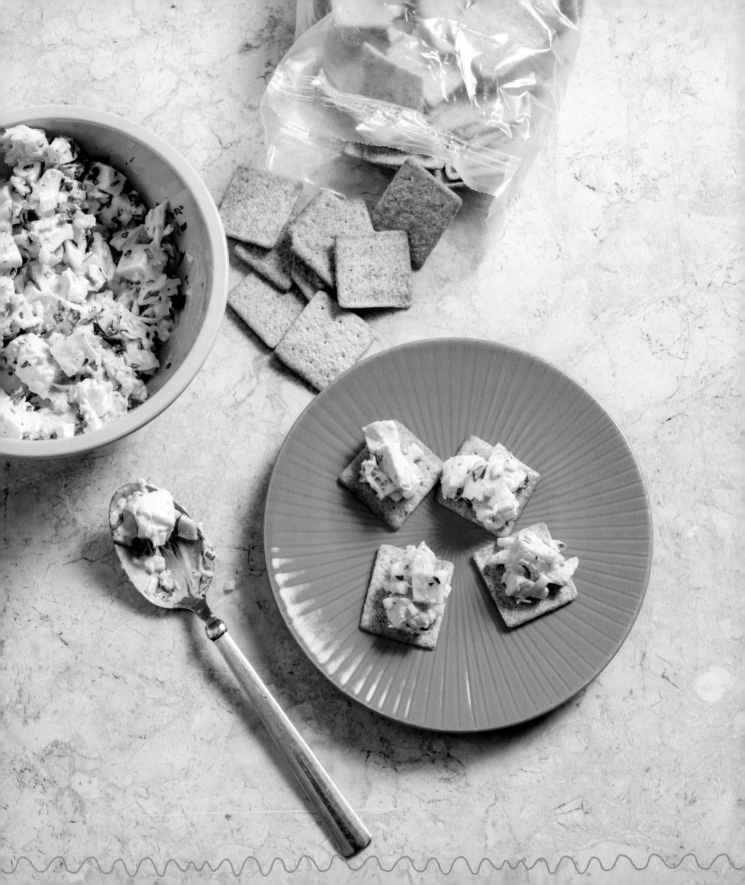

Chicken Salad

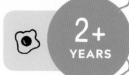

2+
YEARS

Makes about 2½ cups
Total Time: 1 hour and 10 minutes

Why This Recipe Works

Use this recipe to introduce your child to chicken salad and you'll create a lifetime fan. Instead of using dry, leftover chicken, we poach boneless, skinless breasts gently, which ensures the meat retains moisture. A little mayo (for creaminess), lemon juice and Dijon mustard (for a flavor pop), celery and shallot (for crunch), and parsley (for green), and you're ready for preschool.

✳ **STORAGE INFORMATION**
Salad can be refrigerated for up to 2 days.

To ensure that the chicken cooks through, start with cold water in step 1 and don't use breasts that weigh more than 8 ounces or are thicker than 1 inch. This salad can be served in a sandwich, with crackers, or spooned over leafy greens.

Salt and pepper
2 (6- to 8-ounce) boneless, skinless chicken breasts, no more than 1 inch thick, trimmed
¼ cup mayonnaise
2 teaspoons lemon juice
½ teaspoon Dijon mustard
1 celery rib, minced
1 tablespoon minced shallot
1 tablespoon minced fresh parsley

1. Dissolve 2 tablespoons salt in 6 cups cold water in Dutch oven. Submerge chicken in water. Heat pot over medium heat until water registers 170 degrees, about 10 to 15 minutes. Turn off heat, cover pot, and let sit until chicken registers 165 degrees, 15 to 17 minutes.

2. Transfer chicken to paper-towel-lined plate. Refrigerate until chicken is cool, about 30 minutes. While chicken cools, whisk mayonnaise, lemon juice, mustard, and ⅛ teaspoon pepper together in large bowl.

3. Pat chicken dry with paper towels and cut into ½-inch pieces. Transfer chicken to bowl with mayonnaise mixture. Add celery, shallot, and parsley and toss to combine. Season with salt and pepper to taste. Serve or pack in lunch box.

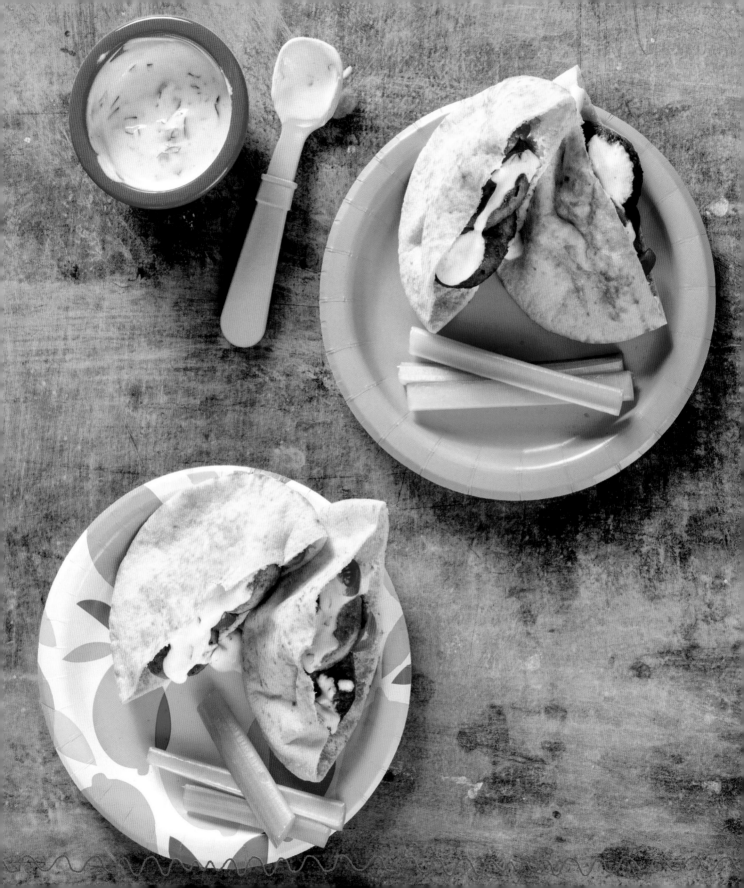

Mini Falafels with Yogurt Sauce

Makes 16 falafel patties
Total Time: 35 minutes

2+ YEARS

Why This Recipe Works

With convenient canned chickpeas and the help of a food processor, we created an easy at-home take on a Mediterranean and Middle Eastern classic: falafel. Pita bread plays a double role in this recipe; not only does it serve as the sandwich base, but we also grind some up and use it as a binder to hold the falafel patties together. A bright yogurt sauce is a key component of this sandwich; you'll have some leftover—we like it as a dipping sauce for veggies.

✳ STORAGE INFORMATION
Cooked and cooled falafel can be refrigerated for up to 3 days or frozen for up to 2 weeks. Yogurt sauce can be refrigerated for up to 3 days.

2 (5-inch) pita breads
1 (15-ounce) can chickpeas, rinsed
¼ cup chopped fresh parsley
1 large egg
1¼ teaspoons ground cumin
Salt and pepper
¼ cup canola oil
¾ cup plain whole-milk yogurt
1 tablespoon lemon juice
2 cherry tomatoes, cut into eighths

1. Tear 1 pita bread into small pieces and process in food processor until finely ground, about 15 seconds. Add chickpeas, 2 tablespoons parsley, egg, 1 teaspoon cumin, ¼ teaspoon salt, and ⅛ teaspoon pepper and pulse until chickpeas are coarsely chopped and mixture is cohesive, about 10 pulses. Transfer mixture to medium bowl.

2. Working with 1 tablespoon chickpea mixture at a time, use your hands to form chickpea mixture into patties about 1½ inches in diameter and ½ inch thick (you should have 16 patties).

3. Heat oil in 12-inch nonstick skillet over medium-high heat until just smoking. Cook patties until well browned on both sides, about 3 minutes per side. Transfer falafel to paper-towel-lined plate to drain briefly.

4. Whisk yogurt, lemon juice, remaining 2 tablespoons parsley, and remaining ¼ teaspoon cumin together in small bowl. Season with salt and pepper to taste. Cut remaining pita in half and stuff each half with 2 falafel patties and tomatoes. Drizzle 1 tablespoon sauce inside each pita. (If packing in lunch box, pack sauce separately.) Serve or pack in lunch box.

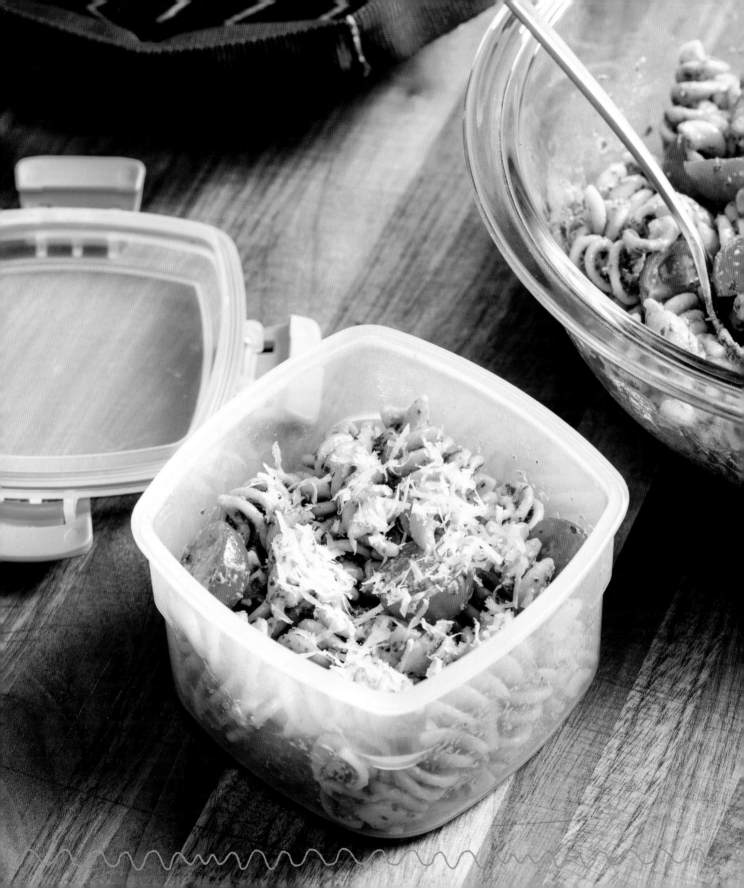

Pesto Pasta Salad

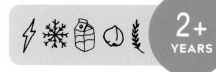

2+ YEARS

Makes 3 cups pasta salad, plus ½ cup extra pesto
Total Time: 40 minutes

Why This Recipe Works

Store-bought pasta salad is usually a disappointing, overpriced mess of overcooked pasta with overdressed, soggy vegetables. For a homemade version that's better, we started by making a kid-friendly pesto sauce by toning down the traditional version's garlicky bite and by adding baby spinach to balance the licorice-like flavor of fresh basil. To create a creamy (and healthy!) dressing for the pasta, we added some yogurt to the pesto, too. This is a lunch you may want to pack up for yourself, so we made sure the recipe makes enough for both your child and you.

✳ STORAGE INFORMATION

Pasta salad can be refrigerated for up to 2 days. This recipe makes enough pesto for two batches of pasta salad. The remaining half of pesto can be kept in airtight container, covered with thin layer of oil (1 to 2 tablespoons), and refrigerated for up to four days or frozen for up to one month—be sure to wait to add yogurt until just before serving.

Penne or farfalle can be substituted for rotini in this recipe. Note that this recipe makes enough pesto for two batches of pasta salad.

6 ounces (2 cups) rotini
Salt and pepper
¼ cup plus 1 teaspoon extra-virgin olive oil
3 cups fresh basil leaves
1 cup baby spinach
⅓ cup pine nuts, toasted
1 garlic clove, minced
1 tablespoon lemon juice
1½ ounces Parmesan cheese, grated (¾ cup), plus extra for serving
3 tablespoons whole-milk plain yogurt
3 ounces (½ cup) cherry tomatoes, halved (optional)

1. Bring 2 quarts water to boil in large saucepan. Add pasta and 1 teaspoon salt and cook, stirring often, until tender. Reserve ¼ cup cooking liquid, then drain pasta and transfer to rimmed baking sheet. Toss pasta with 1 teaspoon oil, then spread in even layer. Let pasta and reserved cooking water cool to room temperature, about 15 minutes.

2. Meanwhile, process basil, spinach, pine nuts, garlic, lemon juice, and ½ teaspoon salt in food processor until smooth, about 30 seconds, scraping down sides of bowl as needed. Add Parmesan and remaining ¼ cup oil and process until thoroughly combined, about 30 seconds. Transfer ½ cup pesto to large bowl and stir in yogurt to combine. Transfer remaining ½ cup pesto to airtight container and refrigerate (or freeze) for later use.

3. Add cooled pasta to pesto mixture and toss to combine, adding reserved cooking water, 1 tablespoon at a time, until pesto evenly coats pasta. Stir in cherry tomatoes, if using. Season with salt and pepper to taste. Serve or pack in lunch box with extra Parmesan.

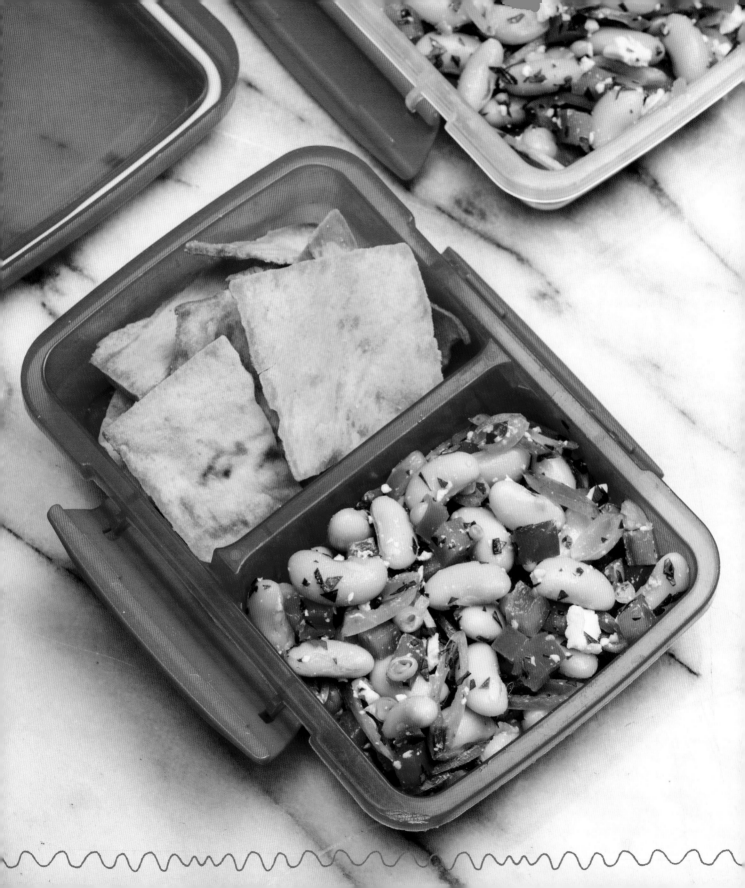

White Bean Salad

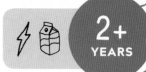

Makes 3 cups
Total Time: 40 minutes

Why This Recipe Works

The key to making this flavorful white bean salad is in the first step: we steep the beans in a garlicky broth. This adds great flavor to the beans and gives you time to chop up some colorful veggies (bell pepper and sugar snap peas). Once the beans are ready to go, this colorful salad comes together in a snap (pea!).

✳ STORAGE INFORMATION

Salad can be refrigerated for up to 2 days.

This salad is great on its own, or try serving it with pita chips.

2 tablespoons plus
    1 teaspoon extra-virgin
    olive oil
2 garlic cloves, peeled and
    smashed
1 cup water
Salt and pepper
1 (15-ounce) can cannellini
    beans, rinsed
1 tablespoon white wine
    vinegar
1 teaspoon minced shallot

1 small red bell pepper,
    stemmed, seeded, and
    cut into ¼-inch pieces
    (¾ cup)
4 ounces sugar snap peas,
    strings removed and
    sliced thin on the bias
    (1 cup)
1 ounce feta cheese,
    crumbled (¼ cup)
2 tablespoons chopped fresh
    parsley

1. Heat 1 teaspoon oil and garlic in small saucepan over medium heat until garlic just begins to brown, about 2 minutes. Slowly add water and ¼ teaspoon salt and bring to simmer. Remove saucepan from heat. Stir in beans, cover, and let sit for 20 minutes. Meanwhile, combine vinegar and shallot in large bowl and let sit for 20 minutes.

2. Drain beans and discard garlic. Add beans, bell pepper, snap peas, feta, parsley, and remaining 2 tablespoons oil to shallot mixture and toss to combine. Season with salt and pepper to taste. Serve or pack in lunch box.

Vegetable Sushi Bites

Makes 20 sushi bites
Total Time: 1 hour

Why This Recipe Works

Sushi is one of our favorite on-the-go lunches (clearly, as we even make a sweet version, see page 239). These avocado, carrot, and cucumber sushi bites are a great way to pack raw vegetables and nutritious nori into a school lunch. No utensils are necessary; sushi bites are a naturally great finger food.

✳ STORAGE INFORMATION

After preparing sushi rolls through step 4, whole rolls can be wrapped in plastic wrap and refrigerated for up to 24 hours. Cut into bites just before serving or packing in lunch box.

Do not substitute other short-grain rices for the sushi rice, or the rice will be mushy.

1 cup water
½ cup sushi rice
¼ teaspoon salt
1½ teaspoons unseasoned rice vinegar
½ teaspoon sugar
2 (8-by-7½-inch) sheets nori

½ avocado, sliced thin
1 small carrot, peeled and cut into 2-inch-long matchsticks
¼ cucumber, peeled, seeded, and cut into 2-inch-long matchsticks

1 Bring water, rice, and salt to boil in small saucepan over medium-high heat. Reduce heat to low, cover, and simmer until rice is tender and water is fully absorbed, about 20 minutes. Transfer rice to medium bowl.

2 Stir vinegar and sugar into rice and let mixture cool to room temperature, about 20 minutes.

3 Place nori on cutting board, long sides parallel to counter. Spread half of cooled rice evenly over each nori sheet (see "Assembling Sushi Bites," right). Divide avocado slices between nori sheets, arranging slices horizontally over rice and leaving 1-inch border between bottom of nori sheet and avocado. Then layer carrot and cucumber on top of avocado.

4 Working with 1 sheet nori at a time, fold bottom edge of nori sheet up and over vegetable filling, then continue to roll tightly into cylinder. Place both rolls seam side down.

5 Cut each roll into 10 bites, each about ¾ inch wide. Serve or pack in lunch box.

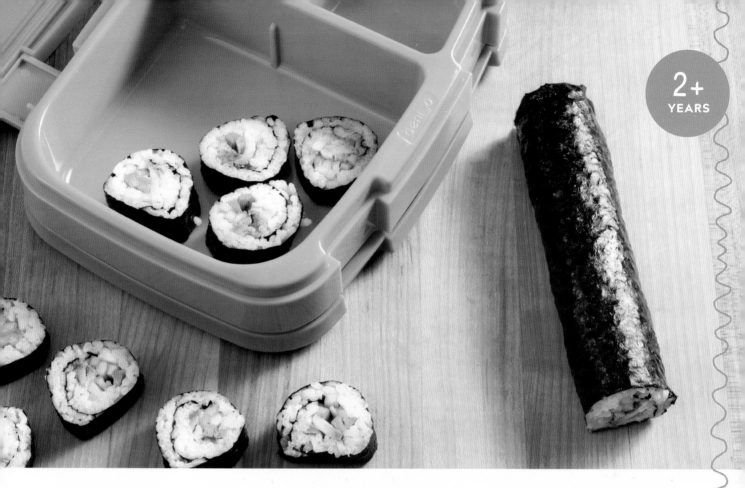

ASSEMBLING SUSHI BITES

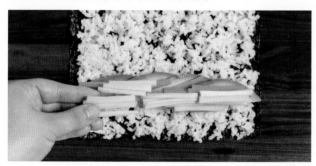

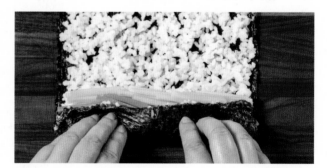

(1) Place nori sheets on cutting board, long sides parallel to counter. Spread half of cooled rice evenly over each nori sheet. Divide avocado slices between nori sheets, arranging slices horizontally over rice and leaving 1-inch border between bottom of nori sheet and avocado. Then layer carrot matchsticks and cucumber matchsticks over avocado.

(2) Fold bottom edge of each nori sheet up and over vegetable filling, then continue to roll tightly into cylinder. Place both rolls seam side down.

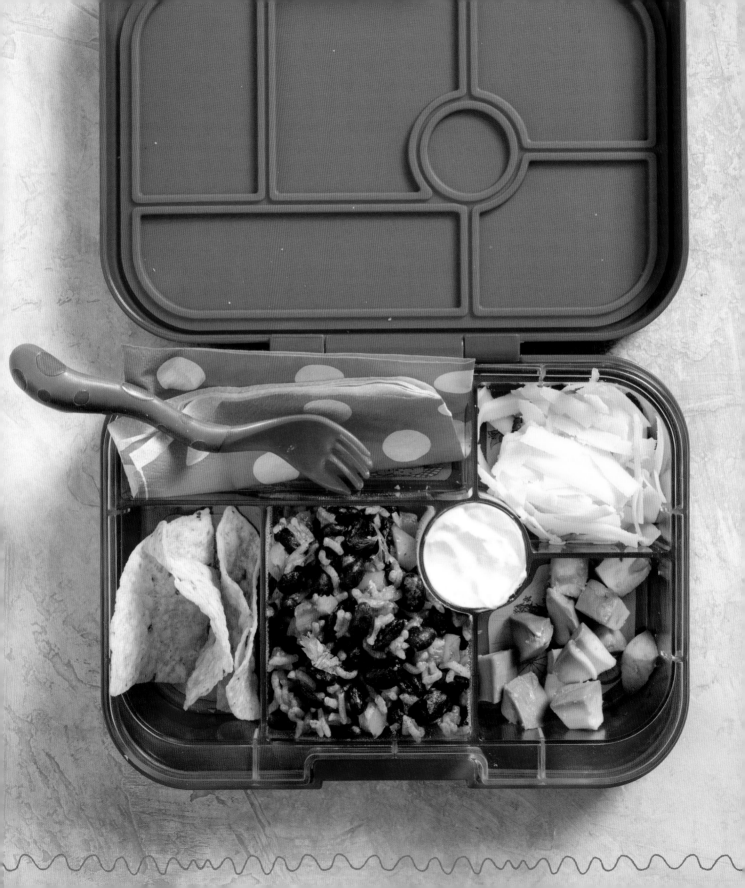

Rice and Bean Toddler Taco Bowl

2+ YEARS

Makes 3½ cups
Total Time: 45 minutes

Why This Recipe Works

Does life at preschool get any better than lunchtime with a taco bowl? Probably not. Especially because you can dress this taco bowl up any way you like with your toddler's favorite toppings. To streamline the cooking process, we cook the rice and beans together in one skillet after blooming the spices and garlic in oil. The result is a super-tasty, one-pan lunch that can be served hot (break out the thermos!) or at room temperature. (And, happily, this recipe makes enough for a few days of your toddler's lunch—or enough to pack for your lunch, too!)

✳ STORAGE INFORMATION

Rice and bean mixture can be refrigerated for up to 2 to 3 days.

You will need a nonstick 10-inch skillet with a tight-fitting lid for this recipe. Toppings are pretty much limitless, but we like diced avocado, shredded cheese, lime wedges, sour cream, and/or tortilla chips.

1 tablespoon canola oil
1 small yellow bell pepper, stemmed, seeded, and cut into ¼-inch pieces
1 garlic clove, minced
1 teaspoon chili powder
½ teaspoon ground cumin
Salt and pepper
1 tablespoon tomato paste
1 (15-ounce) can black beans, rinsed
1¼ cups chicken broth
½ cup long-grain white rice, rinsed
1 tablespoon minced fresh cilantro, optional

1. Heat oil in 10-inch nonstick skillet over medium heat until shimmering. Add bell pepper, garlic, chili powder, cumin, and ¼ teaspoon salt and cook until pepper has softened, about 3 minutes. Stir in tomato paste and cook until fragrant and starting to brown, about 1 minute.

2. Stir beans, broth, and rice into skillet, scraping up any browned bits, and bring to simmer. Cover skillet, reduce heat to low, and cook until liquid is absorbed, and rice is tender, 22 to 26 minutes, stirring once halfway through cooking. Stir in cilantro, if using, and season with salt and pepper to taste. Serve with your favorite toppings or pack in lunch box or thermos.

Indian-Style Potato Hand Pies

Makes 8 hand pies
Total Time: 1 hour and 40 minutes, 15 minutes cooling time

Why This Recipe Works

This potato-and-pea hand pie has just the right amount of cumin, ginger, and turmeric to remind us of a tasty Indian samosa while still being mild enough for young taste buds. Plus, the pie dough wrapper makes it perfectly packable for a lunch box (just pack a little yogurt sauce on the side!). This recipe takes a bit more up-front work, but it will give you multiple lunches.

Pillsbury Refrigerated Pie Crusts are our winning store-bought dough. There are two crusts in one package.

HAND PIES

1 large russet potato (12 ounces), peeled and cut into ½-inch chunks (2 cups)
1¼ teaspoons salt
1½ tablespoons canola oil
1 shallot, chopped fine
2 garlic cloves, minced
1 teaspoon ground cumin
½ teaspoon ground ginger
¼ teaspoon ground turmeric
¼ cup frozen peas, thawed
2 tablespoons minced fresh cilantro
1 package store-bought pie dough

SAUCE – – – – – – – – – – – – – – –

⅓ cup plain whole-milk yogurt
1 teaspoon lemon juice
1 teaspoon minced fresh cilantro
¼ teaspoon ground cumin
⅛ teaspoon salt

1 FOR THE HAND PIES: Place potatoes and 1 teaspoon salt in large saucepan and add water to cover by 1 inch. Bring to boil over high heat, then reduce heat to medium-low and simmer until potatoes are tender and paring knife can be inserted into potatoes with little resistance, 8 to 10 minutes. Drain potatoes.

2 Heat 1 tablespoon oil in now-empty saucepan over medium heat until shimmering. Add shallot and remaining ¼ teaspoon salt and cook until shallot is softened, about 3 minutes. Stir in garlic, cumin, ginger, and turmeric, and cook until fragrant, about 30 seconds. Stir in cooled potatoes and cook until well coated with spice mixture, about 2 minutes. Stir in ¼ cup water and peas, scraping up any browned bits from bottom of saucepan with wooden spoon.

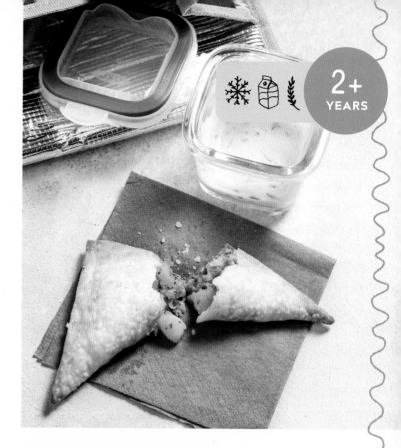

3. Transfer potato mixture to bowl and let cool slightly, then refrigerate until completely cool, about 30 minutes. Stir in cilantro.

4. **FOR THE SAUCE:** Meanwhile, stir all ingredients together. Refrigerate until ready to serve.

5. Adjust oven rack to middle position and heat oven to 400 degrees. Line rimmed baking sheet with parchment paper.

6. Cut each pie crust into an 8-inch square, then cut each square into four 4-inch squares (you will have 8 squares total). Discard dough scraps.

7. Arrange dough squares on cutting board or counter. Place 2 tablespoons potato filling in center of each square (see "Assembling Hand Pies," right). Brush edges of dough squares with water. Working with one square at a time, fold dough over filling into triangle shape. Pinch edges together to seal. Arrange triangles on prepared sheet and brush triangles with remaining ½ tablespoon oil.

8. Bake hand pies until golden, 18 to 20 minutes, rotating sheet halfway through baking. Transfer hand pies to wire rack and let cool for 15 minutes. Serve with sauce or pack in lunch box, packing sauce separately.

ASSEMBLING HAND PIES

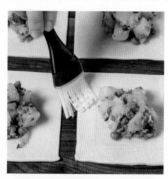

1. Arrange dough squares on cutting board or counter. Place 2 tablespoons potato filling in center of each square. Brush edges of dough squares with water.

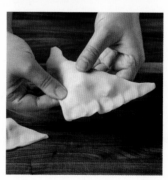

2. Working with one square at a time, fold dough over filling into triangle shape. Pinch edges together to seal.

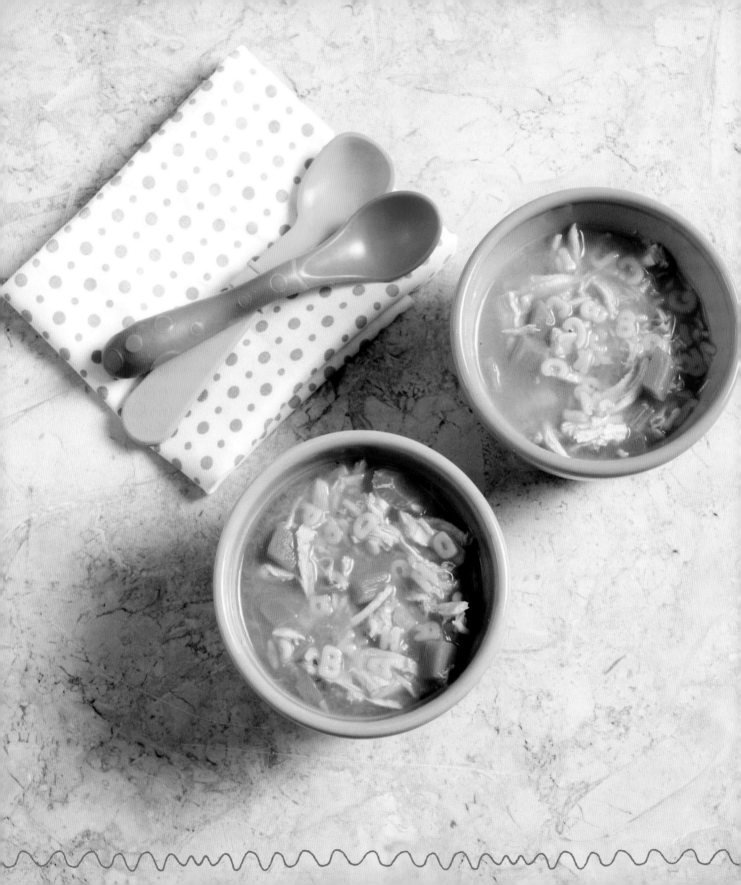

Alphabet Soup with Chicken

⚡ 🌾 **2+ YEARS**

Makes 3 cups
Total Time: 45 minutes

Why This Recipe Works

Break out the thermos for this comforting, kid-favorite soup. It has all the familiar flavors of chicken noodle soup with an added boost from tomato paste and a couple of garlic cloves. The chicken cooks gently and remains tender and juicy even when shredded into the soup. Your kiddo can try to find his or her name in the soup—now that spells fun!

✳ STORAGE INFORMATION

Soup can be refrigerated for up to 2 days.

Ditalini or orzo can be substituted for the alphabet pasta.

1 (6-ounce) boneless, skinless chicken breast, trimmed
Salt and pepper
1 tablespoon canola oil
1 carrot, peeled and cut into ¼-inch pieces
1 celery rib, cut into ¼-inch pieces
1 tablespoon tomato paste
2 garlic cloves, minced
1 teaspoon minced fresh thyme
3 cups chicken broth
¼ cup alphabet pasta

1. Pat chicken dry with paper towels and season with salt and pepper. Heat oil in large saucepan over medium-high heat until just smoking. Brown chicken lightly on both sides, 2 to 3 minutes per side; transfer chicken to plate.

2. Add carrot and celery to now-empty saucepan, reduce heat to medium, and cook until softened, about 5 minutes. Stir in tomato paste, garlic, and thyme and cook until fragrant, about 1 minute. Stir in broth, scraping up any browned bits.

3. Add browned chicken and any accumulated juices to saucepan and bring to simmer. Cover and cook until chicken registers 165 degrees, 8 to 10 minutes. Transfer chicken to cutting board, let cool slightly, then shred into bite-size pieces.

4. Meanwhile, stir pasta into soup and cook until tender, 7 to 9 minutes. Stir in shredded chicken and season with salt and pepper to taste. Serve or pack in thermos.

Snacks and Sides to Pack in Your Lunch Box

Here are some fun snack ideas to pack in your child's lunch box along with the recipes in this chapter.

Ants on a Log
Spread nut butter on a celery stick, and top with a line of raisins.

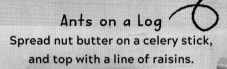

Ants on a Slope
Spread cream cheese on a celery stick and top with a line of raisins.

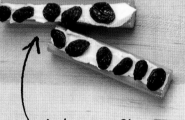

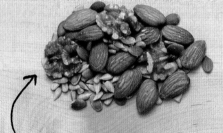

Nut and Seed Mix
Mix together 1 tablespoon almonds, 1 tablespoon walnuts, 1 teaspoon sunflower seeds, and 1 teaspoon pepitas.

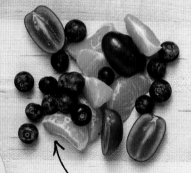

Fruit
Mix together halved or quartered grapes, peeled and sectioned mandarin oranges or clementines, and blueberries.

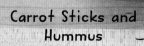

Carrot Sticks and Hummus
Pack hummus in a small container and add carrot slices on the side.

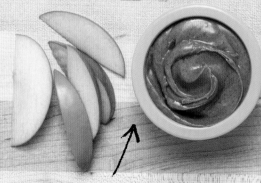

Apples with Nut Butter
Pack sliced Granny Smith apples with a nut butter for dipping.

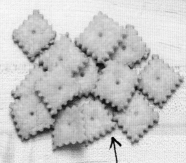

Cheese Crackers
(page 112)

Edamame
Thaw a handful of frozen shelled
edamame beans and pat dry.
Toss with pinch of salt, if desired.

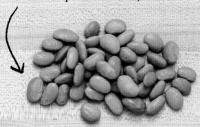

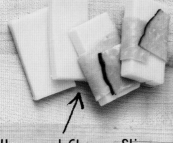

Ham and Cheese Slices
Wrap ½ piece of deli ham
around each slice of cheddar
(or simply pack sliced cheddar
cheese alone).

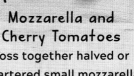

**Whole-Wheat
Sesame Crackers**
(page 224)

**Mozzarella and
Cherry Tomatoes**
Toss together halved or
quartered small mozzarella
balls (or ciliegine or bocconcini)
and halved or quartered cherry
tomatoes. Drizzle with extra-
virgin olive oil and season with
salt and pepper to taste.

**Raw Fruit and
Nut Bars**
(page 111)

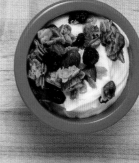

**Tiny Carrot
Muffins**
(page 107)

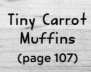

**Yogurt and
Granola**
Add a container of
yogurt to the lunch box,
and add some granola
in a small container (see
page 203 for Almond-
Raisin Granola).

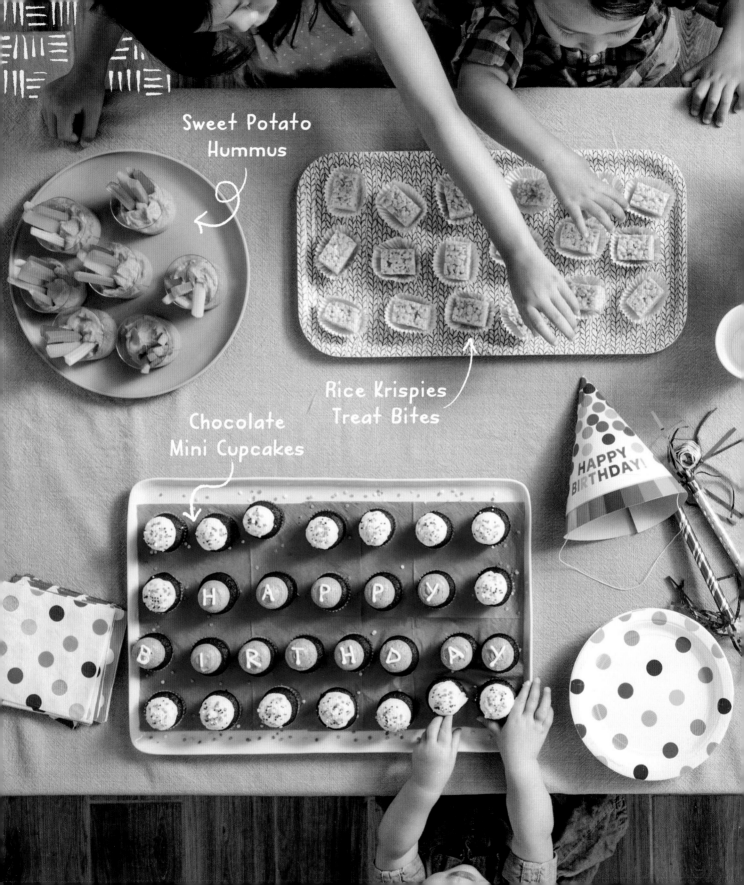

Sweet Potato Hummus

Rice Krispies Treat Bites

Chocolate Mini Cupcakes

HAPPY BIRTHDAY!

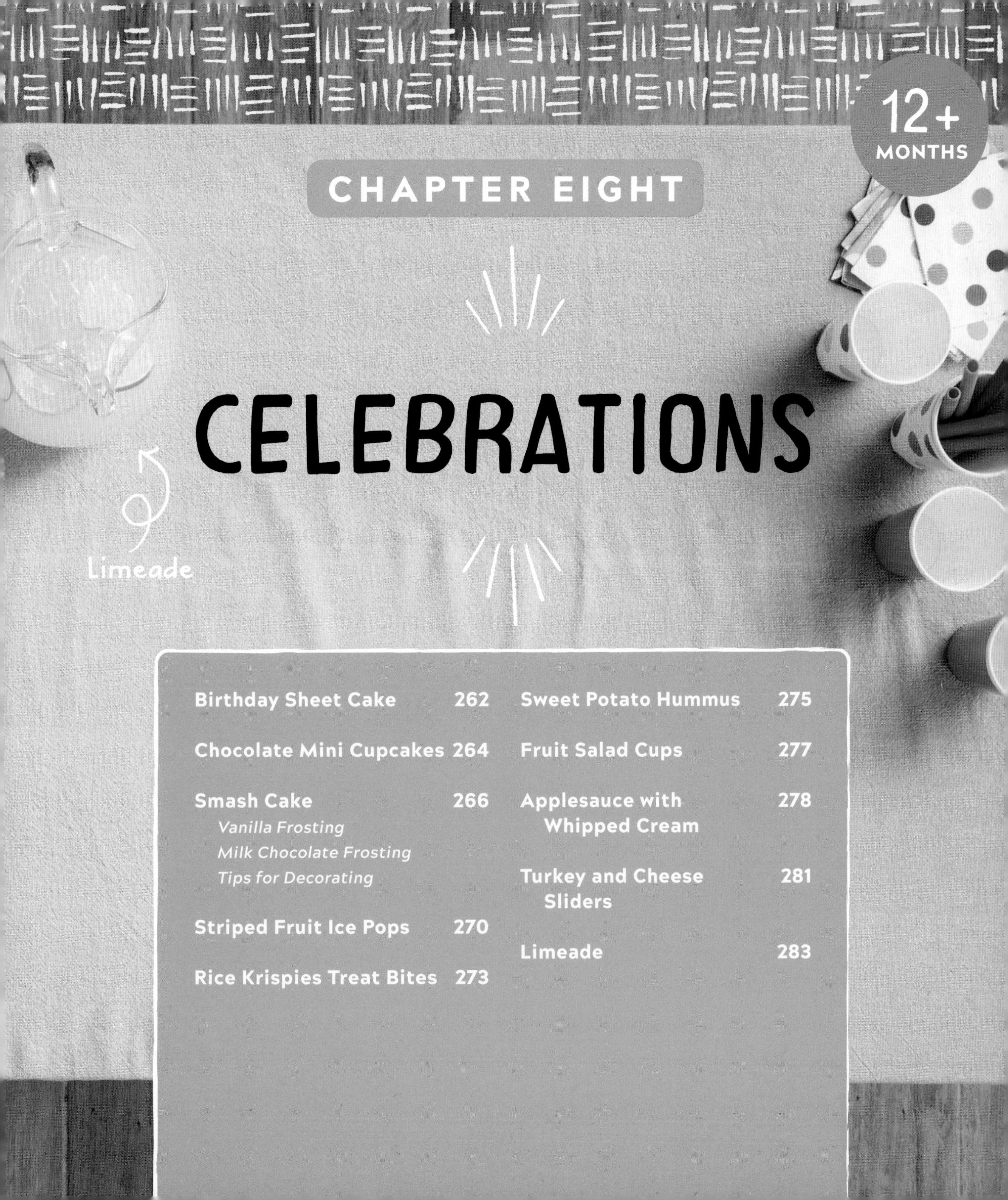

CHAPTER EIGHT

CELEBRATIONS

Limeade

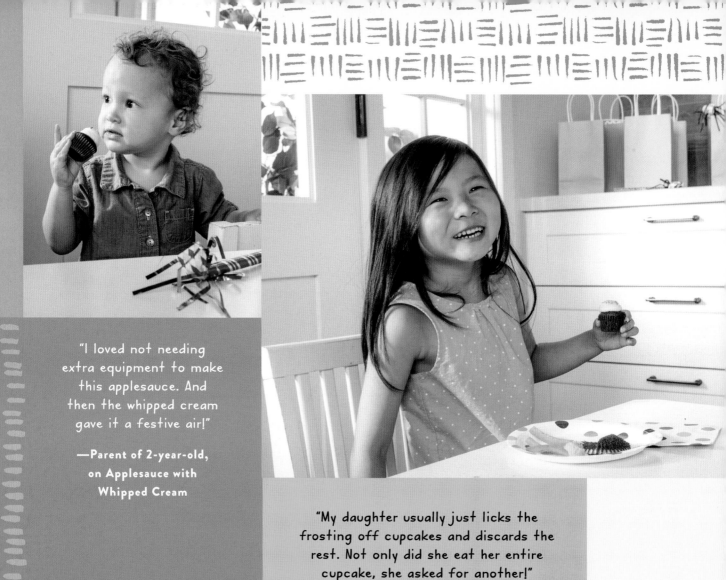

"I loved not needing extra equipment to make this applesauce. And then the whipped cream gave it a festive air!"

—Parent of 2-year-old, on Applesauce with Whipped Cream

"My daughter usually just licks the frosting off cupcakes and discards the rest. Not only did she eat her entire cupcake, she asked for another!"

—Parent of 5-year-old, on Chocolate Mini Cupcakes

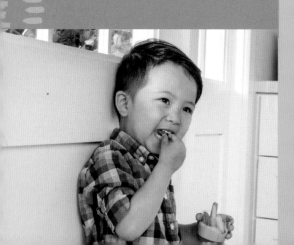

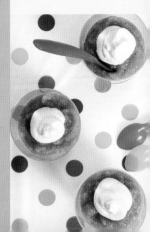

ALL ABOUT CELEBRATIONS

There is a magical moment in the toddler phase: your child suddenly understands the concept of celebrations and how exciting it is to get together with friends and family and have a good time.

This chapter is full of recipes for a gathering. There are options for classic birthdays: Birthday Sheet Cake (page 262) with Vanilla Frosting (page 268). There are options for small treats: Chocolate Mini Cupcakes (page 264) with Milk Chocolate Frosting (page 268). Is it summer? Go for the Striped Fruit Ice Pops (page 270). Are you celebrating a first birthday (or having a tiny gathering)? Yes, we created a recipe for a Smash Cake (page 266). (Your baby will love shoving his or her face into one of the most delicious cakes you've ever made!) See page 269 for tips on decorating cakes (and cupcakes) of all kinds.

We've added some healthy, toddler-friendly options as well, like Sweet Potato Hummus (page 275), Fruit Salad Cups (page 277), and, our personal favorite, Applesauce with Whipped Cream (page 278).

Parties are not easy to execute, no matter how old the attendees. Our advice? Plan ahead. Simplify where possible. Don't forget to schedule around nap time. And when it comes to food, choose the number of recipes that work for *your* schedule, always plan to make a little more food than you think you'll need, and remember that disposable plates are your friends.

Birthday Sheet Cake

Serves 18 to 20 toddlers
Total Time: 1 hour, plus cooling and frosting time

Why This Recipe Works

In our humble opinion, there is only one cake for a birthday party. And that cake is a sheet cake. Sheet cakes are relatively easy to make and don't require a crazy number of ingredients or an obscene amount of time to assemble. You don't even have to take it out of the pan, if you don't want to. For this cake, we adapted a chiffon cake technique, which basically meant using a large number of whipped egg whites to deliver a fluffy texture. For moisture, we used a combination of butter and oil, and for a more tender cake, we substituted buttermilk for milk. Frost it with either Vanilla or Milk Chocolate Frosting (page 268). Be sure to check out our tips for decorating (page 269).

Be sure to bring all the ingredients to room temperature before beginning this recipe. It's perfectly fine to serve this (and any sheet cake, for that matter) straight from the pan, but taking the baked and cooled cake out of the pan is as easy as flipping it onto a rack, peeling off the parchment, and inverting it onto a platter. If you plan to take the cake out of the pan, make sure to grease the pan, line the bottom of the pan with parchment paper, grease the parchment, and then flour the pan, before adding the batter. If using a handheld electric mixer, increase mixing times in step 2 by 1 to 2 minutes.

1 cup buttermilk, room temperature
3 large eggs, separated, plus 3 large yolks, room temperature
10 tablespoons unsalted butter, melted and cooled
3 tablespoons canola oil
2 teaspoons vanilla extract
Pinch cream of tartar
1¾ cups (12¼ ounces) sugar
2½ cups (10 ounces) cake flour
1¼ teaspoons baking powder
¼ teaspoon baking soda
¾ teaspoon salt
3 cups Vanilla or Milk Chocolate Frosting (page 268)

1 Adjust oven rack to middle position and heat oven to 325 degrees. Grease and flour 13-by-9-inch baking pan. Whisk buttermilk, 6 egg yolks, butter, oil, and vanilla together in bowl.

2 Using stand mixer fitted with whisk attachment, whip egg whites and cream of tartar on medium-low speed until foamy, about 1 minute. Increase speed to medium-high and whip egg whites to soft billowy mounds, about 1 minute. Gradually add ¼ cup sugar and whip until glossy, stiff peaks form, 2 to 3 minutes; transfer to separate bowl.

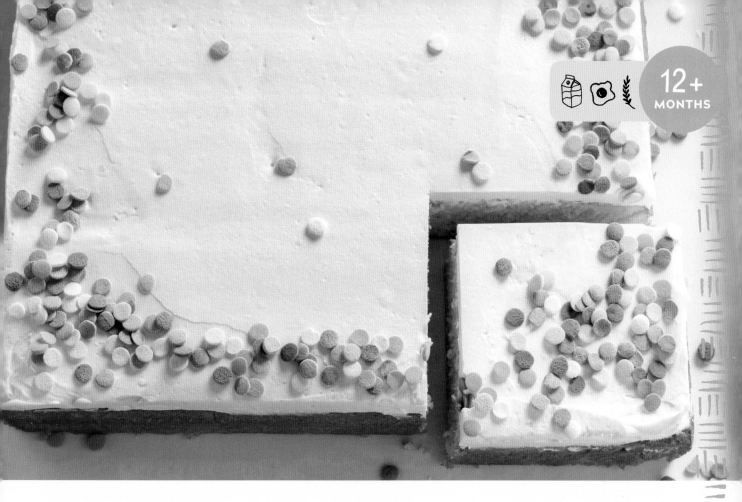

3 Return now-empty bowl to mixer. Add flour, baking powder, baking soda, salt, and remaining 1½ cups sugar, and mix on low speed for 15 seconds to combine. With mixer running, gradually add buttermilk mixture and continue to mix until almost combined (a few streaks of dry flour will remain), about 15 seconds. Scrape down bowl, then mix on medium-low speed until smooth and fully incorporated, 10 to 15 seconds.

4 Using rubber spatula, stir one-third of egg whites into batter. Gently fold remaining egg whites into batter until no white streaks remain. Transfer batter to prepared pan and smooth top with rubber spatula. Gently tap pan on counter to release air bubbles. Bake until toothpick inserted in center comes out clean, 28 to 32 minutes, rotating pan halfway through baking.

5 Let cake cool completely in pan on wire rack, about 2 hours. Spread frosting evenly over top of cake. Serve.

✳ STORAGE INFORMATION

Unfrosted cake can be wrapped tightly in plastic wrap and stored at room temperature for up to 24 hours. Frosted cake can be refrigerated for up to 24 hours. Bring to room temperature before serving.

Chocolate Mini Cupcakes

Makes 24 mini cupcakes
Total Time: 45 minutes, plus cooling and frosting time

Why This Recipe Works

When it comes to cupcakes, the miniature-sized ones come with three added benefits. One, tiny cupcakes are cuter than big cupcakes. Two, consuming a smaller cupcake reduces the risk of an extended sugar high, and then sugar crash. And three: the adults at the party can—and should—eat more than one while their kids are kept in check. For these cupcakes, blooming unsweetened cocoa powder in boiling water and adding chocolate chips delivered deep, rich chocolate flavor—perfect for a cupcake you eat in just a few bites!

✳ STORAGE INFORMATION

Unfrosted cupcakes can be stored at room temperature for up to 24 hours. Frosted cupcakes can be refrigerated for up to 24 hours. Bring to room temperature before serving.

For an accurate measurement of boiling water, bring a full kettle of water to a boil and then measure out the desired amount. Depending on the size of your mini muffin tin, you may have a little extra batter left over. If so, you can discard it, or you can cool the muffin tin and bake off extra cupcakes. If you don't have a mini muffin tin, you can use a standard muffin tin and make 12 standard-size cupcakes; divide batter evenly among 12 muffin cups and bake for 18 to 22 minutes.

1 cup (5 ounces) all-purpose flour
½ teaspoon baking soda
¼ teaspoon salt
½ cup boiling water
⅓ cup (1 ounce) unsweetened cocoa powder
⅓ cup (2 ounces) semisweet chocolate chips

¾ cup (5¼ ounces) sugar
½ cup sour cream
½ cup canola oil
2 large eggs
1 teaspoon vanilla extract
2 cups Vanilla or Milk Chocolate Frosting (page 268)

1 Adjust oven rack to middle position and heat oven to 325 degrees. Line 24-cup mini muffin tin with paper or foil liners.

2 Whisk flour, baking soda, and salt together in medium bowl. Whisk boiling water, cocoa, and chocolate chips in large bowl until smooth. Whisk sugar, sour cream, oil, eggs, and vanilla into cocoa mixture until combined. Whisk in flour mixture until just incorporated. Divide batter evenly among prepared muffin cups, filling to rim (note that there may be extra batter).

3 Bake until toothpick inserted in center comes out with few crumbs attached, 10 to 12 minutes, rotating muffin tin halfway through baking. Let cupcakes cool in muffin tin on wire rack

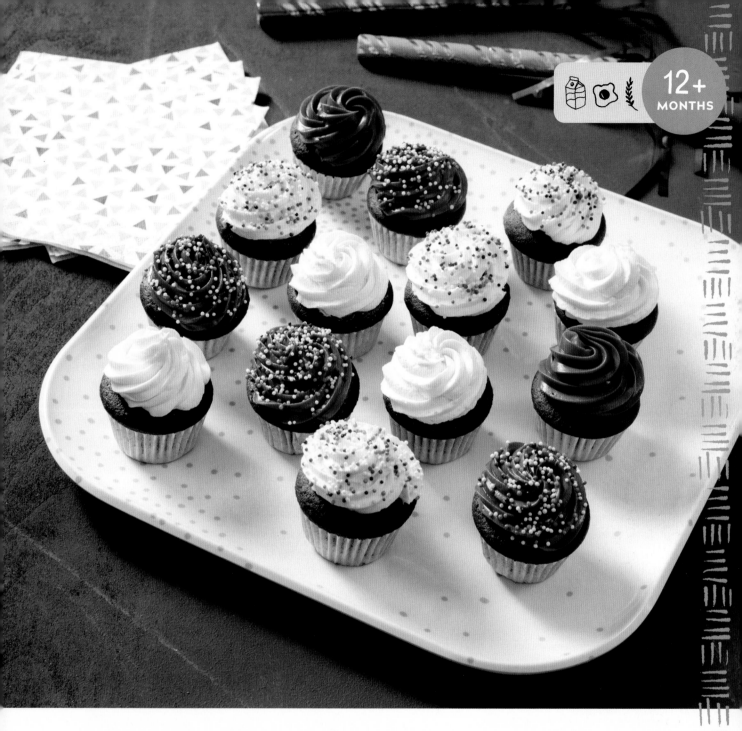

for 10 minutes. Remove cupcakes from muffin tin and let cool completely on rack, about 1 hour. Repeat filling and baking with any remaining batter, if desired.

4 Spread or pipe frosting evenly on cupcakes. Serve.

Smash Cake

Makes one 6-inch cake
Total Time: 45 minutes, plus cooling and frosting time

Why This Recipe Works

A smash cake is a tiny layer cake given to the birthday boy or girl. Oftentimes, this is the toddler's first cake experience. After staring at it for a bit, most toddlers have the impulse to smash his or her face straight into the frosting—hence, "smash" cake. We wanted an easy recipe that would start your kiddo off with their first of many delicious cakes sure to be enjoyed in their lifetime. We wanted a yellow layer cake with the same ethereal texture and supreme fluffiness as the cakes that come from a box without the mysterious chemical additives. Similar to our sheet cake (page 262), we found that whipping egg whites separately and folding them into the batter at the end lightened the cake's texture. A combination of fats (butter plus canola oil) delivered noticeable butter flavor while improving the moistness of the cake. You pick: Vanilla or Milk Chocolate Frosting (page 268). Be sure to check out our tips for decorating (page 269).

Be sure to bring all the ingredients to room temperature before beginning this recipe. You will need two 6-inch round cake pans for this recipe. We recommend using a small offset spatula to easily and neatly frost the cake. If using a handheld electric mixer, increase all mixing times 1 to 2 minutes.

⅓ cup buttermilk, room temperature
2 large egg yolks plus 1 large white, room temperature
3 tablespoons unsalted butter, melted and cooled
1 tablespoon canola oil
¾ teaspoon vanilla extract

½ cup (3½ ounces) sugar
¾ cup (3 ounces) cake flour
½ teaspoon baking powder
⅛ teaspoon baking soda
¼ teaspoon salt
2½ cups Vanilla or Milk Chocolate Frosting (see page 268)

1. Adjust oven rack to middle position and heat oven to 350 degrees. Grease two 6-inch round cake pans, line with parchment paper, grease parchment, and flour pans. Whisk buttermilk, egg yolks, butter, oil, and vanilla together in bowl.

2. Using stand mixer fitted with whisk attachment, whip egg white on medium-low speed until foamy, about 1 minute. Increase speed to medium-high and whip white to soft, billowy mounds, about 1 minute. Gradually add 2 tablespoons sugar and beat until glossy, stiff peaks form, 1 to 2 minutes; transfer to separate bowl.

3. Return now-empty bowl to mixer. Add flour, baking powder, baking soda, salt, and remaining 6 tablespoons sugar, and mix on low speed for 15 seconds to combine. With mixer running, gradually add buttermilk mixture and continue to mix until almost combined (a few streaks of dry flour will remain), about

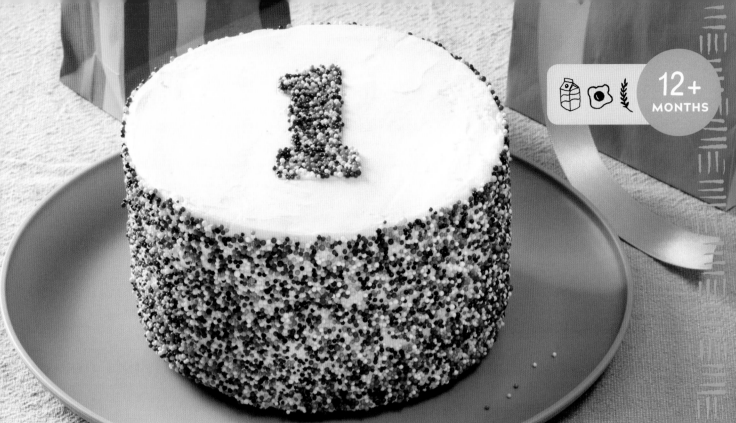

15 seconds. Scrape down bowl, then mix on medium-low speed until smooth and fully incorporated, 10 to 15 seconds.

4   Using rubber spatula, stir one-third of egg whites into batter. Gently fold remaining egg whites into batter until no white streaks remain. Divide batter evenly between prepared pans and smooth tops with rubber spatula. Gently tap each pan on counter to release air bubbles. Bake cakes until toothpick inserted in center comes out clean, 16 to 18 minutes, rotating pans halfway through baking.

5   Let cakes cool in pans on wire rack for 10 minutes. Remove cakes from pans, discarding parchment, and let cool completely on rack, about 1 hour.

6   Place 1 cake layer on platter. Spread ½ cup frosting evenly over top, right to edge of cake. Top with second cake layer, press lightly to adhere, then spread ½ cup frosting evenly over top. Spread remaining 1½ cups frosting evenly over sides of cake. To smooth frosting, run edge of offset spatula around cake sides and over top. (See page 269 for tips on decorating.) Serve.

✳ STORAGE INFORMATION

Unfrosted cakes can be wrapped tightly in plastic wrap and stored at room temperature for up to 24 hours. Frosted cake can be refrigerated for up to 24 hours. Bring to room temperature before serving.

VANILLA FROSTING

Makes 3 cups
Total Time: 15 minutes

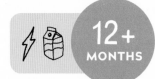

For colored frosting, stir in drops of food coloring at the end, but be sure to use a light hand—a little goes a long way. If using a handheld electric mixer, increase mixing times 1 to 2 minutes.

20 tablespoons (2½ sticks) unsalted butter, each stick cut into quarters and softened
2 tablespoons heavy cream
2 teaspoons vanilla extract
⅛ teaspoon salt
2½ cups (10 ounces) confectioners' sugar

1. Using stand mixer fitted with paddle, beat butter, cream, vanilla, and salt on medium-high speed until smooth, about 1 minute.

2. Reduce speed to medium-low, slowly add sugar, and beat until incorporated and smooth, about 4 minutes.

3. Increase speed to medium-high and beat until frosting is light and fluffy, about 5 minutes.

✳ STORAGE INFORMATION

Frosting can be refrigerated for up to 3 days; let soften at room temperature, about 2 hours, then rewhip on medium speed until smooth, 2 to 5 minutes.

MILK CHOCOLATE FROSTING

Makes 3 cups
Total Time: 25 minutes,
plus chilling time

Our favorite brand of milk chocolate is Dove Silky Smooth Milk Chocolate.

1 pound milk chocolate, chopped
⅔ cup heavy cream
16 tablespoons unsalted butter, cut into 16 pieces and softened

1. Combine chocolate and cream in large microwave-safe bowl. Microwave at 50 percent power until melted, 2 to 3 minutes, stirring occasionally.

2. Add butter, whisking once or twice to break up pieces. Let mixture sit for 5 minutes to finish melting butter, then whisk until completely smooth. Refrigerate frosting, without stirring, until cooled and thickened, 30 minutes to 1 hour.

3. Once cool, whisk frosting until smooth. (Whisked frosting will lighten in color and hold its shape on whisk.)

✳ STORAGE INFORMATION

Frosting can be refrigerated for up to 3 days; let soften at room temperature, about 2 hours, then rewhisk until smooth.

TIPS FOR DECORATING

Once you have frosted your cake with a smooth, even coating, you have a blank canvas for showcasing decorations. Here are some of our favorite ways to dress up a cake or cupcakes.

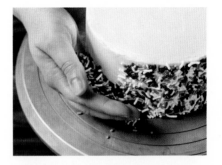

ADD COATING: Coating the sides with small adornments like sprinkles, chocolate shavings, or crushed candies or cookies is an easy way to add visual appeal. (If decorating a smash cake for a little one, keep in mind the size of your adornments; crushed candies or cookies could be choking hazards.) Simply take a small amount of your ingredient of choice in your hand and press it against the sides of the cake.

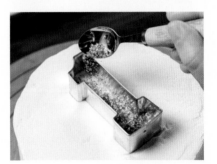

BRING SPARKLE: When you want to add your own special touch to the top of the cake (or cupcakes), press a simply shaped cookie cutter into smooth frosting on top of the cake. Using a cookie cutter as a guide, fill the shape with sprinkles, colored sugar, or another confection of a contrasting color. Carefully remove the cookie cutter, leaving behind the festive decoration.

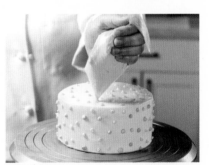

ADD DOTS: To create dot patterns using colored frosting, you will need an extra ½ cup of vanilla frosting. Divide frosting into 2 or 3 bowls and tint each with the food coloring of your choice. Place each frosting in a separate zipper-lock bag. Cut off one small corner from each bag. Working with one bag at a time, hold the bag perpendicular to the surface of the cake. Pipe out a small amount of frosting and then stop piping and pull bag straight away from the cake to ensure neat dots that hold their shape.

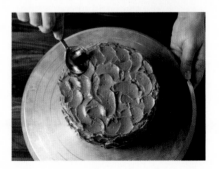

MAKE SWIRLS: One of the simplest ways to decorate a cake is to give the frosting some texture. For artful swoops, press into the frosting using a soupspoon and then twirl as you lift it away.

Striped Fruit Ice Pops

Makes 12 ice pops
Total Time: 30 minutes, plus chilling time

Why This Recipe Works

Striped, fruity ice pops win the party-food game. Stripes are festive! You get multiple flavors in one handheld treat! Plus, this is a light and cool dessert for a summer party. (Though who would say no to a striped ice pop even in winter?) We created an ultra-flavorful, naturally sweetened pop with two bright berry layers (raspberry and blueberry) and a light middle layer (with lemon and a bit of cream) to make the red and purple stand out.

For clean, well-defined stripes, be sure to let each layer freeze completely before adding the next layer, and be careful not to spill the mixture onto the sides of the molds when pouring. This recipe was developed using 3-ounce disposable paper cups, but you can use 3-ounce molds if you have them.

RASPBERRY LAYER

8 ounces (1½ cups) raspberries
½ cup water
2 tablespoons honey
Pinch salt

BLUEBERRY LAYER

8 ounces (1½ cups) blueberries
½ cup water
2 tablespoons honey
Pinch salt

LEMON LAYER

½ cup water
6 tablespoons heavy cream
2 tablespoons honey
1 tablespoon lemon juice
Pinch salt

1. **FOR THE RASPBERRY LAYER:** Process all ingredients in food processor until smooth, about 1 minute. Place twelve 3-ounce disposable paper cups in shallow baking pan. Using 1-tablespoon measuring spoon, carefully pour 2 tablespoons raspberry mixture evenly into each cup, being careful to keep walls of cups free from drips. Cover cups and freeze until firm, about 4 hours.

2. **FOR THE LEMON LAYER:** Whisk all ingredients together in bowl. Using 1-tablespoon measuring spoon, carefully pour 2 tablespoons lemon mixture into each cup on top of raspberry layer. Cover cups tightly with aluminum foil. Push wooden stick through foil into center of each mold until tip hits frozen raspberry mixture. Freeze until firm, about 4 hours.

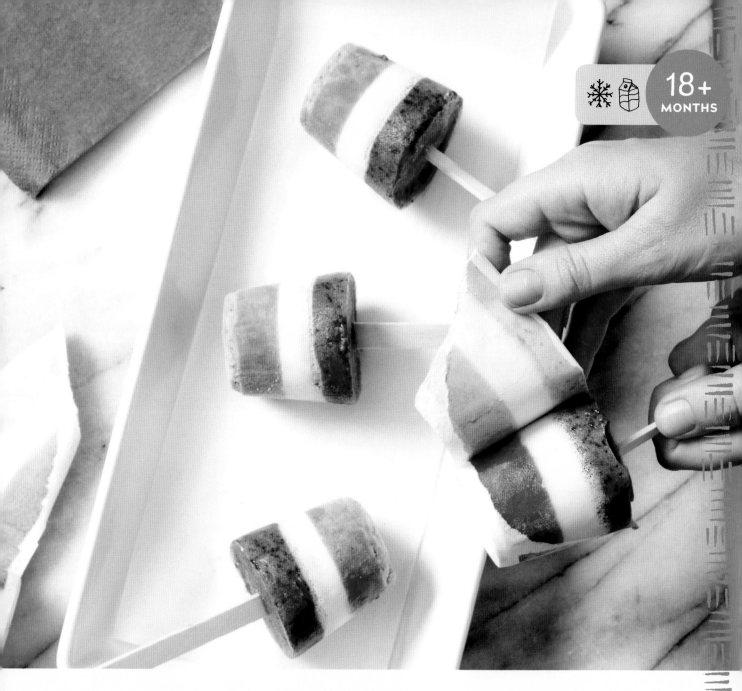

3   **FOR THE BLUEBERRY LAYER:** Process all ingredients in food processor until smooth, about 1 minute. Using 1-tablespoon measuring spoon, carefully pour 2 tablespoons blueberry mixture into each cup on top of lemon layer. Cover cups with foil and freeze until solid, at least 6 hours or up to 5 days.

4   To serve, let ice pops sit at room temperature for 1 minute, then gently pull out from cups. (Alternatively, paper cups can be peeled away from pops.)

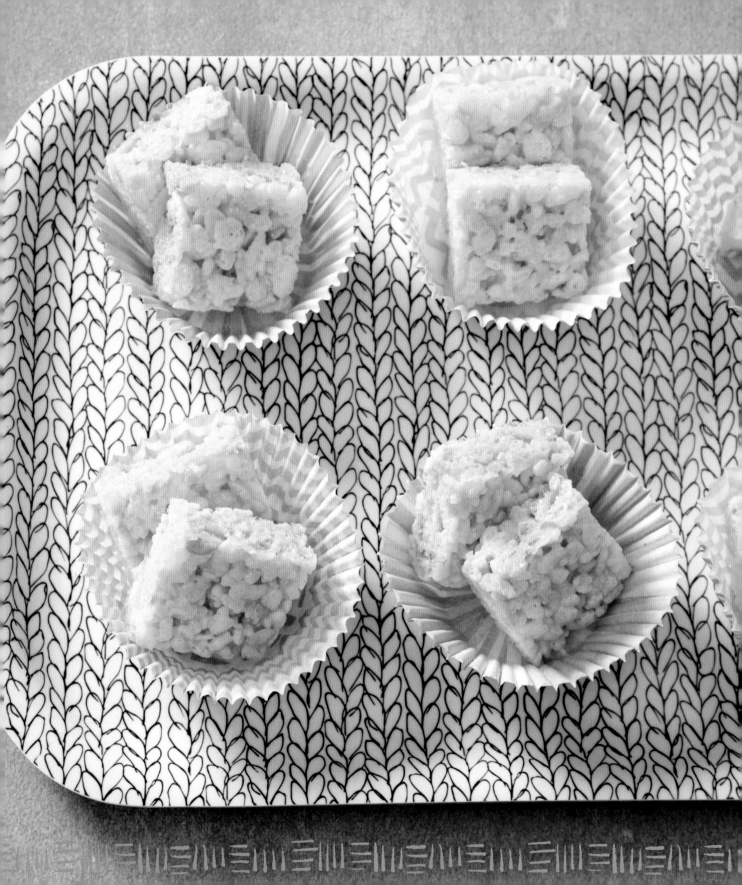

Rice Krispies Treat Bites

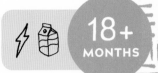

Makes 28 treats
Total Time: 20 minutes, plus cooling time

Why This Recipe Works

While many of the kids attending your celebration may already know how to use technology better than you (we're not judging), there is at the least this point of common ground from generation to generation: a love for Rice Krispies Treats. Almost everyone is familiar with the classic, from-the-box version. Our recipe has the perfect balance of marshmallow, butter, and cereal for a bar with the sticky chew that kids love and that adults remember fondly. The basic procedure is the same as the back-of-the box recipe: melt butter and marshmallows, mix in cereal, and press into a pan—it couldn't be simpler. Adding a little salt to the mix kept sweetness in check.

To ensure neat, easy-to-cut squares, grease the knife before slicing the bars. Any brand of toasted rice cereal will work in this recipe. We like to serve these in mini muffin tin liners.

3 tablespoons unsalted butter
10 ounces marshmallows
½ teaspoon vanilla extract
¼ teaspoon salt
5 cups (5 ounces) crisped rice cereal

1   Make foil sling for 13-by-9-inch baking pan by folding 2 long sheets of aluminum foil; first sheet should be 13 inches wide and second sheet should be 9 inches wide. Lay sheets of foil in pan perpendicular to each other, with extra foil hanging over edges of pan. Push foil into corners and up sides of pan, smoothing foil flush to pan. Grease foil.

2   Melt butter in Dutch oven over low heat. Add marshmallows, vanilla, and salt and cook, stirring constantly, until melted and smooth, about 6 minutes. Off heat, stir in cereal until incorporated. Transfer mixture to prepared pan and press into even layer with greased spatula. Let treats cool for 30 minutes.

3   Using foil overhang, remove treats from pan. Cut into 1-by-1½-inch bites to make 28 bites. Serve.

✳ STORAGE INFORMATION

Rice Krispies Treat Bites can be wrapped tightly in plastic wrap and stored at room temperature for up to 5 days.

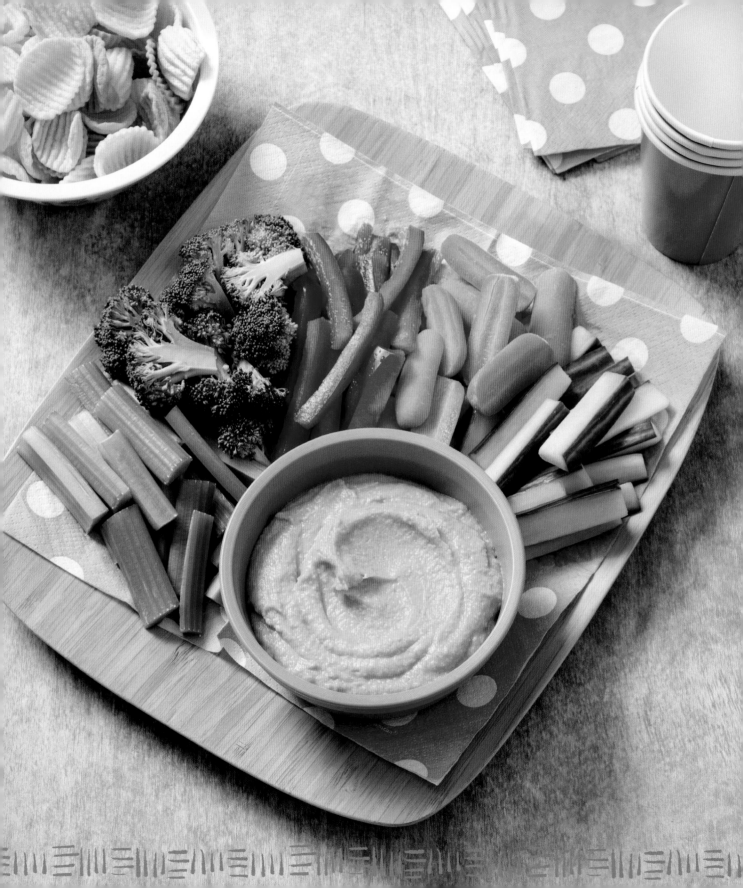

Sweet Potato Hummus

Makes about 3½ cups (serves 12 toddlers)
Total Time: 1 hour

Why This Recipe Works

Celebrations need healthy snacks, too. We wanted to give the usual hummus platter a fun twist, so we added bright, creamy sweet potato. Instead of roasting the sweet potato (which takes over an hour), we simply microwaved the spud. A bit of earthy tahini, clove of garlic, and warm spices (paprika, coriander, and cinnamon) rounded this hummus out.

✳ STORAGE INFORMATION

Hummus can be refrigerated for up to 5 days; bring to room temperature before serving and stir in 1 tablespoon warm water to loosen, if necessary.

Serve with vegetables, whole-grain crackers, or vegetable chips.

1 large sweet potato (about 1 pound), unpeeled
¾ cup water
2 tablespoons lemon juice
¼ cup tahini
2 tablespoons extra-virgin olive oil, plus extra for drizzling
1 (15-ounce) can chickpeas, rinsed
1 small garlic clove, minced
1 teaspoon paprika
1 teaspoon salt
½ teaspoon ground coriander
⅛ teaspoon ground cinnamon

1. Prick sweet potato several times with fork, place on plate, and microwave until very soft, about 12 minutes, flipping halfway through microwaving. Slice potato in half lengthwise, let cool, then scrape sweet potato flesh from skin and transfer to food processor; discard skin.

2. Combine water and lemon juice in small bowl. In separate bowl, whisk tahini and oil together.

3. Process sweet potato, chickpeas, garlic, paprika, salt, coriander, and cinnamon in food processor until almost fully ground, about 15 seconds. Scrape down bowl with rubber spatula. With machine running, add lemon juice mixture in steady stream. Scrape down bowl and continue to process for 1 minute. With machine running, add tahini mixture in steady stream and process until hummus is smooth and creamy, about 15 seconds, scraping down bowl as needed.

4. Transfer hummus to serving bowl. Cover with plastic wrap and let sit at room temperature until flavors meld, about 30 minutes. Drizzle with extra olive oil to taste before serving.

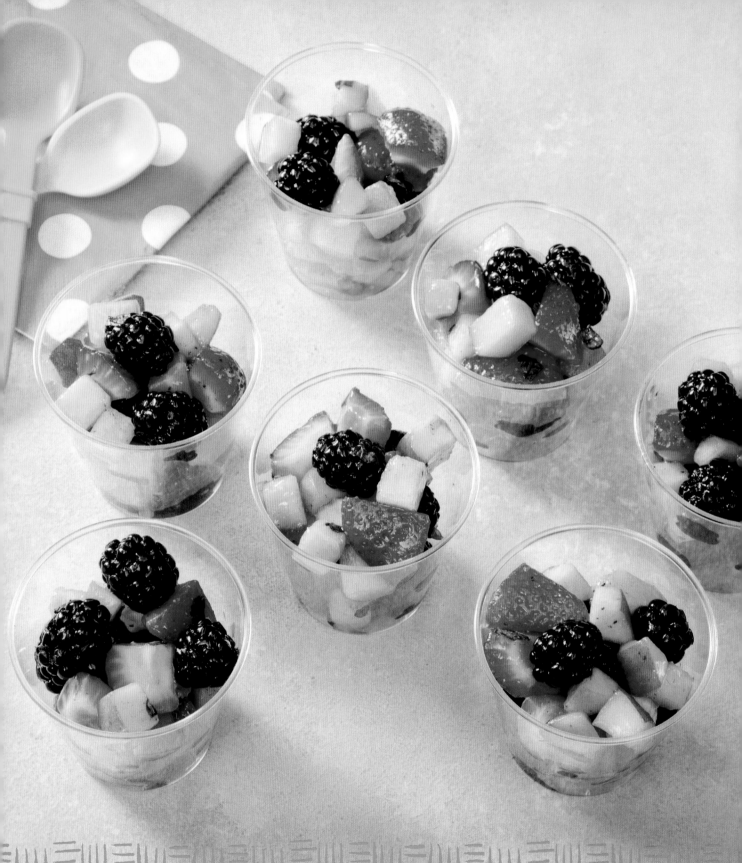

Fruit Salad Cups

⚡ **12+ MONTHS**

Makes about 6 cups (serves 12 toddlers)
Total Time: 25 minutes

Why This Recipe Works

We wanted an easy-eating fruit salad with balanced flavor and sweetness. A combination of peaches, blackberries, and strawberries not only offered a range of complementary flavors but also looked beautiful. A small amount of sugar encouraged the fruit to release its juices, creating a more cohesive salad. Mashing the sugar with fresh mint before stirring it into the fruit ensured even distribution of flavor throughout the salad.

Blueberries can be substituted for the blackberries. Nectarines can be substituted for the peaches.

4 teaspoons sugar
2 tablespoons chopped fresh mint
3 peaches, halved, pitted, and cut into ½-inch pieces
2 cups (10 ounces) blackberries
2 cups (10 ounces) strawberries, hulled and quartered
1 tablespoon lime juice, plus extra juice if needed

1 Combine sugar and mint in large bowl. Using rubber spatula, press mixture into side of bowl until sugar becomes damp, about 30 seconds. Add peaches, blackberries, and strawberries and gently toss to combine.

2 Let sit at room temperature, stirring occasionally, until fruit releases its juices, 15 to 30 minutes. Stir in lime juice and season with extra lime juice to taste. Divide fruit evenly into 12 small individual cups or bowls, if desired, and serve.

Applesauce with Whipped Cream

Makes 4 cups (serves 12 toddlers)
Total Time: 50 minutes

Why This Recipe Works

We wanted to create a vibrant, pink applesauce—the kind of color (and flavor) that only comes naturally when applesauce is made with the apple skins. But we didn't want to use extra equipment (i.e., a food mill). We cooked the apple peels and cores separately from the apple flesh, coaxed out all the flavor and color, and then we pressed the pulpy peel-core mixture through a sieve into the mashed cooked apples. Our favorite party trick: serving the sauce in tiny cups with a dollop of whipped cream on top.

We like the tart flavor and vibrant color of McIntosh apples in this recipe, but if they are unavailable, Jonagold or Pink Lady apples may be substituted. Choose the reddest apples you can find. You may mash this applesauce until it's smooth or leave it chunky for more rustic results. If using a handheld electric mixer for the whipped cream, increase mixing time 1 to 2 minutes.

3 pounds McIntosh apples, peeled and cored, peels and cores reserved
1½ cups water
Pinch salt

Pinch ground cinnamon (optional)
Sugar (optional)
½ cup heavy cream, chilled
½ teaspoon vanilla extract

1. Bring peels and cores and 1 cup water to boil in small saucepan over medium-high heat.

2. Reduce heat to medium, cover, and cook, mashing occasionally with potato masher, until mixture is deep pink in color and cores have broken down, about 15 minutes.

3. While peels and cores cook, cut apples into quarters and place in large saucepan. Add remaining ½ cup water, salt, and cinnamon, if using, and bring to boil over medium-high heat. Reduce heat to medium, cover, and cook, stirring occasionally with rubber spatula, until all apples are soft and about half are completely broken down, about 15 minutes. Using potato masher, mash apples to desired consistency.

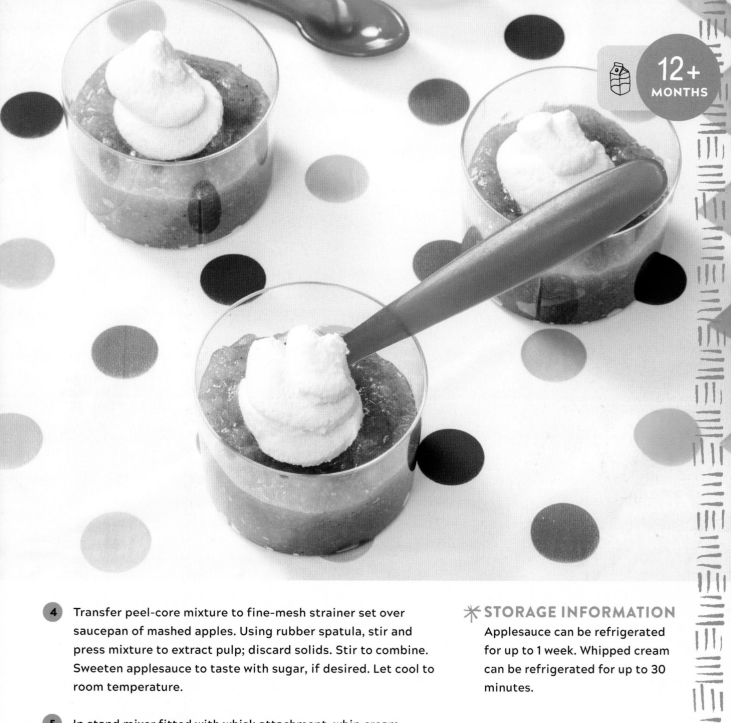

4 Transfer peel-core mixture to fine-mesh strainer set over saucepan of mashed apples. Using rubber spatula, stir and press mixture to extract pulp; discard solids. Stir to combine. Sweeten applesauce to taste with sugar, if desired. Let cool to room temperature.

5 In stand mixer fitted with whisk attachment, whip cream, 1½ teaspoons sugar, and vanilla on medium-low speed until foamy, about 1 minute. Increase speed to high and whip until soft peaks form, 1 to 3 minutes. Divide applesauce evenly between 12 small cups, dollop with whipped cream, and serve.

✳ STORAGE INFORMATION
Applesauce can be refrigerated for up to 1 week. Whipped cream can be refrigerated for up to 30 minutes.

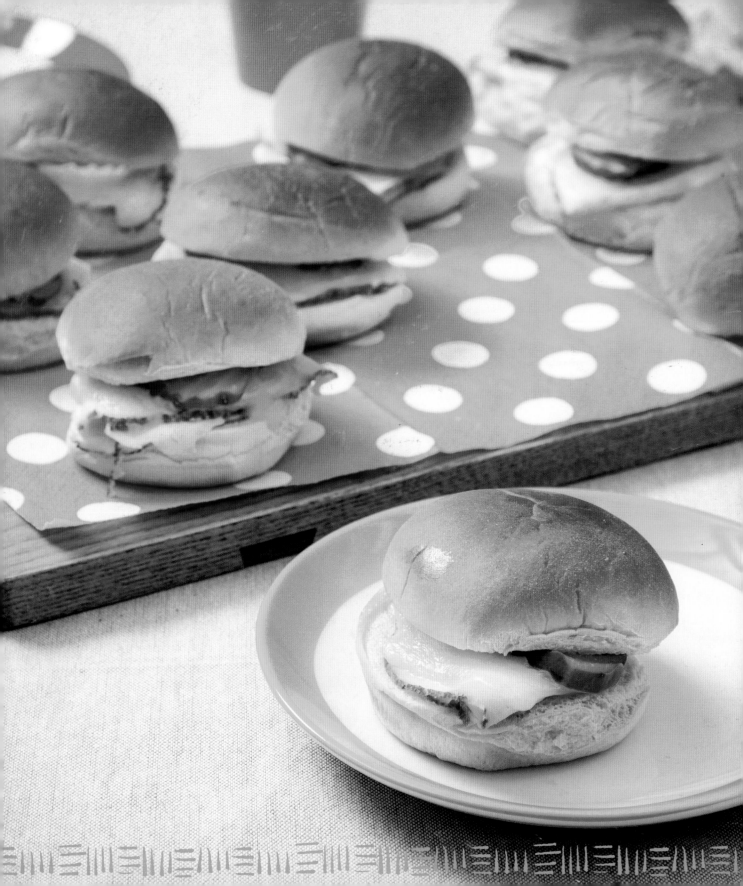

Turkey and Cheese Sliders

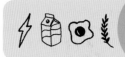

12+ MONTHS

Makes 12 sliders
Total Time: 20 minutes

Why This Recipe Works

Take your turkey and cheese sandwich to the next level by turning it into a slider. Fluffy potato dinner rolls (which are much smaller than a regular sandwich roll) are just the right size for this few-bites commitment. Heating these small sandwiches in the oven makes the rolls nice and toasty and the cheese melty and gooey.

You can also make these sliders in a toaster oven if you have one.

3 tablespoons mayonnaise
12 small potato dinner rolls, sliced open
12 slices deli turkey
24 dill pickle chips (optional)
6 slices deli cheddar cheese, cut in half

1 Adjust oven rack to middle position and heat oven to 400 degrees. Line rimmed baking sheet with parchment paper.

2 Spread mayonnaise evenly over insides of rolls. Layer 1 slice turkey, 2 pickle chips, if using, and ½ slice cheese, folding as needed. Top with bun tops and press down gently.

3 Arrange sliders on prepared sheet. Bake until cheese has melted, about 5 minutes. Serve.

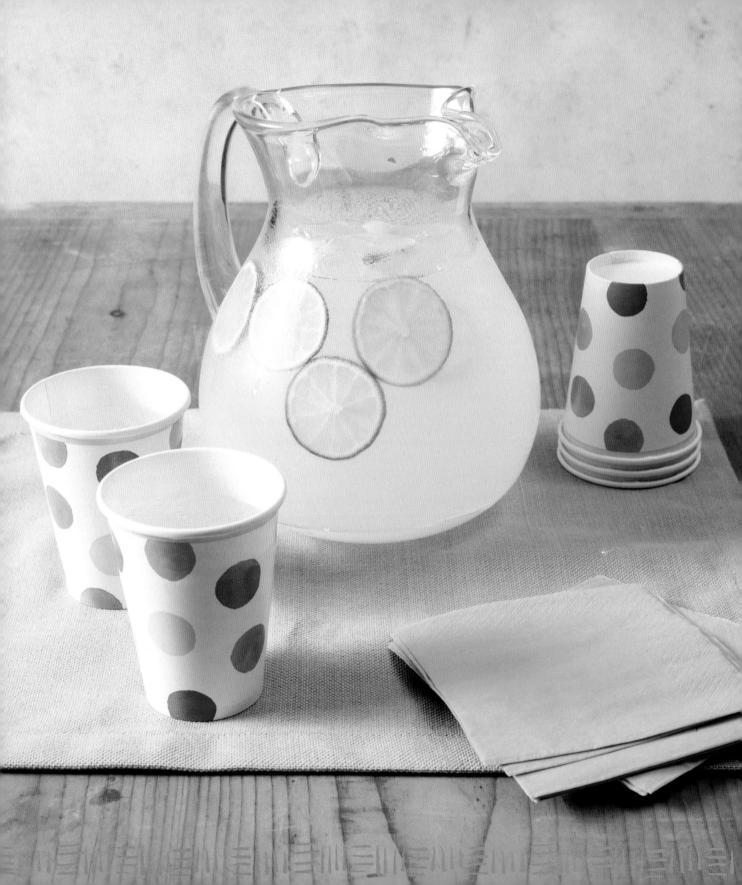

Limeade

Makes about 10 cups (serves 20 toddlers)
Total Time: 15 minutes, plus chilling time

Why This Recipe Works

Homemade limeade is easier to make than you might think. We simply mashed (or muddled) lime slices with granulated sugar to extract the oils contained in the peel and heighten the lime flavor. We then whisked in some water and freshly squeezed lime juice—no simple syrup needed. A bit of whisking was all that was needed to dissolve the sugar. All that's left is to strain the mixture and chill it for an hour before serving.

✳ STORAGE INFORMATION
Limeade can be refrigerated for up to 24 hours.

Limes are commonly waxed to prevent moisture loss, increase shelf life, and protect the fruit from bruising during shipping. Scrub them with a vegetable brush under running water to remove wax or buy organic limes, which are not waxed. Don't worry about seeds getting into the extracted juice; the entire juice mixture is strained at the end of the recipe. Serve with ice, if desired. Note that we recommend chilling the limeade for 1 hour prior to serving.

1½ cups sugar
2 limes, sliced thin, ends discarded, plus 1½ cups juice (15 limes)
7 cups cold water

1. Using potato masher, mash sugar and half of lime slices in large bowl until sugar is completely wet, about 1 minute.

2. Add water and lime juice and whisk until sugar is completely dissolved, about 1 minute. Strain mixture through fine-mesh strainer set over large bowl or pitcher, pressing on solids to extract as much juice as possible. Discard solids.

3. Add remaining lime slices to strained limeade and chill for at least 1 hour or up to 1 day. Serve.

YES, YOU CAN USE A MICROWAVE

We developed each recipe in our puree chapters (page 1 and page 37) to maximize flavor of the ingredients. Often, roasting or steaming gave us the purest, most intense flavor of the fruit or vegetable. But sometimes you don't want to take out the pots and pans, or you just want to make it as fast as possible. That's why we're including this microwave time chart. Follow the directions below to cook your fruit or vegetable speedily in the microwave, and proceed with the blending instructions in the original recipe as desired.

Microwave Directions

Combine prepared fruit or vegetable and water in bowl (except sweet potato) and cover. Microwave following times given below, until fruit or vegetable is tender. Transfer mixture to blender and puree as directed in recipe.

	PREPARE FRUIT OR VEGETABLE	WATER	MICROWAVE TIME	YIELD
Apple	2 pounds Fuji, Gala, or Golden Delicious apples, peeled, cored, and cut into 1-inch pieces	1 cup	10 minutes	2½ cups
Broccoli	4½ cups broccoli florets (12 ounces), cut into 1-inch pieces	1½ cups	8 minutes	2½ cups
Carrot	1 pound carrots, peeled and cut into ½-inch pieces	1½ cups	10 minutes	2½ cups
Cauliflower	4½ cups cauliflower florets (12 ounces), cut into 1-inch pieces	1 cup	8 minutes	2½ cups
Green Bean	1 pound green beans, trimmed and cut into 1-inch pieces	1 cup	10 minutes	2½ cups
Pea	1½ pounds frozen peas	1 cup	5 minutes	2½ cups
Peach	2 pounds peaches, peeled, pitted, and cut into 1-inch pieces	⅓ cup	5 minutes	2½ cups
Pear	2 pounds ripe Bartlett or Anjou pears, peeled, halved, cored, and cut into 1-inch pieces	⅓ cup	5 minutes	2½ cups
Butternut Squash	1 butternut squash (2½ pounds), peeled, seeded, and cut into 1-inch pieces	1 cup	5 minutes	2½ cups
Sweet Potato	3 small sweet potatoes (8 ounces each), pricked all over and placed on plate		12 minutes, flipping potatoes halfway through microwaving, then scoop out flesh	2½ cups

TODDLER SERVING SIZE

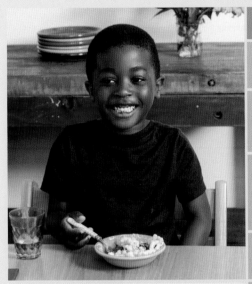

FOOD GROUP	DAILY SERVINGS	1 SERVING EQUALS...
Milk and milk products	6	½ cup milk or yogurt ½ ounce cheese
Meat and other protein foods	2	1 to 3 tablespoons beef, pork, poultry, or fish 2 to 4 tablespoons beans or chopped nuts 1 small egg
Grains	6	¼ to ½ slice bread ¼ to ½ bagel or bun ⅓ to ½ cup ready-to-eat cereal ¼ to ½ cup cooked cereal ¼ to ⅓ cup rice or pasta
Vegetables	2 to 3	¼ to ⅓ cup cooked, canned, or fresh chopped vegetables ¼ to ⅓ cup juice
Fruits	2 to 3	½ small fruit ¼ to ⅓ cup cooked, canned, or fresh chopped fruit ¼ to ⅓ cup juice ⅓ to ½ cup berries
Fats and oils	3	1 teaspoon added butter, margarine, or oil

Not surprisingly, toddlers eat less than adults. Toddlers tend to eat when they're hungry and refuse to eat when not. Here are some basic recommendations on toddler (ages 1 to 3) serving size, from the Academy of Nutrition and Dietetics.

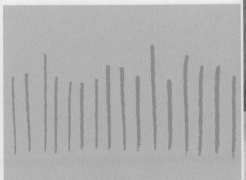

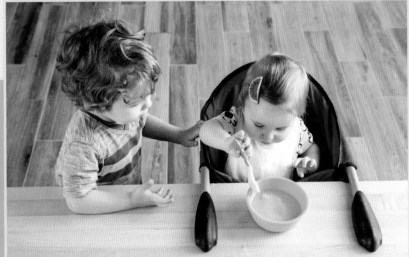

NUTRIENTS

We all know vitamins and minerals are essential for our bodies—and our children's bodies—to function, but what do they actually do? Here is a snapshot of their key roles, and some of the best food sources of each.

VITAMIN	KEY FUNCTIONS AND BENEFITS	COMMONLY FOUND IN
A	Immune function Healthy vision Organ maintenance and cell growth	Broccoli, cherries, cheddar cheese, grapefruit, dates, dark leafy greens, red cabbage, sweet potatoes, winter squash, carrots, tomatoes, mango, peas, milk, red bell peppers, legumes, sardines, eggs
B1 THIAMINE	Energy production Nervous system support	Lentils, green peas, rice, bread, fortified breakfast cereal, pork, pecans, spinach, oranges, cantaloupe, milk, eggs
B2 RIBOFLAVIN	Energy production Antioxidant protection	Eggs, green vegetables, milk products, meat, mushrooms, almonds
B3 NIACIN	Heart and skin health Energy production	Yeast, meat, poultry, red fish (e.g., tuna, salmon), cereal, legumes, seeds, milk, green leafy vegetables, coffee, tea
B5 PANTOTHENIC ACID	Energy metabolism Essential for breaking down nutrients for fuel and fat storage	Animal livers and kidneys, fish, shellfish, pork, poultry, egg yolks, milk, yogurt, legumes, mushrooms, avocado, broccoli, sweet potatoes, whole grains
B6	Brain development and function Energy production	Fortified breakfast cereals, pork, poultry, beef, bananas, chickpeas, potatoes, pistachios, salmon, avocados, spinach, dried plums, nuts
B7 BIOTIN	Energy production	Avocado, legumes, salmon, sardines, eggs, organ meats, almonds, yeast, cauliflower, cheddar cheese, pork, raspberries, whole-wheat bread
B9 FOLIC ACID/FOLATE	DNA synthesis and repair Cell growth	Dark leafy greens, broccoli, cauliflower, brussels sprouts, eggplant, avocado, asparagus, legumes, seeds, rice, red bell peppers, strawberries, eggs, avocado, citrus fruit, enriched grains, beets, lettuce herbs, nuts
B12	Nerve and blood cell health Metabolism	Fish, shellfish, eggs, poultry, beef, milk products, mushrooms, fermented foods
C	Immune function Protein metabolism and wound healing Collagen production Absorption of plant-based iron Antioxidant properties	Berries, cherries, pomegranates, apples, citrus, dark leafy greens, broccoli, cauliflower, brussels sprouts, red cabbage, sweet potatoes, butternut squash, carrots, eggplant, avocado, tomatoes, red bell peppers, artichokes, asparagus, onions, green beans, edamame, tropical fruits, currants, melons, cabbage, potatoes, grapes, stonefruit
D	Bone growth and remodeling Cell growth and development Neuromuscular and immune function Calcium and phosphorus absorption	Fortified milk products (milk, yogurt, kefir, infant formula), tuna and salmon (especially canned), white fish, eggs, cod liver oil, mackerel, sardines, liver
E	Immune function Antioxidant activity	Dark leafy greens, broccoli, avocado, asparagus, eggs, nuts, seeds, vegetable oils, butter, mayonnaise, fish, oysters
K	Blood clotting Bone metabolism	Dark leafy greens, broccoli, cauliflower, brussels sprouts, cabbage, avocado, asparagus

MINERAL	KEY FUNCTIONS AND BENEFITS	COMMONLY FOUND IN
CALCIUM	Bone growth and maintenance Required by heart, muscles, and nerves Aids in digestive health Aids in production and function of blood cells	Milk products, oranges, figs, dates, dark leafy greens, broccoli, sweet potatoes, legumes, salmon (especially canned), sardines, trout, fortified soy products, almonds
COPPER	Building strong tissue Maintaining blood volume Energy production Facilitating some antioxidant activity	Seafood, shellfish, organ meats, whole grains, legumes, chocolate, nuts, seeds
IRON	Hemoglobin and red blood cell production Protein metabolism	Red meat, oysters, lentils, beans, poultry, fish, leafy green vegetables, watercress, tofu, chickpeas, black-eyed peas, molasses
MAGNESIUM	Protein synthesis and nerve function Blood pressure regulation Energy metabolism	Nuts, seeds, chocolate, legumes, whole grains/flours, halibut, leafy green vegetables, tofu, quinoa, lentils, oatmeal, milk
MANGANESE	Bone health Antioxidant properties	Dark leafy greens, sweet potatoes, legumes, nuts, oats, pepitas, whole grains, brown rice, pineapple, teas
PHOSPHORUS	Helps build strong bones and teeth Involved in metabolism and the conversion of food into energy	Legumes, fish, tofu, poultry, beef, nuts, whole grains, milk products
POTASSIUM	Blood pressure regulation Electrolyte balance and fluid regulation Muscle function (helps muscles contract)	Bananas, potatoes, prunes, oranges, tomatoes, raisins, artichokes, lima beans, acorn squash, spinach, sunflower seeds, almonds, molasses
SELENIUM	DNA synthesis and thyroid production Anti-inflammatory and antioxidant properties	Fish and shellfish, poultry, beef, Brazil nuts
ZINC	Cell metabolism Immune function Protein synthesis Wound healing	Legumes, shellfish (especially oysters), beef, milk products, pork, poultry (dark meat), nuts

CONVERSIONS AND EQUIVALENTS

Some say cooking is a science and an art. We would say that geography has a hand in it, too. Flours and sugars manufactured in the United Kingdom and elsewhere will feel and taste different from those manufactured in the United States. So we cannot promise that the loaf of bread you bake in Canada or England will taste the same as a loaf baked in the States, but we can offer guidelines for converting weights and measures. We also recommend that you rely on your instincts when making our recipes. Refer to the visual cues provided. If the dough hasn't "come together in a ball" as described, you may need to add more—even if the recipe doesn't tell you to. You be the judge.

The recipes in this book were developed using standard U.S. measures following U.S. government guidelines. The charts below offer equivalents for U.S. and metric measures. All conversions are approximate and have been rounded up or down to a whole number.

EXAMPLE:

1 teaspoon = 4.9292 milliliters, rounded up to 5 milliliters
1 ounce = 28.3495 grams, rounded down to 28 grams

— — - VOLUME CONVERSIONS — — -

US	METRIC
1 teaspoon	5 milliliters
2 teaspoons	10 milliliters
1 tablespoon	15 milliliters
2 tablespoons	30 milliliters
¼ cup	59 milliliters
⅓ cup	79 milliliters
½ cup	118 milliliters
¾ cup	177 milliliters
1 cup	237 milliliters
1 ¼ cup	296 milliliters
1½ cup	355 milliliters
2 cups (1 pint)	473 milliliters
2½ cups	591 milliliters
3 cups	710 milliliters
4 cups (1 quart)	0.946 liter
1.06 quarts	1 liter
4 quarts (1 gallon)	3.8 liters

— — WEIGHT CONVERSIONS — — -

OUNCES	GRAMS
½	14
¾	21
1	28
1½	43
2	57
2½	71
3	85
3½	99
4	113
4½	128
5	142
6	170
7	198
8	225
9	255
10	283
12	340
16 (1 pound)	450

CONVERSIONS FOR COMMON BAKING INGREDIENTS

Baking is an exacting science. Because measuring by weight is far more accurate than measuring by volume, and thus more likely to produce reliable results, in our recipes we provide ounce measures in addition to cup measures for many ingredients. Refer to the chart below to convert these measures into grams.

INGREDIENT	OUNCES	GRAMS
Flour		
1 cup all-purpose flour*	5	142
1 cup cake flour	4	113
1 cup whole-wheat flour	5½	156
Sugar		
1 cup granulated (white) sugar	7	198
1 cup packed brown sugar (light or dark)	7	198
1 cup confectioners' sugar	4	113
Cocoa Powder		
1 cup cocoa powder	3	85
Butter†		
4 tablespoons (½ stick or ¼ cup)	2	57
8 tablespoons (1 stick or ½ cup)	4	113
16 tablespoons (2 sticks or 1 cup)	8	227

* U.S. all-purpose flour, the most frequently used flour in this book, does not contain leaveners, as some European flours do. These leavened flours are called self-rising or self-raising. If you are using self-rising flour, take this into consideration before adding leaveners to a recipe.

† In the United States, butter is sold both salted and unsalted. We generally recommend unsalted butter. If you are using salted butter, take this into consideration before adding salt to a recipe.

OVEN TEMPERATURE

FAHRENHEIT	CELSIUS	GAS MARK
225	105	¼
250	120	½
275	135	1
300	150	2
325	165	3
350	180	4
375	190	5
400	200	6
425	220	7
450	230	8
475	245	9

CONVERTING TEMPERATURES FROM AN INSTANT-READ THERMOMETER

We include doneness temperatures in many of the recipes in this book. We recommend an instant-read thermometer for the job. Refer to the table above to convert Fahrenheit degrees to Celsius. Or, for temperatures not represented in the chart, use this simple formula:

Subtract 32 degrees from the Fahrenheit reading, then divide the result by 1.8 to find the Celsius reading.

EXAMPLE:
"Roast chicken until thighs register 175 degrees."

TO CONVERT:
175°F − 32 = 143°
143° ÷ 1.8 = 79.44°C, rounded down to 79°C

INDEX